HUMAN
SECTIONAL
ANATOMY

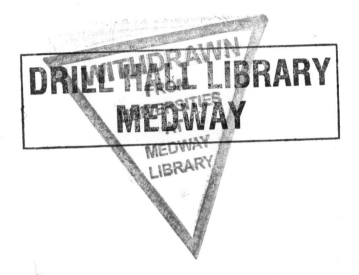

HUMAN SECTIONAL ANATOMY

Pocket atlas of body sections, CT and MRI images

THIRD EDITION

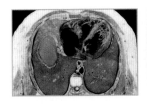 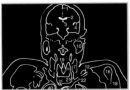 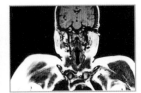 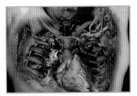

● **HAROLD ELLIS**
CBE MA DM MCh FRCS
FRCOG

Professor
Applied Clinical Anatomy
Group
Applied Biomedical Research
Guy's Hospital
London, UK

● **BARI M LOGAN**
MA FMA Hon MBIE
MAMAA

Formerly University Prosector
Department of Anatomy
University of Cambridge
Cambridge, UK
and
Formerly Prosector
Department of Anatomy
The Royal College of Surgeons
of England
London, UK

● **ADRIAN K DIXON**
MD FRCP FRCR FRCS
FMedSci

Professor
Department of Radiology
University of Cambridge
and
Honorary Consultant
Radiologist
Addenbrooke's Hospital
Cambridge, UK
and
Fellow, Peterhouse

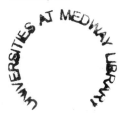
CRC Press
Taylor & Francis Group
Boca Raton London New York

CRC Press is an imprint of the
Taylor & Francis Group, an **informa** business

CRC Press
Taylor & Francis Group
6000 Broken Sound Parkway NW, Suite 300
Boca Raton, FL 33487-2742

© 2009 by Harold Ellis, Bari M. Logan and Adrian K. Dixon

CRC Press is an imprint of Taylor & Francis Group, an informa business

Printed and bound in India by Replika Press Pvt. Ltd.

No claim to original U.S. Government works
Printed on acid-free paper
International Standard Book Number: 978-0-340-98516-8 3rd edition   (Softcover)
First edition published in 1994 in Great Britain by Butterworth-Heinemann

**Library of Congress Cataloging-in-Publication Data and
The British Library Cataloging in Publication Data are available**

**Visit the Taylor & Francis Web site at
http://www.taylorandfrancis.com**

**and the CRC Press Web site at
http://www.crcpress.com**

- *Preface*   *viii*
- *Introduction*   *ix*
  The importance of cross-sectional anatomy   ix
  Orientation of sections and images   xi
  Notes on the atlas   xii
- *References*   *xiii*
- *Acknowledgements*   *xiv*
- *Interpreting cross-sections: helpful hints for medical students*   *xv*

▓ BRAIN   Series of Superficial Dissection [A–H]   2
            Selected images
            3D Computed Tomograms [A–C]   8

■ HEAD   Axial sections [1–19 Male]   10
            Selected images
            Axial Magnetic Resonance Images [A–C]   48
            Coronal sections [1–13 Female]   50
            Sagittal section [1 Male]   76
            TEMPORAL BONE/INNER EAR
            Coronal sections [1–2 Male]   78
            Selected images
            Axial Computed Tomogram [A] Temporal Bone/Inner Ear   80

■ NECK   Axial sections [1–9 Female]   82
            Sagittal section [1 Male]   100

■ THORAX   Axial sections [1–10 Male]   102
            Axial sections [1] Female Breast   122
            Selected images
            Reconstructed Computed Tomograms, Images [A–C]   124
            Axial Computed Tomograms [A–D] Mediastinum   126
            Coronal Magnetic Resonance Images [A–C]   128
            Reconstructed Computed Tomograms, Images [A–E]   130
            Reconstructed 3D Computed Tomograms, Images [A–B]   132

■ ABDOMEN   Axial sections [1–8 Male]   134

Axial sections [1–2 Female]   150

Selected images

3D Computed Tomography Colonogram [A]   154

Coronal Computed Tomograms [A–C]   156

Axial Computed Tomograms [A–F] Lumbar Spine   158

Coronal Magnetic Resonance Images [A–B] Lumbar Spine   160

Sagittal Magnetic Resonance Images [A–D] Lumbar Spine   162

■ PELVIS

MALE – Axial sections [1–11]   164

Selected images

Coronal Magnetic Resonance Images [A–C]   186

FEMALE – Axial sections [1–7]   188

Selected images

Axial Magnetic Resonance Images [A–B]   202

Coronal Magnetic Resonance Images [A–C]   204

Sagittal Magnetic Resonance Image [A]   206

■ LOWER LIMB

HIP – Coronal section [1 female]   208

Selected images

3D Computed Tomograms Pelvis [A–B]   210

THIGH – Axial sections [1–3 Male]   212

KNEE – Axial sections [1–3 Male]   215

KNEE – Coronal section [1 Male]   218

KNEE – Sagittal sections [1–3 Female]   220

LEG – Axial sections [1–2 Male]   226

ANKLE – Axial sections [1–3 Male]   228

ANKLE – Coronal section [1 Female]   232

ANKLE/FOOT – Sagittal section [1 Male]   234

FOOT – Coronal section [1 Male]   236

■ UPPER LIMB

SHOULDER – Axial section [1 Male]   238

SHOULDER – Coronal section [1 Male]   240

Selected images

3D Computed Tomograms Shoulder [A–B]   242

ARM – Axial section [1 Male]   244

ELBOW – Axial sections [1–3 Male]   245

ELBOW – Coronal section [1 Female]   248

FOREARM – Axial sections [1–2 Male]   250

WRIST – Axial sections [1–3 Male]   252

WRIST/HAND – Coronal section [1 Female]   256

WRIST/HAND – Sagittal section [1 Female]   258

HAND – Axial sections [1–2 Male]   260

• *Index*   262

Preface

The study of sectional anatomy of the human body goes back to the earliest days of systematic topographical anatomy. The beautiful drawings of the sagittal sections of the male and female trunk and of the pregnant uterus by Leonardo da Vinci (1452–1519) are well known. Among his figures, which were based on some 30 dissections, are a number of transverse sections of the lower limb. These constitute the first known examples of the use of cross-sections for the study of gross anatomy and anticipate modern technique by several hundred years. In the absence of hardening reagents or methods of freezing, sectional anatomy was used seldom by Leonardo (O'Malley and Saunders, 1952). Andreas Vesalius pictured transverse sections of the brain in his *Fabrica* published in 1543 and in the seventeenth century portrayals of sections of various parts of the body, including the brain, eye and the genitalia, were made by Vidius, Bartholin, de Graaf and others. Drawings of sagittal section anatomy were used to illustrate surgical works in the eighteenth century, for example those of Antonio Scarpa of Pavia and Peter Camper of Leyden. William Smellie, one of the fathers of British midwifery, published his magnificent *Anatomical Tables* in 1754, mostly drawn by Riemsdyk, which comprised mainly sagittal sections; William Hunter's illustrations of the human gravid uterus are also well known.

The obstacle to detailed sectional anatomical studies was, of course, the problem of fixation of tissues during the cutting process. De Riemer, a Dutch anatomist, published an atlas of human transverse sections in 1818, which were obtained by freezing the cadaver. The other technique developed during the early nineteenth century was the use of gypsum to envelop the parts and to retain the organs in their anatomical position – a method used by the Weber brothers in 1836.

Pirogoff, a well-known Russian surgeon, produced his massive five-volume cross-sectional anatomy between 1852 and 1859, which was illustrated with 213 plates. He used the freezing technique, which he claimed (falsely, as noted above) to have introduced as a novel method of fixation.

The second half of the nineteenth century saw the publication of a number of excellent sectional atlases, and photographic reproductions were used by Braun as early as 1875.

Perhaps the best known atlas of this era in the United Kingdom was that of Sir William Macewen, Professor of Surgery in Glasgow, published in 1893. Entitled *Atlas of Head Sections*, this comprised a series of coronal, sagittal and transverse sections of the head in the adult and child. This was the first atlas to show the skull and brain together in detail. Macewen

intended his atlas to be of practical, clinical value and wrote in his preface 'the surgeon who is about to perform an operation on the brain has in these cephalic sections a means of refreshing his memory regarding the position of the various structures he is about to encounter'; this from the surgeon who first proved in his treatment of cerebral abscess that clinical neurological localization could be correlated with accurate surgical exposure.

The use of formalin as a hardening and preserving fluid was introduced by Gerota in 1895 and it was soon found that thorough perfusion of the vascular system of the cadaver enabled satisfactory sections to be obtained of the formalin-hardened material. The early years of the twentieth century saw the publication of a number of atlases based on this technique. Perhaps the most comprehensive and beautifully executed of these was *A Cross-Section Anatomy* produced by Eycleshymer and Schoemaker of St Louis University, which was first published in 1911 and whose masterly historical introduction in the 1930 edition provides an extensive bibliography of sectional anatomy.

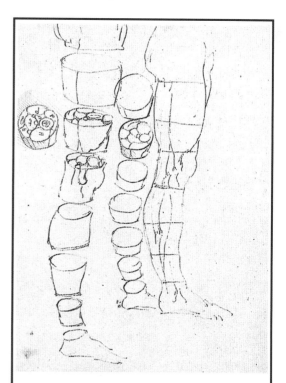

Leonardo da Vinci. The right leg of a man measured, then cut into sections (Source: The Royal Collection © 2007 Her Majesty Queen Elizabeth II).

Introduction

▓ The importance of cross-sectional anatomy

Successive authors of atlases on sectional anatomy have emphasized the value to the anatomist and the surgeon of being able to view the body in this dimension. It is always difficult to consider three dimensions in the mind's eye; to be able to view the relationships of the viscera and fascial planes in transverse and vertical section helps to clarify the conventional appearances of the body's structure as seen in the operating theatre, in the dissecting room and in the textbook.

The introduction of modern imaging techniques, especially ultrasound, computed tomography (CT) and magnetic resonance imaging (MRI), has enormously expanded the already considerable importance of sectional anatomy. The radiologist, neurologist, internist, chest physician and oncologist, as well as specialists in the various fields of surgery, have had to re-educate themselves in the appearances and relationships of anatomical structures in transverse and vertical section. Indeed, precise diagnosis, as well as the detailed planning of therapy (for example, the ablative surgery of extensive cancer) and of interventional radiology, often depends on the cross-sectional anatomical approach.

This atlas combines three presentations of cross-sectional anatomy – that of the dissecting room, CT and MRI. The series are matched to each other as closely as possible on opposite pages. Students of anatomy, surgeons, clinicians and radiologists should find the illustrations of anatomical cross-sections (obtained by the most modern techniques of preparation and photographic reproduction) and the equivalent cuts on imaging (obtained on state-of-the-art apparatus) both interesting and rewarding.

Preservation of cadavers

Preservation of the cadavers used for the sections in this atlas was by standard embalming technique, using two electric motor pumps set at a maximum pressure rate of 15 p.s.i. Preservative fluid was circulated through the arterial system via two cannulae inserted into the femoral artery of one leg. A partial flushing of blood was effected from the accompanying femoral vein by the insertion of a large-bore drainage tube.

After the successful acceptance of 20 L of preservative fluid, local injection by automatic syringe was carried out on those areas that remained unaffected. On average, approximately 30 L of preservative fluid was used to preserve each cadaver.

Following preservation, the cadavers were stored in thick-gauge polythene tubes and refrigerated to a temperature of 10.6 °C at 40 per cent humidity for a minimum of 16 weeks before sectioning. This period allowed the preservative solution to saturate the body tissues thoroughly, resulting in a highly satisfactory state of preservation.

The chemical formula for the preservative solution (Logan *et al.*, 1989) is:

Methylated spirit 64 over proof	12.5 L
Phenol liquefied 80%	2.5 L
Formaldehyde solution 38%	1.5 L
Glycerine BP	3.5 L
Total	**= 20 L**

The resultant working strengths of each constituent is:

Methylated spirit	55%
Glycerine	12%
Phenol	10%
Formaldehyde solution	3%

The advantages of this particular preservative solution are that (i) a state of soft preservation is achieved; (ii) the low formaldehyde solution content obviates excessive noxious fumes during dissection; (iii) a degree of natural tissue colour is maintained, which benefits photography; and (iv) mould growth does not occur on either whole cadavers thus preserved or their subsequent prosected and stored parts.

Safety footnote

Since the preparation of the anatomical material for this book, in 1988, there have been several major changes to health and safety regulations concerning the use of certain chemical constituents in preservative (embalming) fluids. It is important, therefore, to seek local health and safety guidance if intending to adopt the above preservative solution.

Sectioning

In order to produce the 119 cross-sections illustrated in this atlas, five preserved cadavers, two male and three female, were utilised in addition to five upper and five lower separate limbs and two temporal bone specimens.

The parts to be sectioned were deep-frozen to a temperature of −40 °C for a minimum of 3 days immediately before sectioning.

Sectioning was carried out on a purpose-built AEW 600 stainless-steel bandsaw (AEW Delford Systems, Gresham House, Pinetrees Business Park, Salhouse Road, Norwich, Norfolk, NR7 9BB, England). The machine is equipped with a 10 horse power, three-phase electric motor capable of producing a constant blade speed of 6000 feet/minute.

A fine-toothed (four skip) stainless-steel blade was used, 19 mm in depth and precisely 1 mm in thickness (including tooth set).

The design and precision manufacture of the machine results, during operation, in the loss of only 1 mm of material between each section.

Sections were taken from the cadavers to the following thickness of cut:

Head	1 cm serial
Temporal bones	at selected levels
Neck	1.5 cm serial
Thorax	2 cm serial
Abdomen	2 cm serial
Pelvis male	2 cm serial
Pelvis female	2 cm serial
Lower limb	at selected levels
Upper limb	at selected levels

Computed tomography

Since the invention of CT by Hounsfield (1973), there has been renewed interest in sectional anatomy. Despite the high cost, CT systems are now used widely throughout more affluent countries. Radiologists in particular have had to go through a rapid learning process. Several excellent sectional CT anatomy books have been written. More modern CT technology allows a wider range of structures to be demonstrated with better image quality, due mainly to improved spatial resolution and shorter data-acquisition times. Spiral CT techniques have lowered data acquisition time further still, allowing a volume acquisition during a single breath-hold – hence, the justification for yet another atlas that correlates anatomical and CT images. The development of multidetector CT allows multiple thin sections to be acquired during a single breath-hold. The computer can then assimilate this volume of data, from which coronal, sagittal and 3D images can be extracted.

Most of the images in this volume have been obtained on Siemens (Forchheim, Germany) CT systems in Addenbrooke's Hospital, Cambridge. Imaging protocols have continued to evolve from the original descriptions (e.g. Dixon, 1983a), particularly with the advent of spiral data acquisition. Oral contrast medium is often given for abdominopelvic studies; thus, the stomach and small bowel sometimes appear opaque. Intravenous contrast medium provides additional information and thus, in some sections, vessels appear opaque.

Precise correlation between the cadaveric sections and the clinical images is very difficult to obtain in practice. No two patients are quite the same shape. The distribution of fat, particularly in the abdomen, varies from patient to patient and between the sexes (Dixon, 1983b). Furthermore, there are the inevitable physiological discrepancies between cadaveric slices and images obtained in vivo. These are especially noticeable in the juxta-diaphragmatic region. In particular, the vertebral levels do not quite correlate because of the effect of inspiration; all intrathoracic structures are better displayed on images obtained at suspended inspiration. Furthermore, in order to obtain as precise a correlation as possible, some CT images may not be quite of optimal quality. A further difficulty encountered when attempting to correlate the two sets of images is caused by the fact that CT involves ionizing radiation. The radiation dose has to be kept to the minimum that answers the clinical problem; thus, it is not always possible to find photogenic examples of the anatomy shown in the cadavers for all parts of the body.

Some knowledge of the X-ray attenuation of normal structures is useful to assist interpretation of the images. The Hounsfield scale extends from air, which measures −1000 HU (Hounsfield units), through pure water at 0 HU, to beyond +1000 HU for dense cortical bone. Most soft tissues are in the range +35 to +70 HU (kidney, muscle, liver, etc.). Fat provides useful negative contrast at around −100 HU. The displayed image can appear very different depending on the chosen window width (the spread of the grey scale) and the window level (the centre of the grey scale). These differences are especially apparent in Axial section 8 of the thorax, where the images are displayed both at soft-tissue settings (window 400, level +20 HU) and at lung settings (window c.1250, level −850 HU). Such image manipulation merely requires alteration of the stored electronic data at the viewing console, where any parameters can be chosen. The hard-copy photographic record of the electronic data is always a rather poor representation. Indeed, in clinical practice, it may be difficult to display all structures and some lesions on hard-copy film.

Magnetic resonance imaging

The evolution of MRI to its present status from long-established chemical magnetic resonance techniques has been gradual. A key milestone occurred when Lauterbur (1973) first revealed the imaging potential of MRI. Clinical images followed quickly, initially from Aberdeen and Nottingham (e.g. Hawkes *et al.*, 1980). Research by various manufacturers led to a plethora of techniques, moving towards shorter and shorter acquisition times, which are now approaching those of CT. Most of the MR images in this volume were obtained on GE (Milwaukee, USA) MR systems in Addenbrooke's Hospital, Cambridge.

The physics of MRI are substantially more complex than CT, even though the principles of picture elements (pixels) derived from volume elements (voxels) within the body are similar, along with the partial volume artefacts that can occur. Much of the computing and viewing software is similar; indeed, many manufacturers allow viewing of CT and MR images on the same viewing console.

Central to an MRI system is a very strong magnet, usually between 0.2 and 3.0 Tesla (T). 1 T = 10 000

Gauss; the earth's magnetic field strength is approximately 0.5 Gauss.

When the patient is in the magnet, the hydrogen protons within the body align their spins according to the strength and direction of the magnetic field. The hydrogen protons within the water of the body are particularly suitable for magnetic resonance techniques. At 1.0 T, protons within hydrogen nuclei resonate at approximately 42.6 MHz. The protons can be excited so that the net magnetism of the spins is flipped by the application of a radiofrequency signal. Gradient magnetic fields are applied to vary the precessional frequency. The emitted signal is detected as an echo to provide spatial information and data about the chemical environment of the protons within the voxel, etc.

Some common imaging sequences are:

- *Proton density images:* conventionally acquired using a long repetition time (TR; *c.*2000 ms between signals) and a short echo time (TE; *c.*20 ms) before readout. These provide a map of the distribution of hydrogen protons (mainly within water).
- *T1-weighted images:* conventionally acquired with short TR (*c.*700 ms) and short TE (*c.*20 ms). They are useful for demonstrating the anatomy. The T1 time of the tissue refers to the time taken for the longitudinal magnetism to decay following the radiofrequency (RF) pulse and involves energy loss to the lattice in the chemical environment.
- *T2-weighted images:* conventionally acquired using long TR (e.g. 2000 ms) and long TE (80+ ms). These images often show oedema and fluid most clearly and are good for demonstrating lesions. The T2 time of the tissue refers to the time taken for the transverse magnetism to decay following the RF pulse. It involves the way in which the spin of one proton interacts with the spins of neighbouring protons.
- *Fast imaging sequences:* in order to complete acquisitions quickly (e.g. within a breath-hold), numerous techniques have been devised. These include gradient echo sequences, whereby the magnetization is never allowed to recover fully. Other techniques involve a rapid succession (train) of RF pulses and echoes, requiring advanced computer processing.
- *Tissue-specific techniques:* the different environments of protons (fat, water, flowing blood, etc.) mean that protocols can be adapted to accentuate certain features. Fat can be suppressed by the application of a RF pulse at the resonant frequency of fat followed by a gradient pulse to null the signal from fat. Images can also be generated to show either static fluid or flowing blood.

Because of the range of possible sequences, the appearances of the resulting images vary considerably. It is important to realize that the grey scale of the image reflects the intensity of the returning signal. There are no absolute values, such as in CT.

In general, fat returns high signal and appears bright (white), unless fat suppression is used (see above).

There is not sufficient water vapour in air to produce a signal. Therefore, air always returns very little signal and appears dark (black). Dense cortical bone also appears black; cortical bone has very tightly bound protons within its structure, and the lack of mobility results in reduced signal. Medullary bone contains a lot of fatty marrow and thus usually appears bright. Sequences can be performed so that blood within the vessels will return high signal; this is the basis of magnetic resonance angiography.

In the magnetic resonance images presented here, the sequence(s) have been chosen to demonstrate certain anatomical features to best effect. Thus, the precise parameters and the appearance vary extensively. On occasions, a proton density image and corresponding T2-weighted image are displayed side by side for optimal demonstration of anatomical features.

■ Orientation of sections and images

A concerted effort over recent years has meant that axial cross-sectional and coronal images are now viewed in a standard conventional manner. Hitherto, there was wide variation, which led to considerable confusion and even medicolegal complications.

All axial cross-sectional images in clinical practice are now viewed as shown in **Figure A**; that is, from 'below' and 'looking up'. This is the logical method, in so far that the standard way in which a doctor approaches the examination of the supine patient is from the right-hand foot end of a couch. The image is thus in the correct orientation for the doctor's palpating right hand. For example, the doctor has to 'reach across' the image in order to find the spleen, exactly as he or she would during the clinical examination of the abdomen. Similarly, for the head, the right eye is the one more accessible for right-handed ophthalmoscopy. Thus, all axial sections should be considered, learned and even displayed with an orientation logo shown in **Figure B**. This is the same orientation as that used for other images (e.g. chest X-ray). Here, again, the right of the patient is on the viewer's left, just as if the clinician was about to shake hands with the patient.

There is now worldwide agreement over this matter with regard to axial imaging. Furthermore, many anatomy books have adopted this approach so that students learn this method from the outset. Ideally, embryologists and members of all other disciplines concerned with anatomical orientation should, ultimately, conform to this method.

The orientation logo in **Figure B** is suitable for the head, neck, thorax, abdomen and pelvis. In the limbs, however, when only one limb is displayed, further clarification is required. All depends on whether a right or left limb is being examined. To

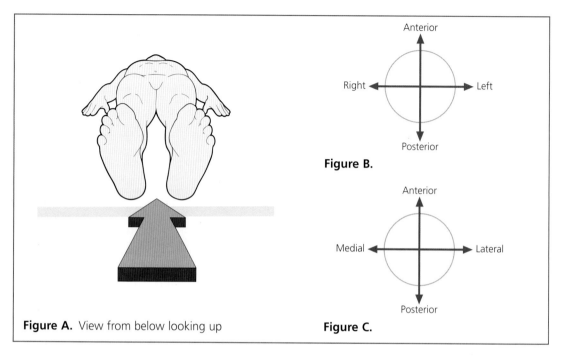

Figure B.

Figure C.

Figure A. View from below looking up

assist this quandary, a medial and a lateral marker is provided in **Figure C**. In this book, a left limb has been used throughout. Again, viewing is as from 'below'.

The orientation of coronal images has also been standardized so that they are viewed with the patient's right on the left, exactly as for a chest X-ray or when talking to the patient face to face.

There is no firm standardization of sagittal images. Various manufacturers display their images in different ways. Although there is a certain logic in viewing from the patient's right side, the visual approach for a clinician examining a patient on a couch, the majority of manufacturers display sagittal images viewed from the left. Thus, in this book most sagittal images are viewed from the left side of the patient.

Figure D, line A: the radiographic baseline used for axial head sections and images in this atlas has been selected as that running from the inferior orbital margin to the external auditory meatus. This allows most of the brain to be demonstrated without excessive bony artefact.

Figure D, line B: for sections and images of the neck and the rest of the body, a true axial plane has been used.

▓ Notes on the atlas

This atlas presents various sections of the cadaver with corresponding radiological images. The logical sequence should enable the student to find the desired anatomical level with ease.

The numbers placed on the colour photographs and on the line drawings that accompany each

radiological image match, and the key to these numbers is given on the accompanying list on each page spread. Where numbers are in coloured boxes on the key, these refer to features that are apparent only on the radiological image.

Brief notes accompany each section and refer to important anatomical and radiological features.

In the majority of sections, bilateral structures have been labelled only on one side. This has been done in order to allow readers to have an unobscured view of

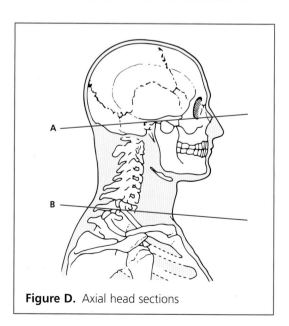

Figure D. Axial head sections

structures and to put their own anatomical knowledge to the test.

A series of views of a minimally dissected brain is provided in order to clarify the orientation of cerebral topography in the series of head sections.

The colour photographs of the brain dissections and of the sections of the upper and lower limb are of natural size. Those of the head and neck sections have been reduced slightly, and still greater reduction has been used in the thorax, abdomen and pelvis series in order to fit the page format.

Several spreads of selected images (e.g. mediastinum) have been included in order to show the features of important anatomical areas in more detail than can be demonstrated easily in cadavers and standard imaging.

Terminology

Terminology conforms to the International Anatomical Terminology – *Terminologia Anatomica* – created in 1988 by the Federative Committee on Anatomical Terminology (FCAT) and approved by the 56 member associations of the International Federation of Associations of Anatomists (IFAA).

Important changes to note are:

The Greek adjective 'peroneal' is now replaced by the Latin 'fibular' for various muscles, vessels, nerves and structures of the lower limb, e.g. Fibularis tertius instead of Peroneus tertius; Fibular artery instead of Peroneal artery; Common fibular nerve instead of Common peroneal nerve.

For this new edition, the term 'peroneal' is included italicized in brackets in order to help identify change, e.g. Common fibular *(peroneal)* nerve.

Note also that flexor accessories is now known as 'quadratus plantae'.

References

Dixon, A.K. (1983a) *Body CT: A Handbook*. Churchill Livingstone, Edinburgh.

Dixon, A.K. (1983b) Abdominal fat assessed by computed tomography: sex difference in distribution. *Clinical Radiology* 34, 189–91.

Eycleshymer, A.C. and Schoemaker, D.M. (1930) *A Cross-Section Anatomy*. Appleton, New York.

Federative Committee on Anatomical Terminology (1988) *Terminologia Anatomica: International Anatomical Terminology*. Thieme, New York.

Hawkes, R.C., Holland, G.N., Moore, W.S and Worthington, B.S. (1980) Nuclear magnetic resonance tomography of the brain. *Journal of Computer Assisted Tomography* 4, 577–80.

Hounsfield, G.N. (1973) Computerized transverse axial scanning (tomography). *British Journal of Radiology* 46, 1016–102.

Lauterbur, P.C. (1973) Image formation by induced local interaction: examples employing nuclear magnetic resonance. *Nature* 242, 190–91.

Logan, B.M., Watson, M. and Tattersall, R. (1989) A basic synopsis of the 'Cambridge' procedure for the preservation of whole human cadavers. *Institute of Anatomical Sciences Journal* 3, 25.

Logan, B.M., Liles, R.P. and Bolton, I. (1990) A photographic technique for teaching topographical anatomy from whole body transverse sections. *Journal of Audio Visual Media in Medicine* 13, 45–8.

O'Malley, C.D. and Saunders, J.B. (1952) *Leonardo da Vinci on the Human Body*. Schuman, New York.

Acknowledgements

▨ Dissecting room staff

For skilled technical assistance in the preservation and sectioning of the cadavers

Mr M Watson, Senior Technician
Mr R Tattersall, Technician
Ms L Nearn, Technician
Mrs C Bester, Technician
Mr M O'Hannan, Porter

Department of Anatomy, University of Cambridge

▨ Audiovisual unit

For photographic expertise

Mr J Bashford
Mr R Liles LMPA
Mr I Bolton
Mr A Newman

Department of Anatomy, University of Cambridge

For the excellent artwork and graphics

Mrs Rachel Chesterton and Ms Emily Evans

▨ Printing of colour photographs

Streamline Colour Labs, Cambridge

▨ Secretarial

For typing of manuscript

Miss J McLachlan
Miss AJJ Burton
Miss S Clark
Mrs K Frans

Departments of Anatomy and Radiology, University of Cambridge

▨ Annotation of central nervous system (brain and head sections)

Professor Roger Lemon

The Sobell Department of Neurophysiology, Institute of Neurology, London

Dr Catherine Horner

Lecturer in Neurobiology, Department of Anatomy, University of Cambridge

▨ Annotation of head and limb sections

Dr Ian Parkin

Clinical Anatomist, Department of Anatomy, University of Cambridge

▨ Computed tomography and magnetic resonance imaging

For performing many of the procedures

Mrs B Housden DCR
Mrs L Clements DCR
Mrs C Sims DCR
Mr D Gibbons DCR

and many other radiographers at Addenbrooke's Hospital, Cambridge.

Many radiological colleagues provided useful advice.

Dan Gibbons also kindly constructed many of the 3D generated CT images.

▨ Production of the atlas

The authors would also like to thank the staff at Hodder Arnold Health Sciences for their help and advice in the production of this atlas, in particular:

Sarah Burrows, Commissioning Editor
Naomi Wilkinson, Development Editor
Francesca Naish, Project Editor
Joanna Walker, Production Manager
Lindsay Smith, Production Controller.

Interpreting cross-sections: helpful hints for medical students

When first confronted with an anatomical cross-section or a corresponding CT/MRI image, students are often overwhelmed by the amount of structural information on display to be identified. This apprehension may be overcome by adopting a logical approach to interpretation by appreciating the 'tight-packed' compartmental composition of a cross-section. The following series of 'build-up' pictures (A–L) of an anatomical axial cross-section have been created in order to illustrate this strategy of thought.

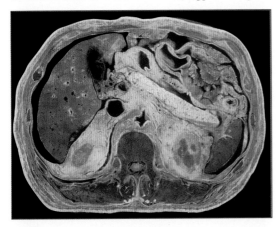

The above is an axial cross-section through the abdomen of an adult male subject.

Many important key structures are displayed, but where to begin identifying them in a logical sequence?

First establish:

1. View:

Is the view looking up or down?
The orientation guide will solve this.

2. Section level:

Where does the slice pass through the body of the subject?
The section level guide will solve this.

Now begin a logical tour of the section, beginning over the page with picture A and build up your knowledge through the sequence of pictures to L.

■ Orientation

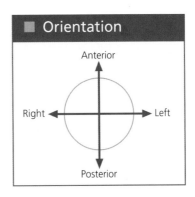

■ Section level

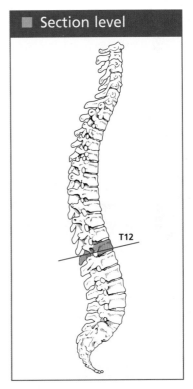

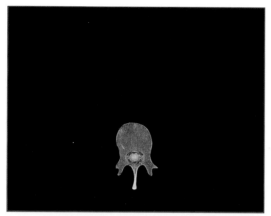

A Vertebral body of twelfth thoracic vertebra, spine, transverse process and laminae, spinal cord within the meninges.

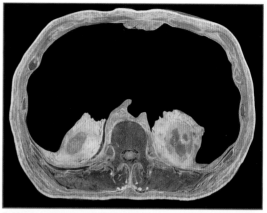

D Para and perirenal (perinephric) fat capsules surrounding the kidneys.

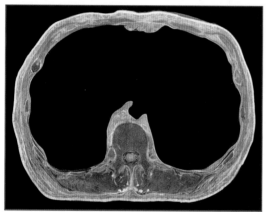

B Outer skin of abdominal wall and back, muscles of the abdominal wall, ribs, intercostal muscles, erector spinae muscles of back, psoas muscles. Appreciate the size of the abdominal cavity.

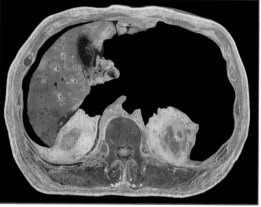

E Liver (green bile staining from the gall bladder), gall bladder, common bile duct, hepatic artery and portal vein (the largest of the three components of the portal triad).

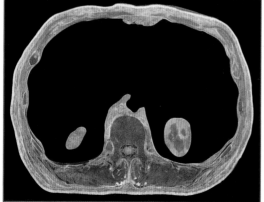

C Left and right kidney; disparate in size because the left is positioned higher than the right within the abdomen.

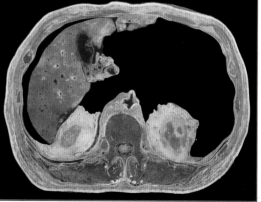

F Aorta (misshapen in this subject due to arteriosclerosis). At this level (T12), it is just emerging behind the median arcuate ligament into the abdominal cavity.

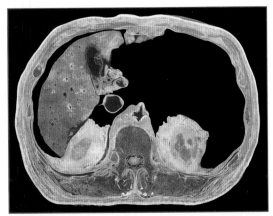

G Inferior vena cava separated from the portal triad by the epiploic foramen (foramen of Winslow).

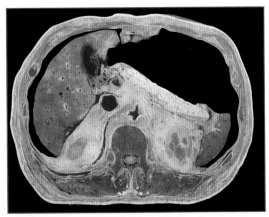

J The pancreas (head, body and tail).

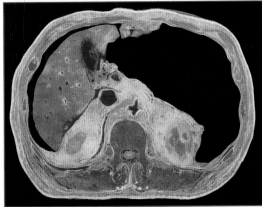

H Adipose tissue containing small blood vessels, lymph nodes, lymphatics and the fine nerves of the sympathetic trunk.

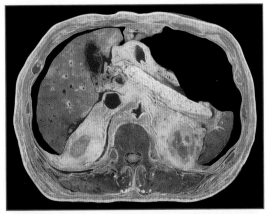

K Stomach, part of pylorus with part of first part of the duodenum, right gastro-epiploic blood vessels within omentum.

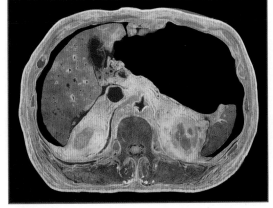

I The spleen.

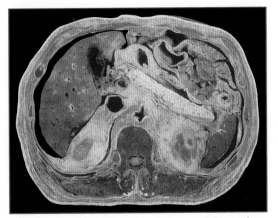

L Large bowel (portion of transverse and descending colon, the splenic flexure), surrounded by greater omentum.

A detailed account of a similar section to this with an accompanying CT can be found on pages 136–139.

HUMAN
SECTIONAL
ANATOMY

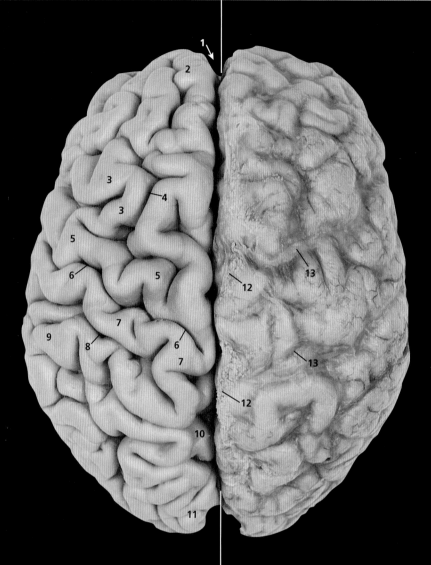

A Left cerebral hemisphere. From above, with the arachnoid mater and blood vessels removed

1 Longitudinal cerebral fissure (arrowed)
2 Frontal pole
3 Middle frontal gyrus
4 Superior frontal sulcus
5 Precentral gyrus
6 Central sulcus
7 Postcentral gyrus
8 Postcentral sulcus
9 Inferior parietal lobe
10 Parieto-occipital fissure
11 Occipital gyri

B Right cerebral hemisphere. From above, with the arachnoid mater and blood vessels intact

12 Arachnoid granulations
13 Superior cerebral veins

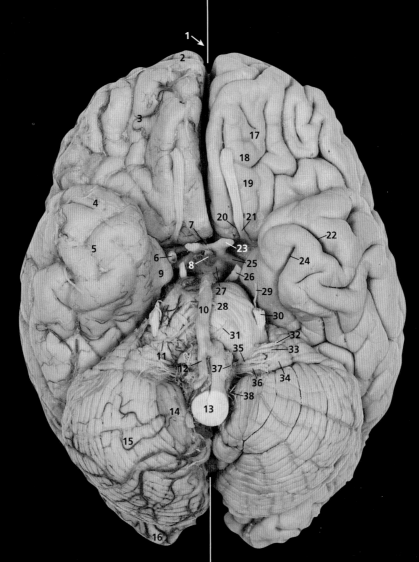

C   Right cerebral hemisphere, cerebellum and brain stem. From below, with the arachnoid mater and blood vessels intact

1 Longitudinal cerebral fissure (arrowed)
2 Frontal pole
3 Inferior surface of frontal pole
4 Temporal pole
5 Inferior surface of temporal pole
6 Internal carotid artery
7 Optic chiasma
8 Infundibulum
9 Parahippocampal gyrus
10 Basilar artery
11 Labyrinthine artery
12 Right vertebral artery
13 Medulla oblongata
14 Tonsil of cerebellum
15 Cerebellar hemisphere
16 Occipital pole

D   Left cerebral hemisphere, cerebellum and brain stem. From below, with the arachnoid mater and blood vessels removed

17 Orbital gyri
18 Olfactory bulb
19 Olfactory tract (I)
20 Medial olfactory stria
21 Lateral olfactory stria
22 Inferior temporal sulcus
23 Optic nerve (II)
24 Collateral sulcus
25 Optic tract
26 Oculomotor nerve (III)
27 Mamillary body
28 Pons

29 Trochlear nerve (IV)
30 Trigeminal nerve (V)
31 Abducent nerve (VI)
32 Facial nerve (VII)
33 Vestibulocochlear nerve (VIII)
34 Flocculus
35 Glossopharyngeal nerve (IX)
36 Vagus nerve (X)
37 Hypoglossal nerve (XII)
38 Accessory nerve (XI)

3

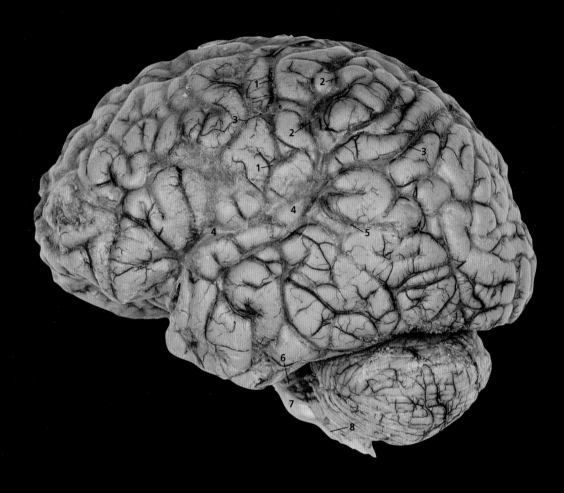

E From the left, with the arachnoid mater and blood
vessels intact

1 Rolandic artery (in central sulcus)
2 Superior anastomotic vein (Troland)
3 Superior cerebral veins
4 Lateral fissure
5 Inferior anastomotic vein (Labbé)
6 Superior cerebellar artery
7 Basilar artery
8 Vertebral artery

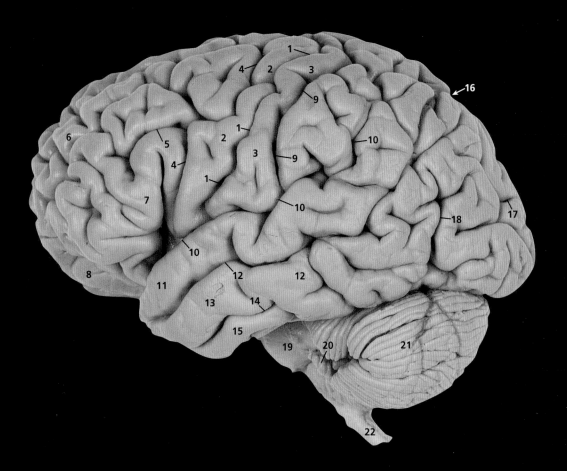

F   From the left, with the arachnoid mater and blood vessels removed

1 Central sulcus	12 Superior temporal sulcus
2 Precentral gyrus	13 Middle temporal gyrus
3 Postcentral gyrus	14 Inferior temporal sulcus
4 Precentral sulcus	15 Inferior temporal gyrus
5 Inferior frontal sulcus	16 Parieto-occipital fissure (arrowed)
6 Superior frontal gyrus	17 Lunate sulcus
7 Inferior frontal gyrus	18 Anterior occipital sulcus
8 Orbital gyri	19 Pons
9 Postcentral sulcus	20 Flocculus
10 Lateral fissure	21 Cerebellar hemisphere
11 Superior temporal gyrus	22 Medulla oblongata

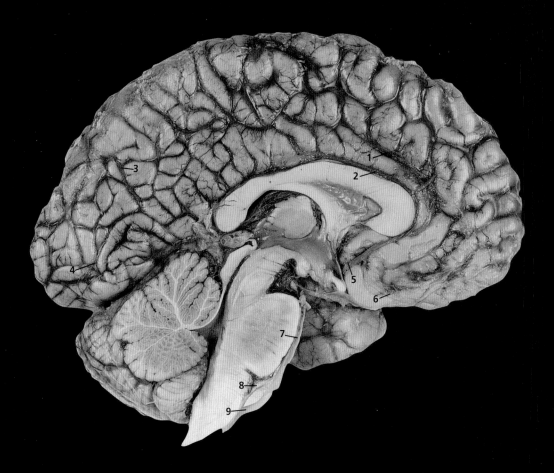

G Median sagittal section. The left half, from the right, with the arachnoid mater and blood vessels intact

1 Callosomarginal artery
2 Pericallosal artery
3 Calcarine artery
4 Posterior inferior
5 Anterior cerebellar artery
6 Orbital artery
7 Basilar artery
8 Anterior inferior cerebellar artery
9 Left vertebral artery

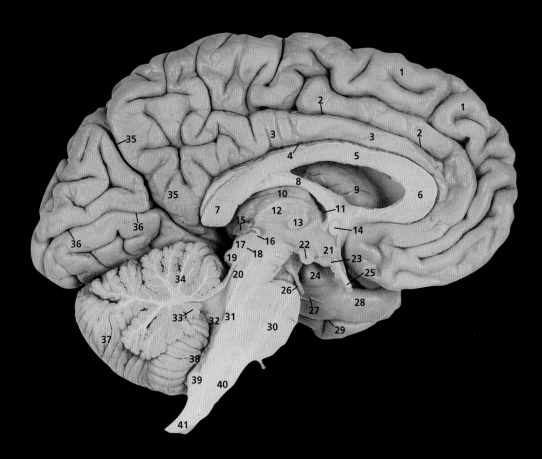

H Median sagittal section. The left half, from the right, with the arachnoid mater and blood vessels removed

  1 Superior frontal gyrus
  2 Cingulate sulcus
  3 Cingulate gyrus
  4 Callosal sulcus
  5 Corpus callosum – body
  6 Corpus callosum – genu
  7 Corpus callosum – splenium
  8 Fornix
  9 Caudate nucleus (head) in wall
     of lateral ventricle
 10 Choroid plexus, third ventricle
 11 Interventricular foramen
     (Monro)
 12 Thalamus
 13 Massa intermedia

 14 Anterior commissure
 15 Pineal body
 16 Posterior commissure
 17 Superior colliculus
 18 Aqueduct (of Sylvius)
 19 Inferior colliculus
 20 Mesencephalon
 21 Hypothalamus
 22 Mamillary body
 23 Infundibulum
 24 Uncus
 25 Optic nerve (II)
 26 Oculomotor nerve (III)
 27 Trochlear nerve (IV)
 28 Parahippocampal gyrus

 29 Rhinal sulcus
 30 Pons
 31 Pontine tegmentum
 32 Fourth ventricle
 33 Nodulus
 34 Anterior lobe of cerebellum
 35 Parieto-occipital fissure
 36 Calcarine sulcus
 37 Cerebellar hemisphere
 38 Tonsil of cerebellum
 39 Inferior cerebellar peduncle
 40 Pyramid
 41 Medulla oblongata

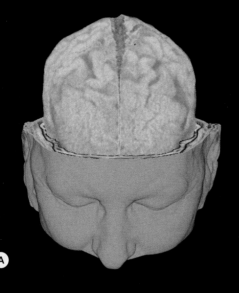

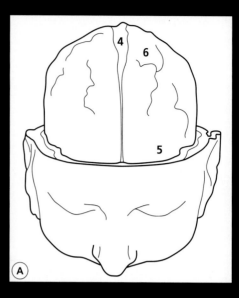

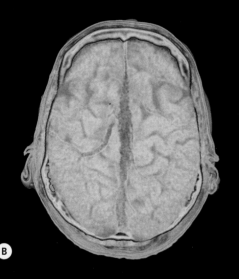

1	Skin and subcutaneous tissue	**4**	Superior sagittal sinus
2	Frontal bone	**5**	Frontal lobe
3	Pinna	**6**	Parietal lobe

■ Notes

These edited 3D CT images neatly show the relationship of the brain to the skull and facial bones. The skin, subcutaneous tissues, scalp and meninges have been stripped away electronically in order to show the relations to best effect. The frontal perspective is self explanatory. The 'axial' image is in effect viewed from 'above'. A few of the appropriate landmarks have been labelled.

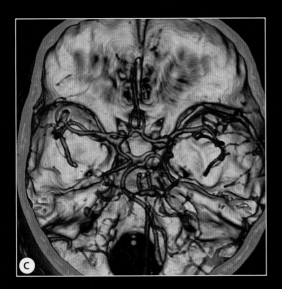

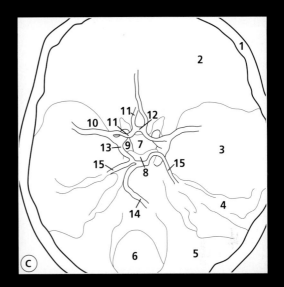

1 Skull vault	**6** Foramen magnum	**11** Anterior cerebral artery
2 Anterior cranial fossa	**7** Pituitary fossa	**12** Anterior communicating artery
3 Middle cranial fossa	**8** Posterior clinoid process	**13** Posterior communicating artery
4 Petrous ridge of temporal bone	**9** Internal carotid artery	**14** Basilar artery
5 Posterior cranial fossa	**10** Middle cerebral artery	**15** Posterior cerebral artery

■ Orientation

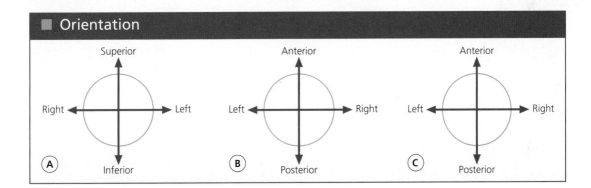

■ Notes

3D CT angiogram showing the vessels forming the circle of Willis in relation to the fossae formed by the base of the skull. This particular type of image is viewed from 'above'. Despite careful technique there is a little contamination with overlying vessels, which slightly confuses the image. Nevertheless the major vessels can be identified clearly and this image reveals how variable the circle of Willis can be. For example one of the two vertebral arteries is dominant as they come through the foramen magnum (**6**) to create the basilar artery (**14**). The right posterior communicating artery (**13**) is large and is the main contributor to the posterior cerebral artery (**15**) on this side. Note the close relation of the circle of Willis to the pituitary fossa (**7**) and posterior clinoid process (**8**). Note also how the internal carotid arteries (**9**) ascend on either side of the pituitary fossa. Aneurysms in this region can affect the pituitary, the optic chiasm and numerous cranial nerves.

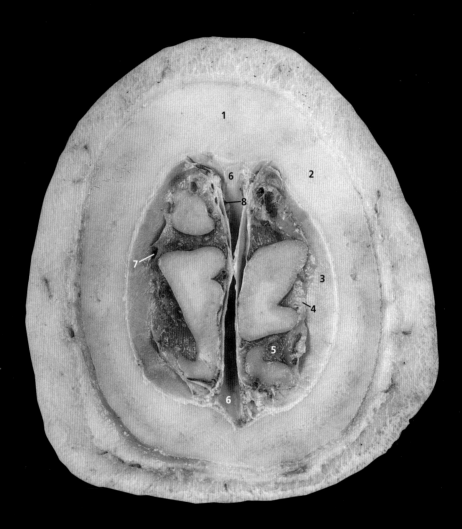

1 Frontal bone
2 Parietal bone
3 Dura mater
4 Arachnoid mater
5 Pia mater
6 Superior sagittal sinus
7 Superior cerebral vein
8 Arachnoid granulation

Section level

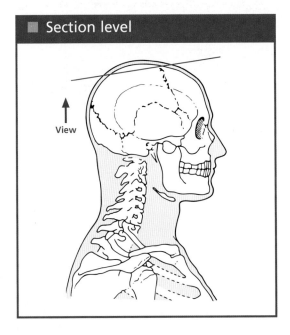

View

Orientation

Anterior

Right ← → Left

Posterior

Notes

This section passes through the apex of the skull vault and traverses the parietal bones (**2**) and the superior portion of the frontal bone (**1**).

Between the inner and outer tables of the bones of the skull vault lie trabecular bone, termed diploe, which contains red bone marrow. This is highly vascular and a common site for blood-borne metastatic tumour deposits and multiple myeloma. Diploic veins (see (**8**) on page 18) occupy channels in this trabecular bone. These are absent at birth but begin to appear at about 2 years of age. They are large and thin-walled, being merely endothelium supported by elastic tissue, and they communicate with meningeal veins, dural sinuses and the pericranial veins. Radiographically they may appear as relatively transparent bands 3–4 mm in diameter.

The dura mater, which lines the inner aspect of the skull, comprises an outer, or endosteal, layer, or endocranium (**3**) (which is, in fact, the periosteum, which lines the inner aspect of the skull) and an inner, or meningeal, layer (**4**). Most of the intracranial venous sinuses are formed as clefts between these two layers, as demonstrated in this section by the superior sagittal sinus (**6**). The exceptions to this rule are the inferior sagittal sinus and the straight sinus, which are clefts within the meningeal layer.

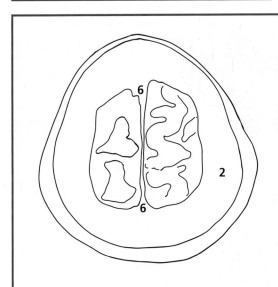

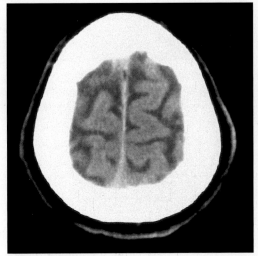

Axial computed tomogram (CT)

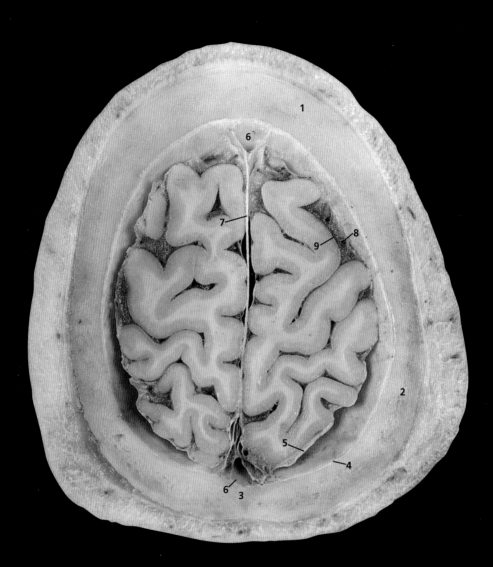

1 Frontal bone
2 Parietal bone
3 Sagittal suture
4 Dura mater
5 Arachnoid mater
6 Superior sagittal sinus
7 Falx cerebri
8 Subarachnoid space
9 Pia mater

■ Section level

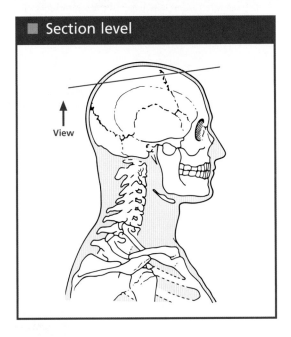

View

■ Orientation

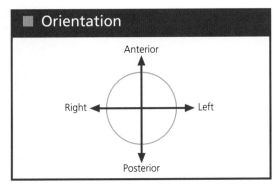

Anterior

Right ←→ Left

Posterior

■ Notes

This section, at a deeper plane through the skull vault, demonstrates the falx cerebri (**7**), which is formed as a double fold of the inner, meningeal, layer of the dura mater (**5**) and which forms the dural septum between the cerebral hemispheres.

The inner layer of the dura is lined by the delicate arachnoid mater. The pia mater (**9**) is vascular and invests the brain, spinal cord, cranial nerves and spinal nerve roots. It remains in close contact with the surface of the brain, including the depths of the cerebral sulci and fissures.

Over the convexities of the brain, the pia and arachnoid are in close contact. Over the cerebral sulci and the cisterns of the brain base, the pia and arachnoid are separated by the subarachnoid space (**8**), which contains cerebrospinal fluid. This space is traversed by a fine spider's web of fibres (*arachnoid*: pertaining to the spider).

The total volume of cerebrospinal fluid in the adult is approximately 150 mL, of which some 25 mL is contained in the ventricular system, 25 mL in the spinal theca and the remaining 100 mL in the cerebral subarachnoid space.

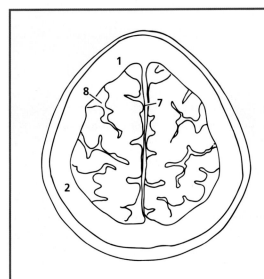

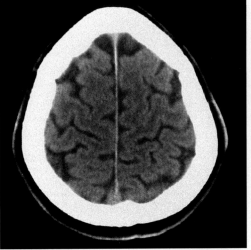

Axial computed tomogram (CT)

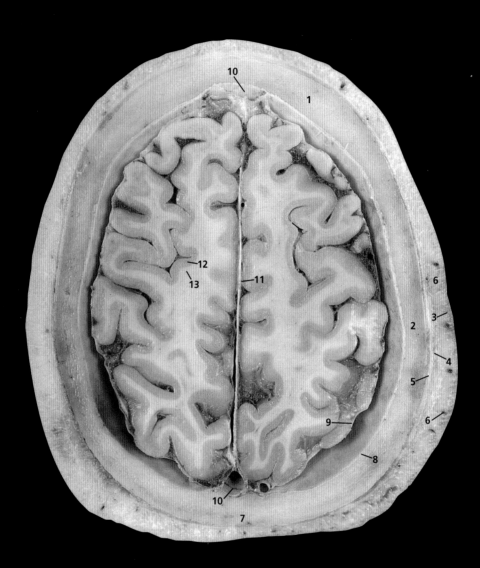

1 Frontal bone
2 Parietal bone
3 Skin and dense subcutaneous
  tissue
4 Epicranial aponeurosis (galea
  aponeurotica)
5 Pericranium
6 Branches of superficial
  temporal artery

7 Sagittal suture
8 Dura mater
9 Arachnoid mater
10 Superior sagittal sinus
11 Falx cerebri
12 Grey matter
13 White matter

Section level

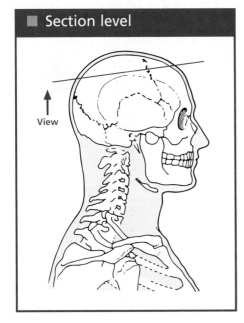

View

Orientation

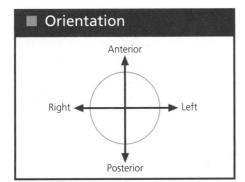

Anterior

Right ◄─────► Left

Posterior

Notes

This section, through the upper parts of the cerebral hemispheres, gives a clear picture of the distinction between the outer grey matter (**12**), which contains nerve cells, and the inner white matter (**13**), made up of nerve fibres. This is in contradistinction to the arrangement of the spinal cord, with the central grey and surrounding white matter.

Note the five layers of the scalp – skin, underlying dense connective tissue (**3**), dense epicranial aponeurosis, or galea aponeurotica (**4**), which is separated by a film of loose areolar connective tissue from the outer periosteum of the skull, the pericranium (**5**). The pericranium is densely adherent to the surface of the skull and passes through the various foramina, where it becomes continuous with the outer endosteal layer of the dura (**8**) and is also continuous with the sutural ligaments that occupy the cranial sutures.

Each of these layers is of clinical significance. The scalp is richly supplied with sebaceous glands and is the commonest site of epidermoid cysts. The connective tissue is made up of lobules of fat bound in tough fibrous septa. The blood vessels of the scalp lie in this layer; when the scalp is lacerated, the divided vessels retract between these septa and cannot be picked up with artery forceps in the usual way – they can be controlled by firm digital pressure against the skull on either side of the laceration. The aponeurotic layer is the occipitofrontalis, which is fibrous over the dome of the scalp but muscular in the occipital and frontal regions (see (**2**) on p. 24 and (**2**) on p. 26). The underlying loose areolar connective tissue accounts for the mobility of the scalp on the underlying bone. It is in this plane that surgical mobilization of scalp flaps is performed. Blood in this layer tracks forward into the orbits to produce periorbital haematomas. The periosteum adheres to the suture lines of the skull, so that a collection of blood or pus beneath this layer outlines the affected bone. This may produce the cephalohaematoma seen in birth injuries involving the skull.

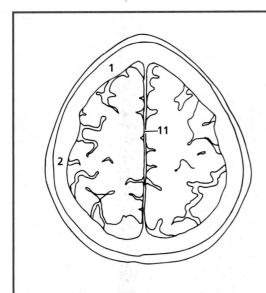

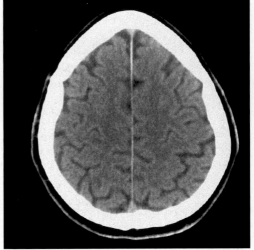

Axial computed tomogram (CT)

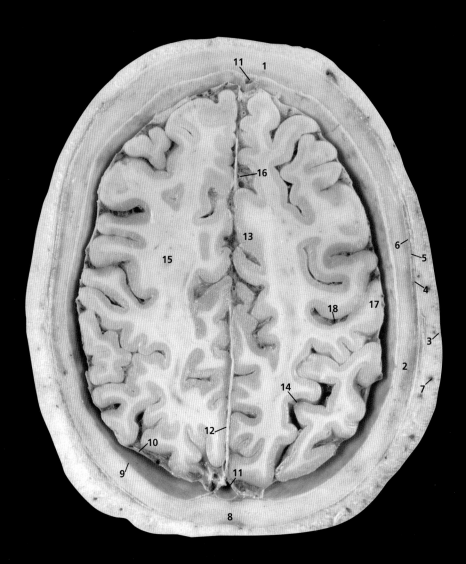

1 Frontal bone
2 Parietal bone
3 Skin and dense
   subcutaneous tissue
4 Epicranial aponeurosis
   (galea aponeurotica)
5 Temporalis
6 Pericranium
7 Branch of superficial
   temporal artery
8 Sagittal suture

9 Dura mater
10 Arachnoid mater
11 Superior sagittal sinus
12 Falx cerebri
13 Cingulate gyrus
14 Parieto-occipital sulcus
15 Corona radiata
16 Anterior cerebral artery
   (branches)
17 Postcentral gyrus
18 Central sulcus

Section level

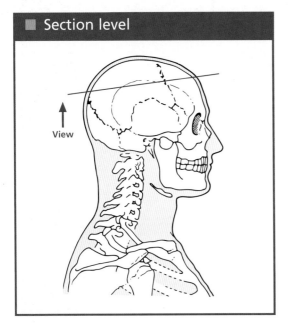

View

Orientation

Anterior

Right ← → Left

Posterior

Notes

This section allows some of the main gyri and sulci of the cerebrum to be identified. Cross-reference should be made to the photographs of the external aspects and sagittal section of the brain for orientation.

The corona radiata (**15**) comprises a fan-shaped arrangement of afferent and efferent projection fibres, which join the grey matter to lower centres. On the computed tomography (CT) image, it appears as a curved linear area of low attenuation termed the centrum semiovale.

The superficial temporal artery, of which the parietal branch can be seen at (**7**), is the smaller terminal branch of the external carotid artery, the other being the maxillary artery. The middle terminal branch can be seen immediately in front of (**4**). The blood supply to the scalp is the richest of all areas of the skin and there are free anastomoses between its various branches. It is for this reason that a partially avulsed scalp flap is usually viable.

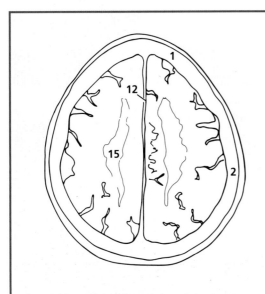

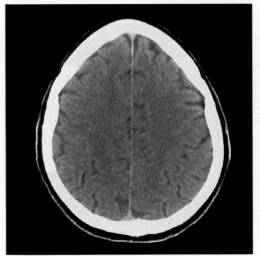

Axial computed tomogram (CT)

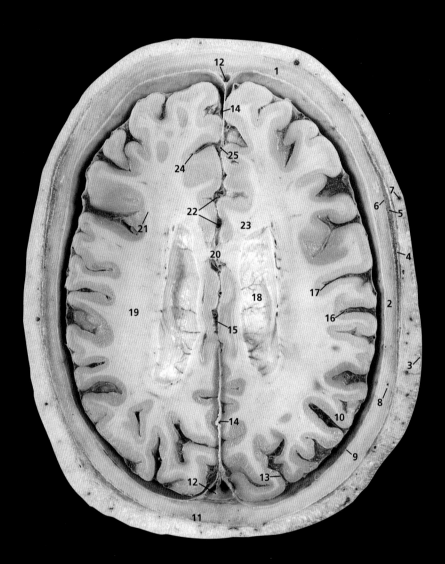

1 Frontal bone
2 Parietal bone
3 Skin and dense subcutaneous tissue
4 Temporal fascia
5 Temporalis
6 Pericranium
7 Branches of superficial temporal artery
8 Diploic vein
9 Dura mater
10 Arachnoid mater
11 Sagittal suture
12 Superior sagittal sinus
13 Lunate sulcus
14 Falx cerebri
15 Cingulate gyrus
16 Postcentral sulcus
17 Central sulcus
18 Roof of body of lateral ventricle
19 Corona radiata
20 Corpus callosum
21 Longitudinal fasciculus (corticocortical fibres)
22 Anterior cerebral artery (branches)
23 Forceps minor
24 Cingulate sulcus
25 Inferior sagittal sinus

Section level

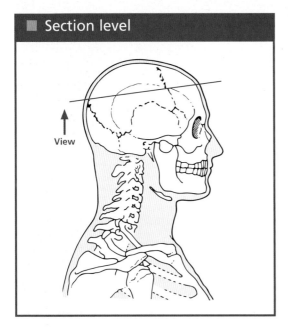

View

Notes

This section passes through the roof of the lateral ventricle (**18**).

The central sulcus, or fissure of Rolando (**17**), is the most important of the sulcal landmarks, since it separates the precentral (motor) gyrus from the postcentral (sensory) gyrus. It also helps demarcate the frontal and parietal lobes of the cerebrum.

Again, the corona radiata (**19**), or centrum semiovale, is well seen in both the section and the CT image.

The corpus callosum (**20**) – and seen also on p. 7, in (**5**), (**6**) and (**7**) – is the largest fibre pathway of the brain. It links the cortex of the two cerebral hemispheres and roofs much of the lateral ventricles. Its anterior portion is termed the genu; its body is termed the trunk, which is arched and convex superiorly. It ends posteriorly as the splenium, which is its thickest part – see p. 20 (**17**). Congenital absence of the corpus callosum, or its surgical division, results in surprisingly little disturbance of function.

Orientation

Anterior

Right — Left

Posterior

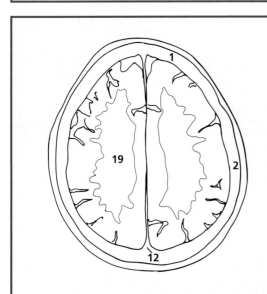

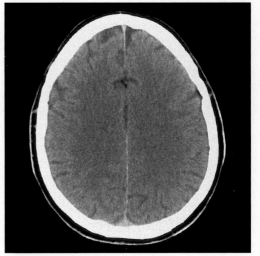

Axial computed tomogram (CT)

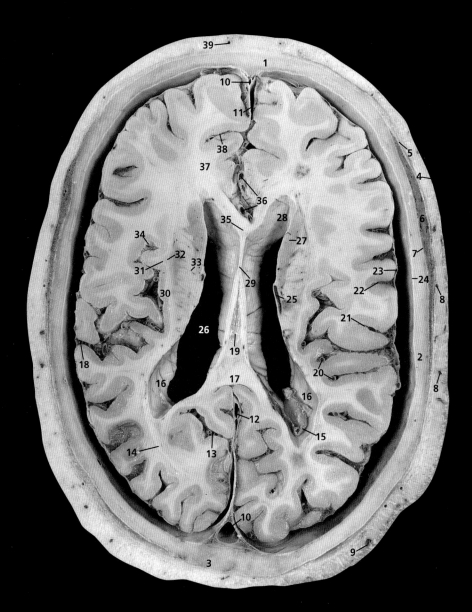

1 Frontal bone
2 Parietal bone
3 Sutural bone
4 Skin and dense subcutaneous tissue
5 Epicranial aponeurosis (galea aponeurotica)
6 Temporalis
7 Pericranium
8 Branches of superficial temporal artery
9 Occipital vein
10 Superior sagittal sinus
11 Falx cerebri
12 Straight sinus
13 Parieto-occipital sulcus
14 Optic radiation
15 Choroid plexus
16 Posterior horn lateral ventricle
17 Splenium of corpus callosum
18 Lateral sulcus (Sylvian fissure)
19 Third ventricle
20 Middle cerebral artery (branches)
21 Postcentral sulcus
22 Central sulcus
23 Arachnoid mater
24 Dura mater
25 Thalamostriate vein
26 Body of lateral ventricle
27 Body of caudate nucleus
28 Frontal horn of lateral ventricle
29 Septum pellucidum
30 Insula
31 Claustrum
32 Putamen
33 Internal capsule
34 Circular sulcus
35 Genu of corpus callosum
36 Anterior cerebral artery (branches)
37 Forceps minor
38 Cingulate sulcus
39 Supra-orbital artery

▪ Section level

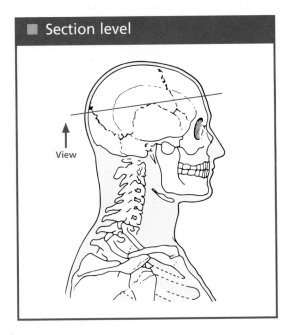

View

▪ Orientation

Anterior

Right ← → Left

Posterior

▪ Notes

This section passes through the bodies of the lateral ventricles (**26**) and the third ventricle (**19**).

The lateral ventricles comprise a frontal horn (**28**) and body (**26**), which continues with the posterior or occipital horn (**16**), which, in turn, enters the inferior horn within the temporal lobe. This will be seen in later sections. The lateral ventricles are separated almost completely from each other by the septum pellucidum (**29**) but communicate indirectly via the third ventricle (**19**), a narrow slit-like cavity.

The choroid plexuses of the lateral ventricles (**15**), which are responsible for the production of most of the cerebrospinal fluid extend from the inferior horn, through the body to the interventricular foramen, where they become continuous with the plexus of the third ventricle.

In addition to the centres of ossification of the named bones of the skull, other centres may occur in the course of the sutures, which give rise to irregular sutural (Wormian) bones (**3**). They occur most frequently in the region of the lambdoid suture, as here, but sometimes they may be seen at the anterior, or more especially, the posterior fontanelle. They are usually limited to two or three in number, but they may occur in greater numbers in congenital hydrocephalic skulls and other congenital anomalies.

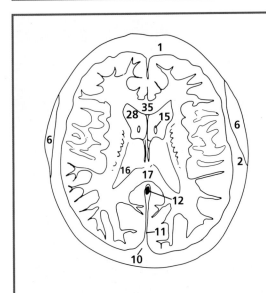

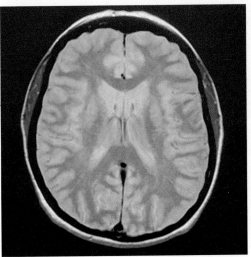

Axial magnetic resonance image (MRI)

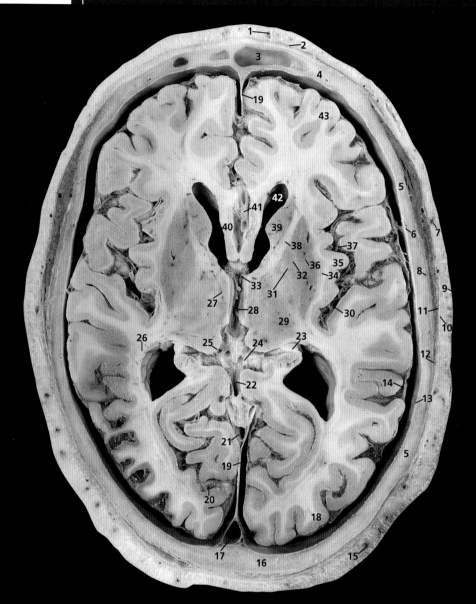

1 Supra-orbital artery
2 Frontal belly of occipitofrontalis
3 Frontal sinus
4 Frontal bone
5 Parietal bone
6 Middle meningeal artery and vein
7 Branch of temporal artery
8 Sliver of squamous part of temporal bone
9 Skin and dense subcutaneous tissue
10 Epicranial aponeurosis (galea aponeurotica)
11 Temporalis
12 Pericranium
13 Dura mater
14 Arachnoid mater

15 Occipital artery
16 Squamous part of occipital bone
17 Superior sagittal sinus
18 Occipital lobe
19 Falx cerebri
20 Calcarine sulcus
21 Straight sinus
22 Great cerebral vein
23 Fornix
24 Internal cerebral vein (branches)
25 Pulvinar of thalamus
26 Optic radiation
27 Medial nucleus of thalamus
28 Third ventricle
29 Ventroposterior thalamic nucleus
30 Circular sulcus

31 Globus pallidus – internal segment
32 Globus pallidus – external segment
33 Choroid plexus in interventricular foramen (Monro)
34 Claustrum
35 Insula
36 Putamen
37 Middle cerebral artery (branches)
38 Anterior limb of internal capsule
39 Caudate nucleus – head
40 Corpus callosum
41 Anterior cerebral artery
42 Frontal horn of lateral ventricle
43 Frontal lobe

Section level

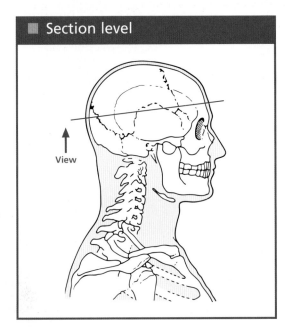

View

Orientation

Anterior

Right   Left

Posterior

Notes

This section passes through the apex of the squamous part of the occipital bone (**16**) and the frontal sinus (**3**). These are paired but are rarely symmetrical, while the septum between them is usually deviated from the midline. They vary greatly in size, as may be appreciated from viewing a number of skull radiographs. Each lies posterior to the supercilliary arch and extends upwards above the medial part of the eyebrow and back on to the medial part of the orbital roof. Sometimes they are divided by incomplete bony septa; rarely, one or both may be absent. Each drains into the anterior part of the middle meatus on the lateral wall of the nasal cavity via the frontonasal duct.

The interventricular foramen of Monro (**33**) is well demonstrated and drains the lateral ventricle on both sides into the third ventricle (**28**), thus providing a linkage between the ventricular systems within the two cerebral hemispheres.

This section also demonstrates the components of the basal ganglia, the claustrum (**34**), and the lentiform nucleus, made up of the globus pallidus (**31**, **32**) and putamen (**36**). The latter is largely separated from the head of the caudate nucleus (**39**) by the anterior limb of the internal capsule (**38**).

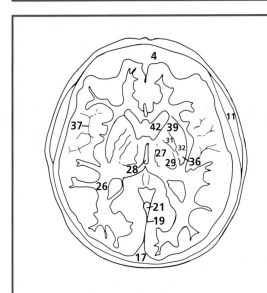

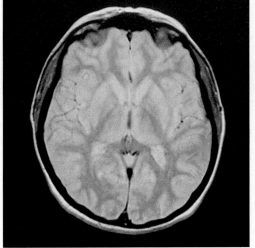

Axial magnetic resonance image (MRI)

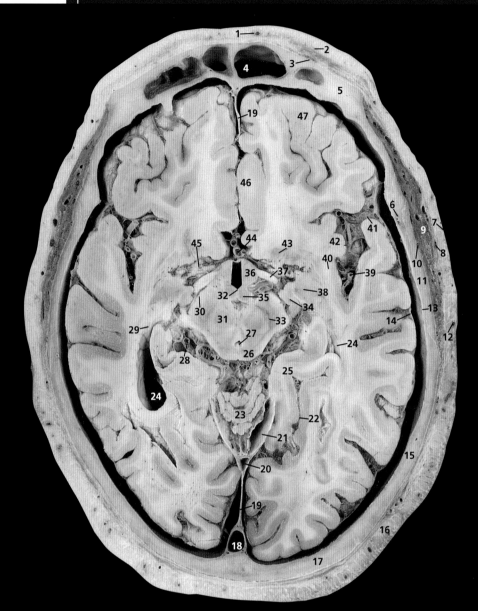

1 Supra-orbital artery
2 Orbital part of occipitofrontalis
3 Frontal belly of occipitofrontalis
4 Frontal sinus
5 Frontal bone
6 Middle meningeal artery and vein
7 Skin and dense subcutaneous tissue
8 Epicranial aponeurosis (galea aponeurotica)
9 Temporalis
10 Pericranium
11 Squamous part of temporal bone

12 Superficial temporal artery
13 Dura mater
14 Arachnoid mater
15 Parietal bone
16 Occipital artery
17 Squamous part of occipital bone
18 Superior sagittal sinus
19 Falx cerebri
20 Straight sinus
21 Tentorium cerebelli
22 Collateral sulcus
23 Vermis of cerebellum
24 Lateral ventricle
25 Parahippocampal gyrus

26 Superior colliculus
27 Aqueduct of Sylvius
28 Posterior cerebral artery
29 Tail of caudate nucleus
30 Cerebral peduncle
31 Red nucleus
32 Third ventricle
33 Substantia nigra
34 Cornu ammonis (hippocampus)
35 Mamillary body
36 Hypothalamus
37 Optic tract
38 Amygdala
39 Middle cerebral artery (branches)

40 Claustrum
41 Lateral sulcus (Sylvius)
42 Insula
43 Nucleus accumbens septi
44 Anterior cerebral artery
45 Anterior perforated substance
46 Cingulate gyrus
47 Orbitofrontal cortex

48 Cisterna ambiens
49 Temporal lobe
50 Interpeduncular cistern

Section level

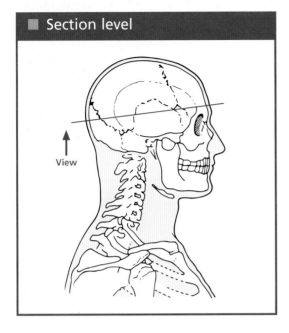

View

Orientation

Anterior

Right ← → Left

Posterior

Notes

This section passes through the upper part of the squamous temporal bone (**11**) and traverses the midbrain at the level of the cerebral peduncle (**30**) and the red nucleus (**31**).

The red nucleus (**31**) has a pinkish tinge, which is visible only in fresh tissue. The colour is produced by a ferric iron pigment present in the neurons of the red nucleus.

The aqueduct of Sylvius (**27**) is the communication between the third ventricle (see Axial section 7) and the fourth ventricle (see Axial section 10).

The colliculi, two superior (**26**) and two inferior, blend to form the tectum over the aqueduct (**27**). This is sometimes termed the quadrigeminal plate, hence an alternative name for the cisterna ambiens (**48**) is the quadrigeminal cistern. Other names for this include superior cistern and cistern of the great cerebral vein. As this cistern contains the great cerebral vein and the pineal body, it is an important anatomical landmark.

The squamous part of the temporal bone (**11**) is the thinnest bone of the calvarium (although, in contrast, its petrous part is the densest). It is, however, 'protected' by the thick overlying temporalis muscle (**9**).

The middle meningeal artery (**6**) is a branch of the maxillary artery, and its accompanying vein, and may be torn, either together or individually, in fractures of the temporal bone. This constitutes the commonest cause of a traumatic extradural haematoma.

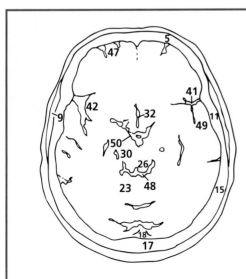

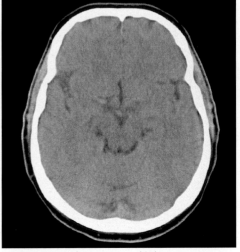

Axial computed tomogram (CT)

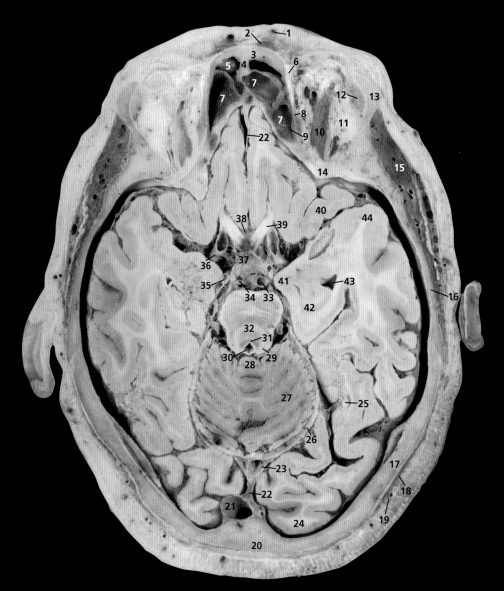

1 Supra-orbital artery
2 Frontal belly of
   occipitofrontalis
3 Frontal bone
4 Frontal crest
5 Frontal sinus
6 Trochlea
7 Ethmoidal air cells
8 Superior oblique
9 Orbital plate of
   ethmoid bone
10 Superior rectus
   underlying levator
   palpebri superioris
11 Orbital fat
12 Lacrimal gland
13 Zygomatic process of
   frontal bone

14 Lesser wing of
   sphenoid bone
15 Temporalis
16 Temporal bone
17 Parietal bone
18 Posterior belly of
   occipitofrontalis
19 Occipital artery
20 Occipital bone
21 Superior sagittal sinus
22 Falx cerebri
23 Straight sinus
24 Occipital pole
25 Floor of lateral
   ventricle (occipital
   horn)
26 Tentorium cerebelli
   (outer edge)

27 Anterior lobe of
   cerebellum
28 Cerebellar vermis
29 Inferior colliculus
30 Aqueduct of Sylvius
31 Locus coeruleus
32 Decussation of
   superior cerebellar
   peduncle
33 Basilar artery
34 Superior cerebellar
   artery
35 Posterior cerebral
   artery
36 Internal carotid artery
37 Pituitary infundibulum
38 Optic chiasma
39 Optic nerve (II)

40 Orbitofrontal cortex
41 Uncus of
   parahippocampal
   gyrus
42 Hippocampus
43 Temporal horn of
   lateral ventricle
44 Temporal pole

45 Vitreous humour
46 Lens
47 Middle cerebral artery

Section level

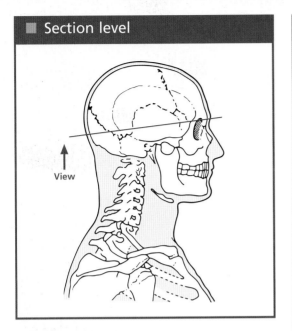

View

Orientation

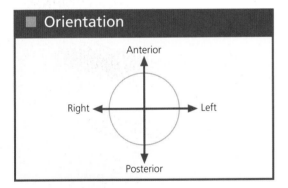

Anterior

Right ←——→ Left

Posterior

Notes

This section traverses the upper part of the orbits, the midbrain at the level of the inferior colliculus (**29**) and the anterior lobe of the cerebellum (**27**).

The straight sinus (**23**) lies in the sagittal plane of the tentorium cerebelli (**26**) at its attachment to the falx cerebri (**22**). It receives both the inferior sagittal sinus and the great cerebral vein, and drains posteriorly, usually into the left, but occasionally into the right, transverse sinus.

The optic nerves (**39**) have an intracranial course of about 10 mm. They unite at the optic chiasma (**38**), which lies immediately anterior to the infundibulum of the hypophysis cerebri, or pituitary gland (**37**). See also Coronal section 8 on p. 64.

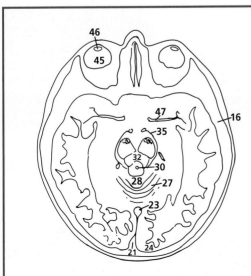

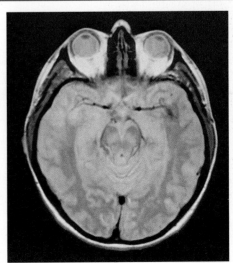

Axial magnetic resonance image (MRI)

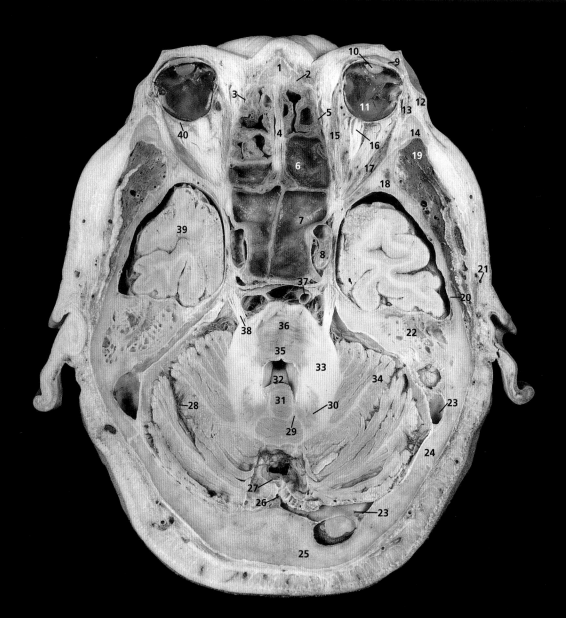

1 Nasal bone
2 Frontal process of maxilla
3 Nasolacrimal duct
4 Perpendicular plate of ethmoid bone
5 Orbital plate of ethmoid bone
6 Posterior ethmoidal air cells
7 Sphenoidal sinus
8 Internal carotid artery within cavernous sinus
9 Cornea
10 Lens
11 Vitreous humour

12 Orbicularis oculi – orbital part
13 Orbicularis oculi – palpebral part
14 Frontal process of zygomatic bone
15 Medial rectus
16 Optic nerve (II)
17 Lateral rectus
18 Greater wing of sphenoid bone
19 Temporalis
20 Squamous part of temporal bone
21 Superficial temporal artery and vein

22 Mastoid air cells
23 Transverse sinus
24 Parietal bone
25 Squamous part of occipital bone
26 Falx cerebelli
27 Superior sagittal sinus
28 Posterolateral fissure
29 Emboliform (interposed) nucleus
30 Dentate nucleus
31 Vermis of cerebellum
32 Fourth ventricle
33 Middle cerebellar peduncle

34 Hemisphere of cerebellum
35 Pontine tegmentum
36 Pontine nuclei
37 Basilar artery
38 Trigeminal nerve (V)
39 Temporal lobe
40 Sclera

41 Crista galli of ethmoid
42 Petrous part of temporal bone
43 Internal auditory meatus

■ Section level

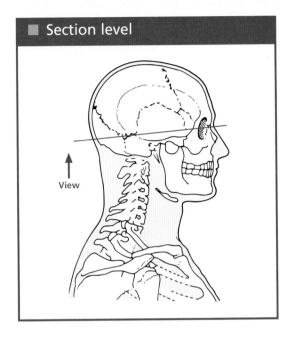

View

■ Orientation

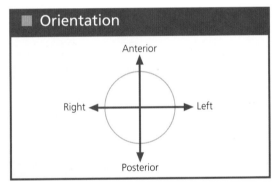

Anterior

Right ← → Left

Posterior

■ Notes

This section transects the eyeballs, the sphenoid sinus (**7**) and the pons (**36**) at the level of the middle cerebellar peduncles (**33**).

The structure of the orbit in horizontal section can be appreciated in this section. The eyeball with its cornea (**9**), lens (**10**) and vitreous humour (**11**) contained within the tough sclera (**40**), and the optic nerve (**16**) lie surrounded by the extrinsic muscles (**15**, **17**). The slit-like nasolacrimal duct (**3**) drains downwards into the inferior meatus.

The fourth ventricle (**32**) lies above the tegmentum of the pons (**35**) and below the vermis of the cerebellum (**31**).

The ethmoidal air cells, or sinuses (**6**), are made up of some eight to ten loculi suspended from the outer extremity of the cribriform plate of the ethmoid bone and bounded laterally by its orbital plate. They thus occupy the upper lateral wall of the nasal cavity. The cells are divided into anterior, middle and posterior groups by bony septa. The middle group bulge into the middle meatus to form an elevation, the bulla ethmoidalis, into which they open. The anterior cells drain into the hiatus semilunaris, which is a groove below the bulla. The posterior cells drain into the superior meatus.

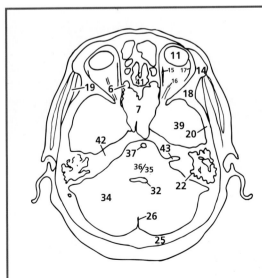

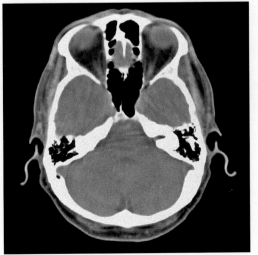

Axial computed tomogram (CT)

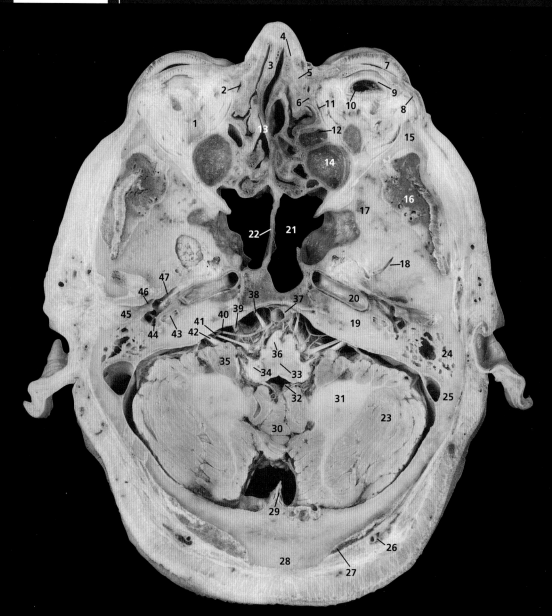

1 Inferior rectus
2 Nasolacrimal duct
3 Cartilage of nasal septum
4 Nasal bone
5 Frontal process of maxilla
6 Lacrimal bone
7 Upper eyelid
8 Orbicularis oculi
9 Sclera
10 Vitreous humour
11 Orbital plate of ethmoid bone
12 Ethmoidal air cells
13 Perpendicular plate of ethmoid bone
14 Apex of maxillary antrum
15 Frontal process of zygomatic bone
16 Temporalis
17 Greater wing of sphenoid bone
18 Middle meningeal artery
19 Petrous part of temporal bone
20 Internal carotid artery
21 Sphenoidal sinus
22 Septum of sphenoidal sinus
23 Cerebellar hemisphere
24 Mastoid air cells
25 Transverse sinus
26 Occipital artery and vein
27 Trapezius
28 External occipital protuberance
29 Falx cerebelli
30 Vermis
31 Middle cerebellar peduncle
32 Fourth ventricle with choroid plexus
33 Medulla oblongata
34 Inferior cerebellar peduncle
35 Flocculus
36 Pyramidal tract
37 Basilar artery
38 Abducent nerve (VI)
39 Trigeminal nerve (V)
40 Labyrinthine artery
41 Facial nerve (VII)
42 Vestibulocochlear (auditory) nerve (VIII)
43 Cochlea
44 Stapes
45 External auditory meatus
46 Tympanic membrane and handle of malleus
47 Auditory tube (Eustachian)

Section level

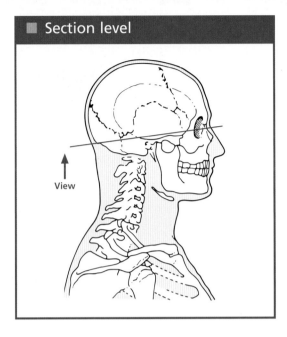

View

Orientation

Anterior

Right ← → Left

Posterior

Notes

This section passes through the upper part of the nasal cavity, the medulla oblongata (**33**) and, posteriorly, through the external occipital protuberance (**28**).

The sphenoidal sinus (**21**) is unusually large in this specimen. It is divided by a median septum (**22**) and drains anteriorly into the nasal cavity at the spheno-ethmoidal recess.

Note the relations of the labyrinthine artery (**40**), a branch of the basilar artery (**37**), the facial nerve (**41**) and the vestibulocochlear (or auditory) nerve (**42**) as they enter the internal auditory meatus of the temporal bone together with the close relationships of the trigeminal nerve (V) (**39**) and the cerebellum (**35**). As an acoustic neuroma of the vestibulocochlear nerve enlarges, it stretches the adjacent cranial nerves V and VII anteriorly and also presses on the cerebellum and brain stem to produce the cerebello-pontine angle syndrome. Rather surprisingly, facial nerve weakness with unilateral taste loss is uncommon – occurring in less than five per cent of cases – although the facial nerve is at risk in surgical removal of the tumour.

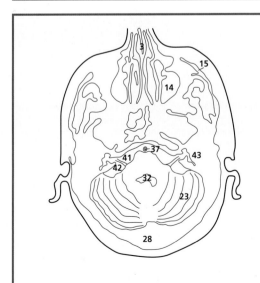

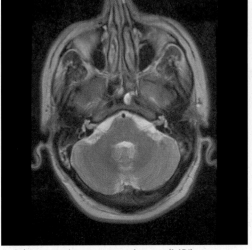

Axial magnetic resonance image (MRI)

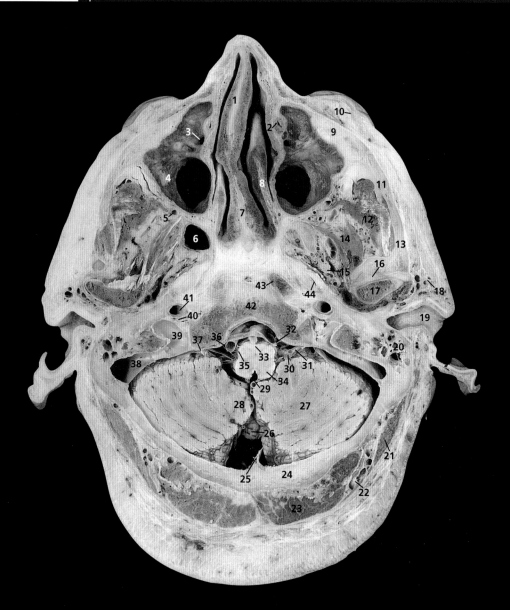

1 Cartilage of nasal septum
2 Nasolacrimal duct
3 Orifice of maxillary sinus
4 Maxillary sinus
5 Maxillary artery
6 Sphenoidal sinus
7 Vomer
8 Middle nasal concha
9 Maxilla
10 Orbicularis oculi
11 Zygomatic bone
12 Temporalis and tendon
13 Zygomatic process of temporal bone
14 Lateral pterygoid

15 Trigeminal nerve (V)
16 Articular disc of temporomandibular joint
17 Head of mandible
18 Superficial temporal artery and vein
19 External auditory meatus
20 Mastoid air cells
21 Sternocleidomastoid
22 Occipital artery and vein
23 Trapezius
24 Occipital bone – squamous part
25 Falx cerebelli

26 Vermis
27 Cerebellar hemisphere
28 Tonsil of cerebellum
29 Fourth ventricle (median aperture of roof)
30 Anterior inferior cerebellar artery
31 Glossopharyngeal nerve (IX)
32 Hypoglossal nerve (XII)
33 Pyramidal tract
34 Medulla
35 Inferior olive
36 Vertebral artery
37 Vagus nerve (X)
38 Sigmoid sinus

39 Bulb of internal jugular vein
40 Glossopharyngeal nerve (IX), vagus nerve (X) and accessory nerve (XI)
41 Internal carotid artery
42 Basi-occiput
43 Longus capitis
44 Auditory (Eustachian) tube

45 Pterygopalatine fossa (apex)
46 Foramen ovale

■ Section level

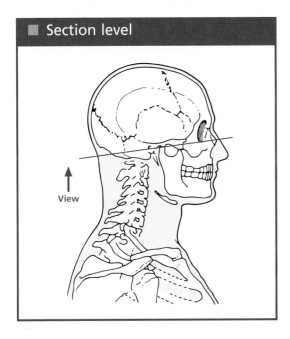

View

■ Orientation

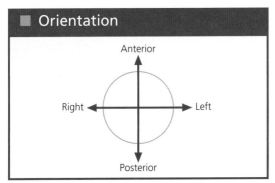

Anterior

Right ◄─────► Left

Posterior

■ Notes

This section transects the maxillary sinus (**4**) and the basi-occiput (**42**) and passes through the external auditory meatus (**19**).

At this level, the vertebral arteries (**36**) are running cranially from their entry into the skull at the foramen magnum to form the basilar artery.

The sigmoid sinus (**38**) runs forward to emerge from the skull at the jugular foramen, at which it becomes the bulb of the internal jugular vein (**39**). Exiting through the jugular foramen anterior to the vein lie, from anterior to posterior, the glossopharyngeal, vagus and accessory cranial nerves (**40**).

The maxillary nerve (Vʲ) passes into the pterygopalatine fossa (**45** on this CT image) having traversed the foramen rotundum. The mandibular nerve (Vʲʲ) leaves the skull via the foramen ovale (**46**).

The maxillary sinus (**4**) is the largest of the air sinuses, is pyramidal in shape and occupies the body of the maxilla. Medially, the sinus drains through its orifice (**3**) into the middle meatus below the middle concha (**8**). The ostium is placed high up on this wall and is thus located inefficiently from a mechanical point of view; drainage depends mainly on the effectiveness of the cilia that line the walls of the sinus.

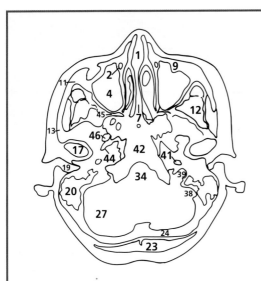

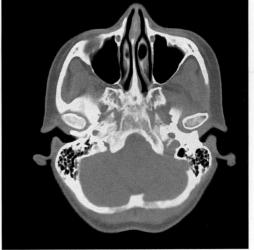

Axial computed tomogram (CT)

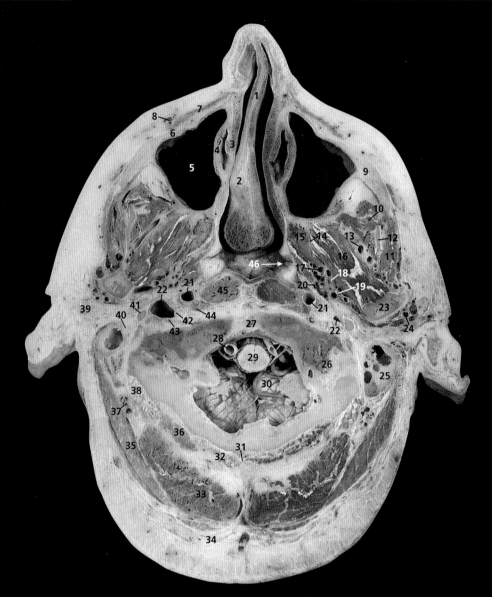

1 Cartilage of nasal septum
2 Vomer
3 Inferior nasal concha
4 Orifice of nasolacrimal duct
5 Maxillary sinus
6 Maxilla
7 Levator labii superioris
8 Facial vein
9 Zygomatic bone
10 Tendon of temporalis
11 Masseter
12 Coronoid process of mandible
13 Maxillary artery and vein

14 Lateral pterygoid plate of sphenoid
15 Medial pterygoid
16 Lateral pterygoid
17 Pterygoid artery and pterygoid venous plexus
18 Lingual nerve (V^{iii})
19 Inferior alveolar nerve (V^{iii})
20 Chorda tympani
21 Internal carotid artery
22 Internal jugular vein
23 Neck of condylar process of mandible
24 Superficial temporal artery
25 Mastoid air cells

26 Base of occipital condyle
27 Basilar part of occipital bone
28 Vertebral artery
29 Spinal cord
30 Tonsil of cerebellum
31 External occipital crest
32 Rectus capitis posterior minor
33 Semispinalis capitis
34 Trapezius
35 Splenius capitis
36 Rectus capitis posterior major
37 Occipital artery and vein

38 Obliquus capitis superior
39 Parotid gland
40 Facial nerve (VII)
41 Styloid process
42 Glossopharyngeal nerve (IX), vagus nerve (X) and accessory nerve (XI)
43 Hypoglossal nerve (XII)
44 Rectus capitis anterior
45 Longus capitis
46 Opening of auditory (Eustachian) tube

47 Nasopharynx
48 Parapharyngeal space
49 Pharyngeal recess

Section level

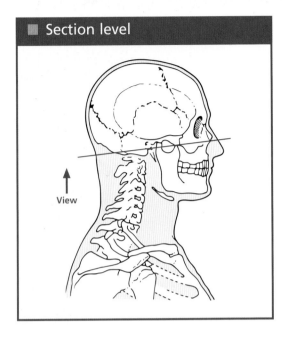

View

Orientation

Anterior

Right ← → Left

Posterior

Notes

This section traverses the nasal septum (**1**) at the level of the inferior nasal concha (**3**), beneath which opens the nasolacrimal duct (**4**). This is the only structure that drains into the inferior meatus of the nasal cavity. Its termination is guarded by a mucosal valve, which prevents reflux from the nose. Posteriorly, the plane passes through the uppermost part of the spinal cord (**29**) and the cerebellar tonsil (**30**).

The internal jugular vein (**22**) in this specimen is small, especially on the left side. The chorda tympani (**20**) is seen here as it emerges from the petrotympanic fissure to join the lingual nerve (**18**) about 2 cm below the base of the skull. It subserves taste sensation to the anterior two-thirds of the tongue and supplies secretomotor fibres to the submandibular and sublingual salivary glands.

The tonsil of the cerebellum (**30**), on the inferior aspect of the cerebellar hemisphere, lies immediately above the foramen magnum. Withdrawal of cerebrospinal fluid at lumbar puncture in a patient with raised intracranial pressure is dangerous as it may result in potentially lethal herniation of the tonsils through this bony ring.

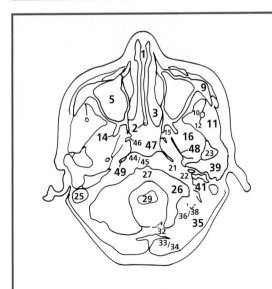

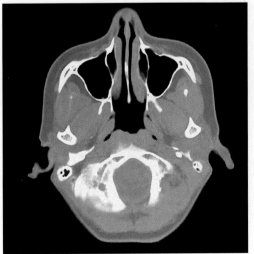

Axial computed tomogram (CT)

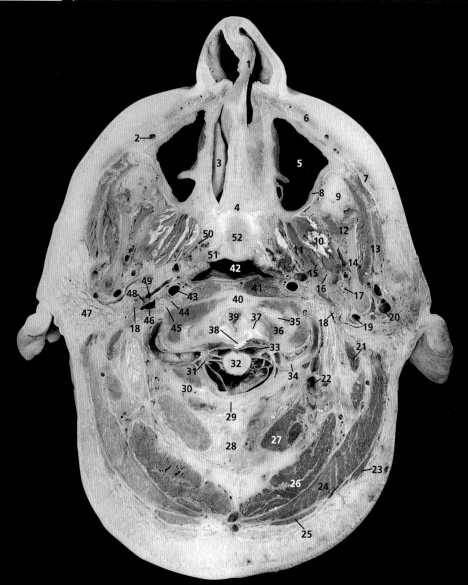

1 Cartilage of nasal septum
2 Facial vein
3 Inferior nasal concha
4 Horizontal plate of palatine bone
5 Maxillary sinus
6 Levator labii superioris
7 Zygomaticus major
8 Maxilla
9 Buccal pad of fat
10 Lateral pterygoid
11 Medial pterygoid
12 Temporalis
13 Masseter
14 Ramus of mandible
15 Lingual nerve (Vⁱⁱⁱ)
16 Inferior alveolar artery vein and nerve (Vⁱⁱⁱ)

17 Maxillary artery
18 Styloid process
19 External carotid artery
20 Retromandibular vein
21 Posterior belly of digastric
22 Anastomotic vertebral vein
23 Sternocleidomastoid
24 Splenius capitis
25 Trapezius
26 Semispinalis capitis
27 Rectus capitis posterior major
28 Ligamentum nuchae
29 Posterior atlanto-occipital membrane
30 Posterior arch of atlas

31 Spinal root of accessory nerve (XI)
32 Spinal cord within dural sheath
33 Spinal dura mater
34 Vertebral artery
35 Atlanto-occipital joint
36 Condyle of occipital bone
37 Alar ligament
38 Transverse ligament of atlas (first cervical vertebra)
39 Dens of axis (odontoid process of second cervical vertebra)
40 Anterior arch of atlas (first cervical vertebra)
41 Longus capitis

42 Nasopharynx
43 Internal carotid artery
44 Glossopharyngeal nerve (IX) and vagus nerve (X)
45 Sympathetic chain
46 Internal jugular vein
47 Parotid gland
48 Stylopharyngeus
49 Accessory nerve (XI)
50 Pterygoid venous plexus
51 Tensor veli palatini
52 Soft palate

53 Pharyngeal recess
54 Parapharyngeal space

Section level

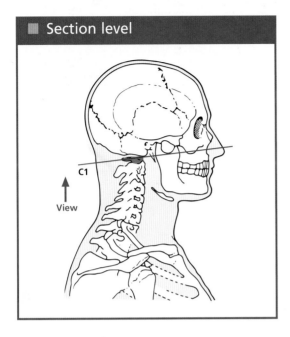

C1

View

Orientation

Anterior

Right ← → Left

Posterior

Notes

This section traverses the nasal cavity through its inferior meatus below the inferior concha (**3**), the hard palate at the horizontal plate of the palatine bone (**4**) and the tip of the dens of the axis, the second cervical vertebra (**39**).

The external carotid artery (**19**) divides at the neck of the mandible into the superficial temporal artery and the maxillary artery (**17**).

Note that the outer endosteal layer of the dura mater of the skull blends with the pericranium at the foramen magnum. The dural sheath surrounding the spinal cord (**32**) represents the continuation of the inner meningeal layer of the cerebral dura (see Axial section 1).

Note that the large vertebral canal of the atlas (first cervical vertebra), demonstrated well in this section between the posterior atlanto-occiptal membrane (**29**) and the anterior arch of the atlas (**40**), and seen well also in the Axial section 15, can be conveniently divided by the 'rule of three' into three roughly equal areas – that occupied by the cervical spinal cord (**32**), that occupied by the dens of the axis (**39**) and that occupied by the dural sheath and the extradural space.

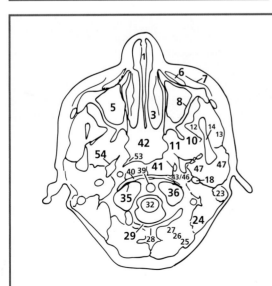

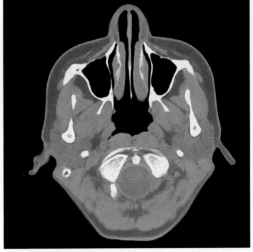

Axial computed tomogram (CT)

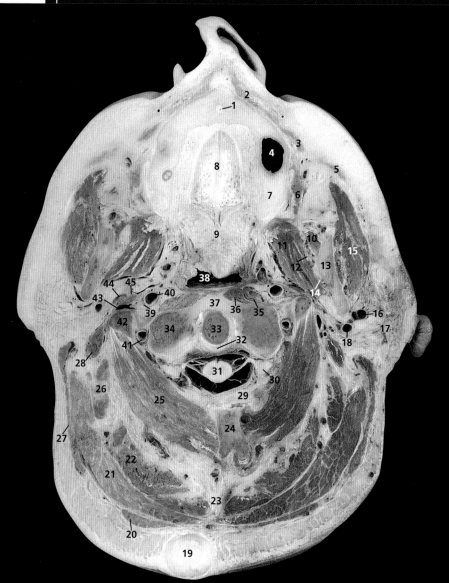

1 Nasopalatine nerve (Vⁱⁱ) within incisive canal
2 Orbicularis oris
3 Levator anguli oris
4 Maxillary antrum
5 Zygomaticus major
6 Buccinator
7 Alveolar process of maxilla
8 Hard palate
9 Soft palate
10 Temporalis
11 Medial pterygoid
12 Lingual nerve (Vⁱⁱⁱ)
13 Ramus of mandible
14 Inferior alveolar artery vein and nerve
15 Masseter

16 Retromandibular vein
17 Parotid gland
18 External carotid artery
19 Dermoid cyst of scalp
20 Trapezius
21 Splenius capitis
22 Semispinalis capitis
23 Ligamentum nuchae
24 Spine of axis
25 Obliquus capitis inferior
26 Longissimus capitis
27 Sternocleidomastoid
28 Posterior belly of digastric
29 Posterior arch of atlas (first cervical vertebra)

30 Dorsal root ganglion of second cervical nerve
31 Spinal cord within dural sheath
32 Transverse ligament of atlas
33 Dens of axis (odontoid process of second cervical vertebra)
34 Lateral mass of atlas (first cervical vertebra)
35 Longus capitis
36 Longus colli
37 Anterior arch of atlas (first cervical vertebra)
38 Nasopharynx
39 Vagus nerve (X) and hypoglossal nerve (XII)

40 Internal carotid artery
41 Vertebral artery
42 Transverse process of atlas (first cervical vertebra)
43 Internal jugular vein
44 Styloid process, with origins of styloglossus and stylohyoid and glossopharyngeal nerve (IX)
45 Stylopharyngeus

46 Levator and tensor veli palatini
47 Parapharyngeal space
48 Inferior nasal concha
49 Cartilage of nasal septum

■ Section level

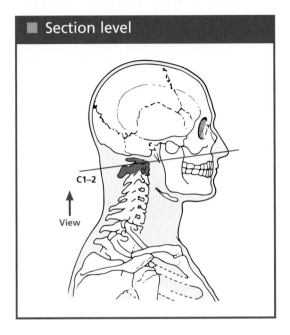

C1–2

View

■ Orientation

Anterior

Right ←→ Left

Posterior

■ Notes

This section traverses the hard (**8**) and soft (**9**) palate, the nasopharynx (**38**), the dens (**33**) and the spine of the axis (**24**). The CT image is rather more cranial.

Flexion and extension of the skull (nodding movements of the head) take place at the atlanto-occipital joint between the upper facet of the lateral mass of the atlas (**34**) and the corresponding facet on the occipital bone. Rotation of the skull (looking to the left and right) takes place at the atlanto-axial articulation between the dens (**33**) and the facet on the anterior arch of the atlas (**37**). The transverse ligament of the atlas (**32**) is dense and is the principal structure in preventing posterior dislocation of the dens.

Obliquus capitis inferior (**25**) forms the lower outer limb of the suboccipital triangle. The vertebral artery (**41**), on emerging from the foramen transversarium of the atlas, enters this triangle on its ascending course to the foramen magnum.

The maxillary antrum, or sinus (**4**), may be somewhat asymmetrical between the two sides – here it projects more inferiorly on the left side. The floor of the sinus relates to the roots of the upper teeth – at least the upper second premolar and first molar. The sinus may extend forwards, however, as far as the canine and behind to the third molar.

Note that this subject has a large dermoid cyst of the scalp (**19**).

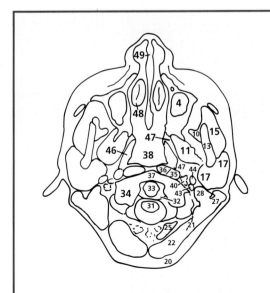

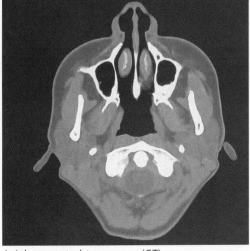

Axial computed tomogram (CT)

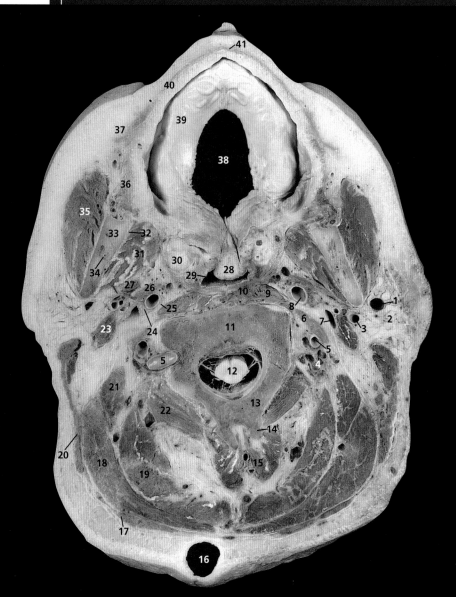

1 Retromandibular vein
2 Parotid gland
3 External carotid artery
4 Vertebral vein
5 Vertebral artery
6 Scalenus medius
7 Internal jugular vein
8 Internal carotid artery
9 Longus capitis
10 Longus colli
11 Body of axis (second cervical vertebra)
12 Spinal cord within dural sheath
13 Lamina of axis (second cervical vertebra)
14 Spine of axis (second cervical vertebra)
15 Semispinalis cervicis
16 Dermoid cyst of scalp
17 Trapezius
18 Splenius capitis
19 Semispinalis capitis
20 Sternocleidomastoid
21 Longissimus capitis
22 Obliquus capitis inferior
23 Posterior belly of digastric
24 Vagus nerve (X) and hypoglossal nerve (XII)
25 Sympathetic chain
26 Stylopharyngeus and glossopharyngeal nerve (IX)
27 Styloglossus and stylohyoid (posteriorly)
28 Base of uvula
29 Nasopharynx
30 Palatine tonsil
31 Medial pterygoid
32 Lingual nerve (V^{iii})
33 Ramus of mandible
34 Inferior alveolar artery, vein and nerve (V^{iii}) within mandibular canal
35 Masseter
36 Buccinator
37 Levator anguli oris
38 Mouth
39 Alveolar margin
40 Orbicularis oris
41 Mucous gland of lip

42 Hard palate
43 Soft palate
44 Styloid process
45 Parapharyngeal space
46 Anterior arch of atlas
47 Dens of axis (odontoid process of second cervical vertebra)
48 Posterior arch of atlas (first cervical vertebra)
49 Foramen transversarium

■ Section level

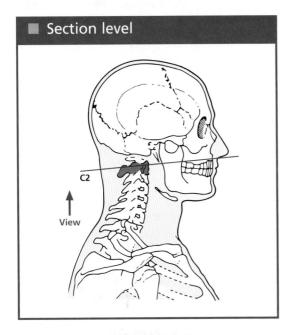

C2

View

■ Orientation

Anterior

Right ← → Left

Posterior

■ Notes

This section passes through the alveolar margin (**39**) of the upper jaw and through the body of the axis (**11**). The CT image is at a more cranial level.

The vertebral artery (**5**) on the right side of this specimen is tortuous and bulges laterally between the transverse processes of the atlas and axis, a not uncommon feature in arteriosclerotic subjects. Each cervical vertebra bears its characteristic foramen transversarium (**49**) within its transverse process. The vertebral artery, with its accompanying vein, ascends through the foramina of C6 to C1 to gain access to the foramen magnum. Not uncommonly, the foramen transversarium is bifid, the larger opening of the two being for the vertebral artery and the smaller for the vein. Sympathetic fibres from the superior cervical ganglion (C1, 2, 3, 4) accompany the artery.

The lips are lined by mucous membrane enclosing orbicularis oris (**40**), the labial vessels and nerves, fibrofatty connective tissue and the labial mucous glands (**41**). These lie between the mucosa and underlying muscle, are about 0.5 cm in diameter and resemble mucous salivary glands. Their ducts drain into the vestibule of the mouth. These glands, like those studded over the oral aspect of the palate, are occasional sites of pleomorphic adenomas, which are similar to those seen more commonly in the parotid gland.

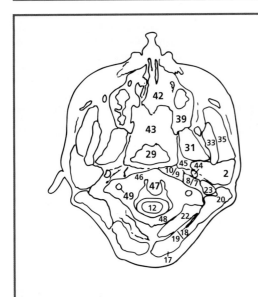

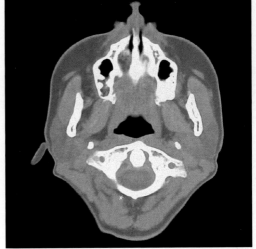

Axial computed tomogram (CT)

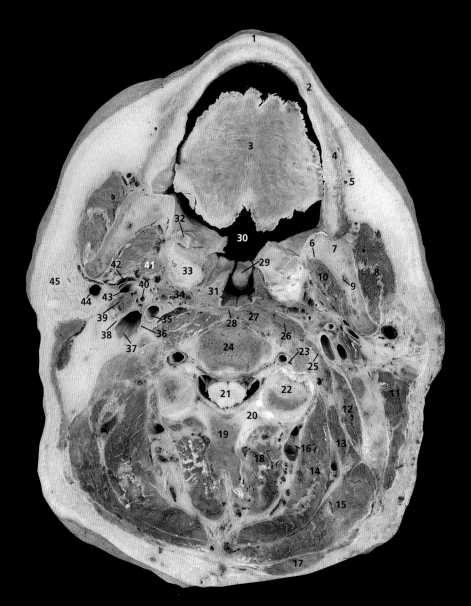

1 Upper lip
2 Orbicularis oris
3 Tongue
4 Buccinator
5 Facial artery and vein
6 Lingual nerve (V^{iii})
7 Ramus of mandible
8 Masseter
9 Inferior alveolar artery vein and nerve (V^{iii}) within mandibular canal
10 Medial pterygoid
11 Sternocleidomastoid
12 Levator scapulae
13 Longissimus capitis
14 Semispinalis capitis

15 Splenius capitis
16 Deep cervical vein
17 Trapezius
18 Semispinalis cervicis
19 Spine of axis (second cervical vertebra)
20 Lamina of axis (second cervical vertebra)
21 Spinal cord within dural sheath
22 Inferior articular process of axis (second cervical vertebra)
23 Vertebral artery and vein
24 Body of axis (second cervical vertebra)

25 Scalenus medius
26 Longus capitis
27 Longus colli
28 Constrictor of pharynx
29 Uvula
30 Oropharynx
31 Palatopharyngeal arch with palatopharyngeal
32 Palatoglossal arch with palatoglossus
33 Palatine tonsil
34 Stylopharyngeus
35 Internal carotid artery
36 Vagus nerve (X)
37 Internal jugular vein
38 Accessory nerve (XI)

39 Digastric (posterior belly)
40 External carotid artery
41 Styloglossus
42 Stylohyoid
43 Posterior auricular artery
44 Retromandibular vein
45 Parotid gland

46 Nasopharynx
47 Parapharyngeal space
48 Alveolar process of maxilla

Section level

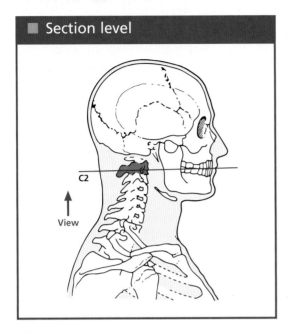

C2

View

Orientation

Anterior

Right ← → Left

Posterior

Notes

This section traverses the upper lip (**1**), the tongue (**3**), the uvula (**29**) and the axis (**19**, **20**, **22**, **24**). The plane of the CT image is slightly more cranial.

The palatine tonsil (**33**) lies in the tonsillar fossa between the anterior and posterior pillars of the fauces. The anterior pillar, or palatoglossal arch (**32**), forms the boundary between the buccal cavity and the oropharynx (**30**); it fuses with the lateral wall of the tongue and contains the palatoglossus muscle. The posterior pillar, or palatopharyngeal arch (**31**), blends with the wall of the pharynx and contains the palatopharyngeus muscle.

The tonsil consists of a collection of lymphoid tissue covered by a squamous epithelium, a unique histological combination that makes it easy to identify it under the microscope. From late puberty onwards, the lymphoid tissue undergoes progressive atrophy.

The prominent deep cervical vein (**16**) is a useful landmark in separating the deeply placed semispinalis cervicis muscle (**18**) from the more superficially placed semispinalis capitis (**14**); this is seen again in Axial section 18.

The intrinsic muscles of the tongue (**3**) are well shown and comprise longitudinal transverse and cervical bands. Acting alone or in combination, they give the tongue its precise and highly varied mobility, which is important in both speech and swallowing.

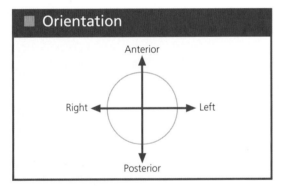

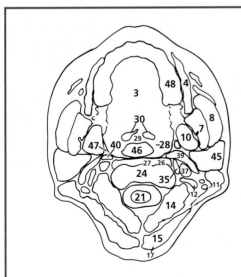

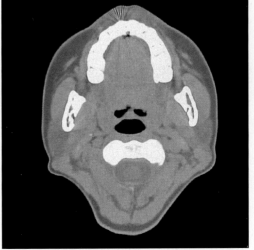

Axial computed tomogram (CT)

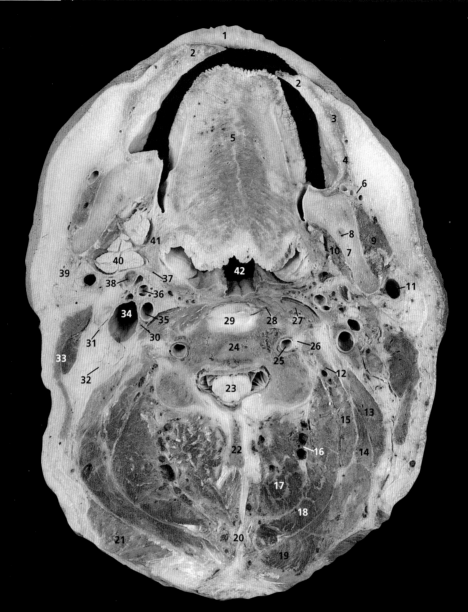

1 Upper lip
2 Lower lip
3 Orbicularis oris
4 Buccinator
5 Transverse intrinsic muscle of tongue
6 Facial artery and vein
7 Ramus of mandible
8 Inferior alveolar artery vein and nerve (V^iii) within mandibular canal
9 Masseter
10 Medial pterygoid
11 Retromandibular vein
12 Scalenus medius

14 Splenius cervicis
15 Longissimus capitis
16 Deep cervical vein
17 Semispinalis cervicis
18 Semispinalis capitis
19 Splenius capitis
20 Ligamentum nuchae
21 Trapezius
22 Spine of third cervical vertebra
23 Spinal cord within dural sheath
24 Body of third cervical vertebra
25 Vertebral artery and vein within foramen

26 Anterior primary ramus of third cervical nerve
27 Longus capitis
28 Longus colli
29 Part of intervertebral disc between second and third cervical vertebrae
30 Vagus nerve (X)
31 Accessory nerve (XI)
32 Deep cervical lymph node
33 Sternocleidomastoid
34 Internal jugular vein
35 Internal carotid artery

37 Stylohyoid
38 Tendon of digastric
39 Parotid gland
40 Submandibular salivary gland
41 Styloglossus entering tongue
42 Oropharynx

43 Genioglossus
44 Constrictor of pharynx
45 Base of tongue
46 Mylohyoid
47 Hyoglossus
48 External jugular vein

Section level

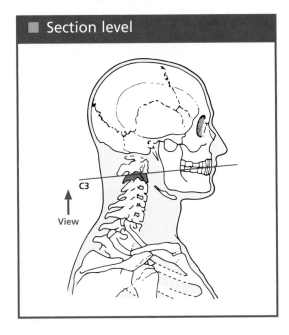

C3

View

Orientation

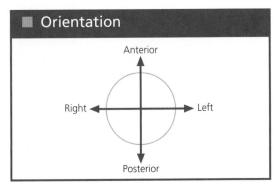

Anterior

Right — Left

Posterior

Notes

This section passes between the lips (**1** and **2**), the body of the third cervical vertebra (**24**) and the spine of the third cervical vertebra (**22**). The CT image is from a different subject and comes from the series that traverse the neck. This is because few cranial CT runs extend as caudal as this level. Moreover, artefacts from the amalgam of dental fillings often obscure this region. Bolus enhancement with intravenous iodinated contrast medium has opacified the major vessels (**34–36**) and assists in their identification.

The submandibular salivary gland (**40**) lies against the ramus of the mandible (**7**) at its angle, separated by the medial pterygoid muscle (**10**). Its close relationship to the parotid gland (**39**) is well demonstrated; it is separated from the latter only by the fascial sheet of the stylomandibular ligament.

The foramen transversarium (**25**), lying within the transverse process, is the characteristic feature of all seven of the cervical vertebrae. That of the seventh cervical vertebra, the vertebra prominens, is often of small size because it transmits only small accessory vertebral veins and not the vertebral artery, which usually enters at the sixth cervical vertebra. The artery is surrounded by a plexus of sympathetic nerve fibres and is accompanied by the smaller vertebral vein. Not infrequently, the foramen transversarium will be seen to be double – the smaller compartment in such examples conveys the vein.

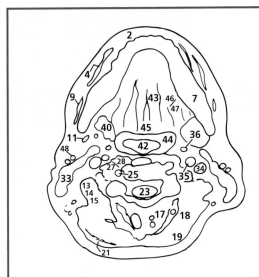

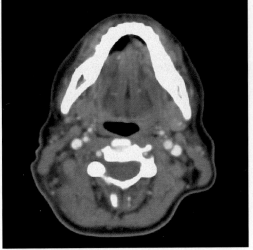

Axial computed tomogram (CT)

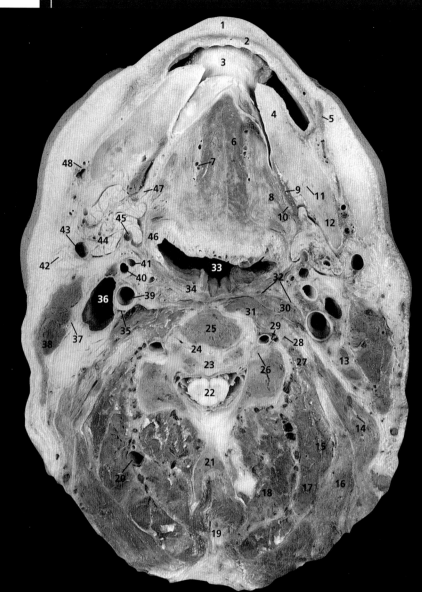

1 Lower lip
2 Orbicularis oris
3 Under surface of tongue
4 Body of mandible
5 Depressor anguli oris
6 Genioglossus
7 Lingual artery and vein
8 Hyoglossus
9 Mylohyoid
10 Lingual nerve (Vⁱⁱⁱ)
11 Inferior alveolar nerve (Vⁱⁱⁱ) within mandibular canal
12 Ramus of mandible
13 Cervical lymph nodes
14 Levator scapulae
15 Splenius cervicis

16 Splenius capitis
17 Semispinalis capitis
18 Semispinalis cervicis
19 Ligamentum nuchae
20 Deep cervical vein
21 Spine of fourth cervical vertebra
22 Spinal cord within dural sheath
23 Part of body of fourth cervical vertebra
24 Part of intervertebral disc between third and fourth cervical vertebrae
25 Part of body of third cervical vertebra
26 Dorsal root ganglion

of fourth cervical nerve
27 Scalenus medius
28 Scalenus anterior origin
29 Vertebral artery and vein within foramen transversarium
30 Longus capitis
31 Longus colli
32 Prevertebral fascia
33 Oropharynx
34 Constrictor muscles of pharynx
35 Vagus nerve (X)
36 Internal jugular vein
37 Accessory nerve (XI)
38 Sternocleidomastoid
39 Internal carotid artery

40 External carotid artery
41 Origin of facial artery
42 Parotid gland
43 Retromandibular vein
44 Submandibular salivary gland – superficial lobe
45 Tendon of digastric
46 Styloglossus
47 Deep lobe of submandibular salivary gland
48 Facial artery and vein

49 Platysma
50 Hyoid bone
51 External jugular vein

46

■ Section level

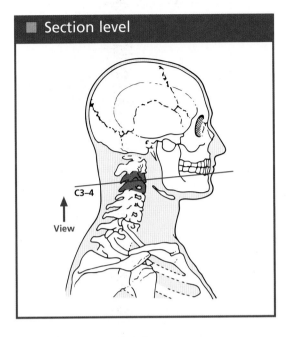

C3–4

View

■ Notes

This section passes through the upper border of the lower lip (**1**), genioglossus at the base of the tongue (**6**) and the cartilaginous disc between the third and fourth cervical vertebrae (**24**).

The prevertebral fascia (**32**) invests the front of the bodies of the cervical vertebrae, the prevertebral muscles (**30**, **31**) and the scalene muscles (**27**, **28**). It forms an almost avascular transverse plane behind the pharynx (**33**) and the great vessels (**36**, **39**). It extends from the skull base above to the superior mediastinum below, where it blends with the anterior longitudinal vertebral ligament. It provides an avascular plane for the anterior surgical approach to the cervical vertebrae. It is deep to this fascia that tuberculous pus will track from an infected cervical vertebra.

The facial artery at its origin from the external carotid artery (**40**) is seen at (**41**). It arches over the submandibular salivary gland (**44**) to cross the lower border of the mandible (**4**), where its pulse is palpable (**48**).

■ Orientation

Anterior

Right   Left

Posterior

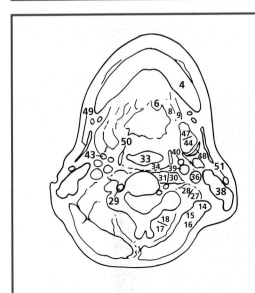

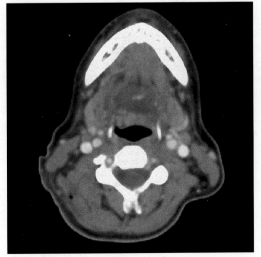

Axial computed tomogram (CT)

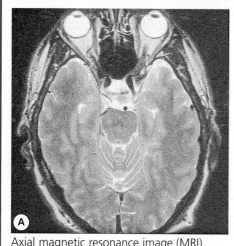
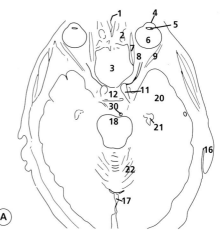

Axial magnetic resonance image (MRI)

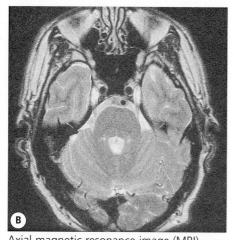
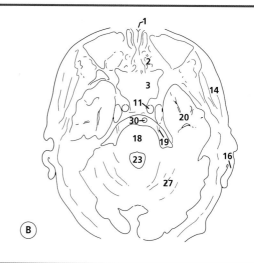

Axial magnetic resonance image (MRI)

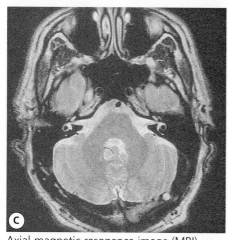
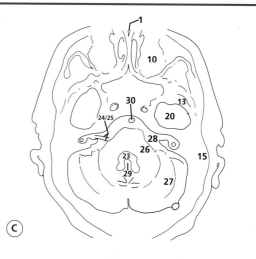

Axial magnetic resonance image (MRI)

■ Section level

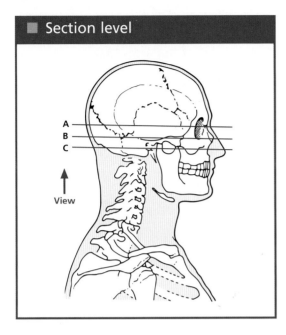

View

■ Orientation

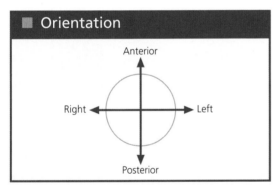

Anterior

Right ←——→ Left

Posterior

■ Notes

These three axial T2-weighted images show many important structures at the base of the brain, along with the orbits and sinuses. The water content of the globe provides good contrast with the lens. On this sequence, the fluid in the globe and cerebrospinal spaces yields similar signal intensity to the fat within the orbit. The T2 weighting also demonstrates the emerging nerves within the cerebrospinal fluid to good effect. Demonstration of a normal VIII (vestibulocochlear) nerve and fluid entering the internal auditory canal (meatus) effectively excludes a neuroma here. Possible lesions at this site (the cerebello-pontine angle) provide one of the commonest referrals for magnetic resonance imaging (MRI). On the spin-echo sequence used here, flowing arterial blood returns no signal and thus appears black; in this way, the internal carotid and basilar arteries are well visualized. Air-containing structures, such as the sphenoidal sinus, also appear black.

The pons is seen well on these images, and areas of infarction and other lesions should be looked for on T2-weighted images. The fourth ventricle is another important landmark in this region; it should be central and symmetrical.

1 Nasal bone	16 Pinna
2 Ethmoidal air cells	17 Straight sinus
3 Sphenoidal sinus	18 Pons
4 Cornea	19 Trigeminal nerve (V)
5 Lens	20 Temporal lobe of brain
6 Vitreous humour	21 Temporal horn of lateral ventricle
7 Medial rectus	22 Anterior lobe of cerebellum
8 Optic nerve (II)	23 Fourth ventricle
9 Lateral rectus	24 Facial nerve (VII)
10 Maxillary sinus	25 Vestibulocochlear (auditory) nerve (VIII)
11 Internal carotid artery – within cavernous sinus (b11)	26 Middle cerebral peduncle
12 Pituitary fossa	27 Cerebellar hemisphere
13 Greater wing of sphenoid bone	28 Internal auditory meatus
14 Temporalis	29 Vermis of cerebellum
15 Mastoid	30 Basilar artery

49

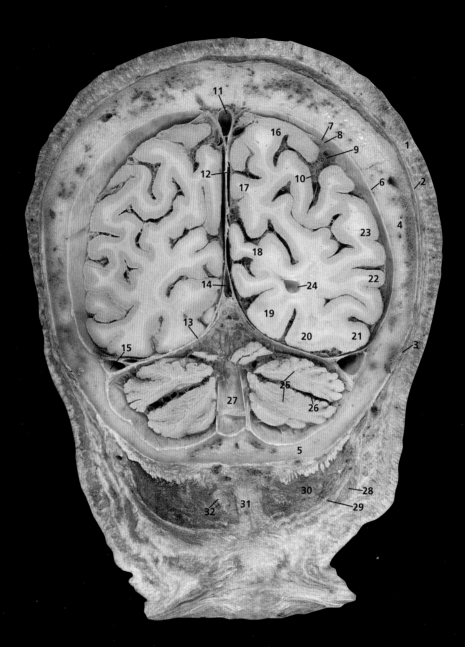

1 Skin and dense subcutaneous
   tissue
2 Epicranial aponeurosis (galea
   aponeurotica)
3 Occipital belly of
   occipitofrontalis
4 Parietal bone
5 Occipital bone
6 Dura mater
7 Subdural space
8 Arachnoid mater
9 Subarachnoid space

10 Pia mater
11 Superior sagittal sinus
12 Falx cerebri
13 Tentorium cerebelli
14 Straight sinus
15 Transverse sinus
16 Superior parietal lobule
17 Precuneus
18 Cuneus
19 Lingual gyrus
20 Medial occipitotemporal gyrus
21 Lateral occipitotemporal gyrus

22 Middle temporal gyrus
23 Inferior parietal lobule
24 Posterior horn of lateral
   ventricle
25 Cerebellar hemisphere
26 Horizontal fissure of cerebellum
27 Internal occipital crest
28 Trapezius
29 Splenius capitis
30 Semispinalis capitis
31 Ligamentum nuchae
32 Greater occipital nerve

■ Section level

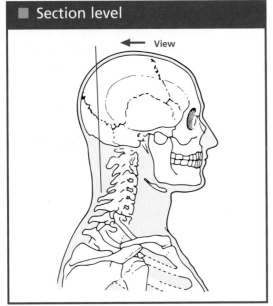

← View

■ Orientation

Superior

Right ← → Left

Inferior

■ Notes

This coronal section passes through the posterior part of the occipital bone (**5**) immediately anterior to the external occipital protuberance. It passes through the posterior extremity of the posterior, or occipital, horn of the lateral ventricle (**24**).

In this, as in all subsequent sections, cross-reference should be made between a coronal section with the photographs of the external aspects and sagittal section of the brain for orientation of the positions of the main sulci and gyri (see pages 2–7).

On this proton-density magnetic resonance image, flowing blood in the venous sinuses appears black (low signal intensity) because the protons that were excited have moved out of the slice before measurement (creating a flow void).

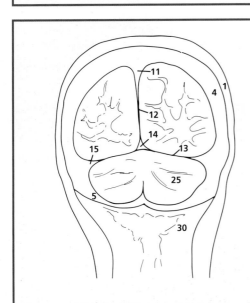

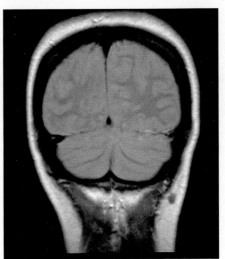

Coronal magnetic resonance image (MRI)

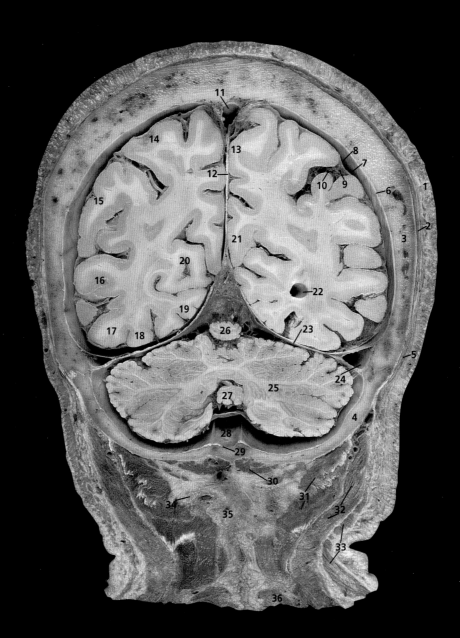

1 Skin and dense subcutaneous tissue
2 Pericranium
3 Parietal bone
4 Occipital bone
5 Occipital belly of occipitofrontalis
6 Dura mater
7 Subdural space
8 Arachnoid mater
9 Subarachnoid space
10 Pia mater
11 Superior sagittal sinus
12 Falx cerebri
13 Precuneus
14 Superior parietal lobule
15 Inferior parietal lobule
16 Middle temporal gyrus
17 Lateral occipitotemporal gyrus
18 Medial occipitotemporal gyrus
19 Lingual gyrus
20 Cuneus
21 Cingulate gyrus
22 Posterior horn of lateral ventricle
23 Tentorium cerebelli
24 Transverse sinus
25 Cerebellar hemisphere
26 Superior vermis
27 Inferior vermis
28 Falx cerebelli
29 Internal occipital crest
30 Rectus capitis posterior minor
31 Semispinalis capitis
32 Splenius capitis
33 Trapezius
34 Greater occipital nerve
35 Ligamentum nuchae
36 Semispinalis cervicis

Section level

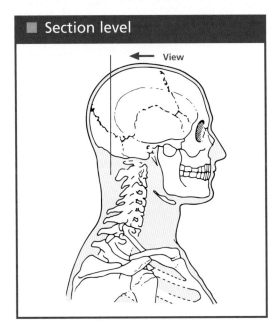

← View

Orientation

Superior

Right ← → Left

Inferior

Notes

The makeup of the layers of the scalp can be appreciated in this and subsequent sections. It comprises hair-bearing skin, lying on dense, highly vascular connective tissue (**1**); note the large vessels seen in many of the sections. This, in turn, is adherent to a tough aponeurosis, which is the aponeurotic sheet joining the occipital belly of occipitofrontalis (**5**) to the frontalis muscle. The former arises from the superior nuchal line, while the latter inserts into the fascia above the eyebrows. The occipital part is supplied by the auricular, and the frontal part by the temporal, branch of the facial nerve (VII). Paralysis of the facial nerve is followed by inability to wrinkle the forehead on the affected side. Beneath the aponeurosis lies a layer of loose areolar tissue, which again can be appreciated in these sections. It is in this plane that avulsion of the scalp can take place in tearing injuries and in which a flap of scalp can be turned down during surgical exposure of the skull. The final layer, the periosteum, is closely adherent to the skull.

This T2-weighted image is through the same position as in the MRI image in coronal section 1. The cerebrospinal fluid in the subarachnoid space (**9**) now yields high signal intensity (white), providing contrast with the gyri.

The various layers of the meninges are demonstrated well (**6**, **8**, **10**). Haemorrhage around these layers is a serious event. An extradural haematoma develops between bone (**3**) and the dura mater (**6**) and usually arises soon after trauma that ruptures a meningeal vessel. A subdural haematoma collects in the subdural space (**7**), usually due to venous bleeding following minor trauma in the elderly. Subarachnoid haemorrhage develops suddenly in the subarachnoid space (**9**), usually following the spontaneous rupture of a cerebral artery, or berry aneurysm.

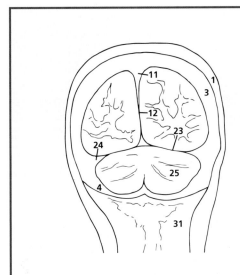

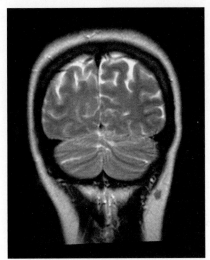

Coronal magnetic resonance image (MRI)

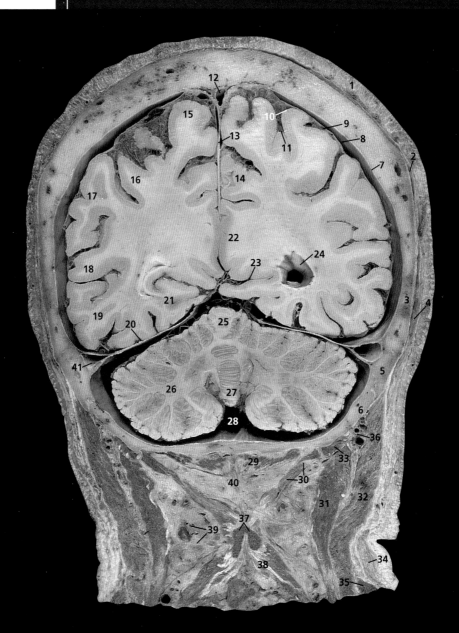

1 Skin and dense subcutaneous tissue	13 Falx cerebri	28 Cerebello-medullary cistern
2 Epicranial aponeurosis (galea aponeurotica)	14 Precuneus	29 Rectus capitis posterior minor
	15 Superior parietal lobule	30 Rectus capitis posterior major
3 Parietal bone	16 Inferior parietal lobule	31 Semispinalis capitis
4 Occipital belly of occipitofrontalis	17 Superior temporal gyrus	32 Splenius capitis
	18 Middle temporal gyrus	33 Superior oblique
5 Occipital margin of temporal bone	19 Inferior temporal gyrus	34 Trapezius
	20 Tentorium cerebelli	35 Levator scapulae
6 Occipital bone	21 Lingual gyrus	36 Occipital artery and vein
7 Dura mater	22 Cingulate gyrus	37 Bifid spine of axis
8 Subdural space	23 Calcarine sulcus	38 Semispinalis cervicis
9 Arachnoid mater	24 Posterior horn of lateral ventricle	39 Occipital lymph nodes
10 Subarachnoid space		40 Ligamentum nuchae
11 Pia mater	25 Superior vermis	41 Transverse sinus
12 Superior sagittal sinus	26 Cerebellar hemisphere	
	27 Inferior vermis	42 Small infarct (see notes)

Section level

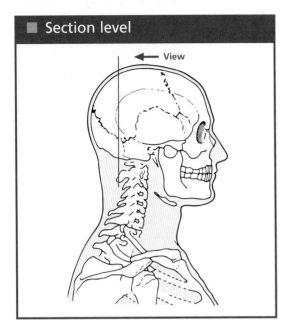

← View

Orientation

Superior

Right ←→ Left

Inferior

Notes

This and neighbouring sections give clear views of the structure of the superior sagittal sinus (**12**) and the transverse sinus (**41**), which are formed as clefts between the outer (endosteal) and inner (meningeal) layers of the dura mater.

The internal structure of the cerebellum (**26**) can be appreciated in this section, with its superficial highly convoluted cortex over a dense core of white matter, which contains the deep cerebellar nuclei. The highly branched appearance of the cerebellum in section is given the fanciful name of 'arbor vitae' – tree of life.

The bifid spine of the axis (**37**) gives attachment to semispinalis cervicis (**38**), rectus capitis posterior major (**30**) and the ligamentum nuchae (**40**), as well as the inferior oblique, which can be seen in the next section.

The small occipital lymph nodes (**39**) are of clinical significance in that they are classically enlarged in rubella (German measles) and some forms of cancer.

This T2-weighted magnetic resonance image shows cerebrospinal fluid (white) in the subarachnoid space (**10**) surrounding the gyri and within the posterior horn of the left lateral ventricle (**24**).

The magnetic resonance image shows a small area of abnormal high signal intensity (**42**) medially in the occipital lobe. The clinical features and radiological features were those of a small infarct.

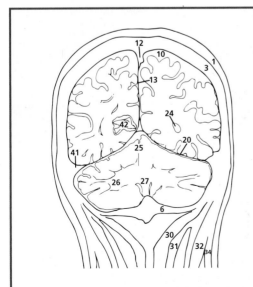

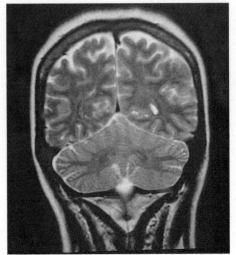

Coronal magnetic resonance image (MRI)

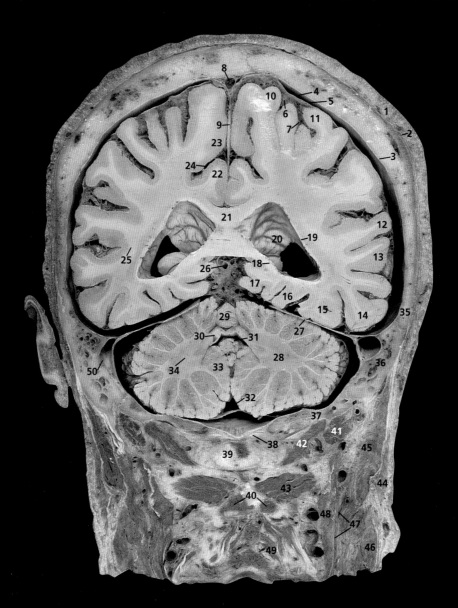

1 Skin and dense subcutaneous tissue
2 Epicranial aponeurosis (galea aponeurotica)
3 Dura mater
4 Subdural space
5 Arachnoid mater
6 Subarachnoid space
7 Pia mater
8 Superior sagittal sinus
9 Falx cerebri
10 Postcentral gyrus
11 Inferior parietal lobule
12 Superior temporal gyrus
13 Middle temporal gyrus
14 Inferior temporal gyrus

15 Lateral occipitotemporal gyrus
16 Medial occipitotemporal gyrus
17 Parahippocampal gyrus
18 Fimbria of hippocampus
19 Tapetum
20 Posterior horn of lateral ventricle
21 Splenium of corpus callosum
22 Cingulate gyrus
23 Paracentral lobule
24 Cingulate sulcus
25 Optic radiation
26 Great cerebral vein

27 Tentorium cerebelli
28 Cerebellar hemisphere
29 Superior vermis
30 Superior medullary vellum
31 Fourth ventricle
32 Cerebello-medullary cistern
33 Tonsil of cerebellum
34 Dentate nucleus
35 Parietal bone
36 Mastoid air cells within petrous part of temporal bone
37 Occipital bone
38 Posterior atlanto-occipital membrane

39 Posterior tubercle of atlas
40 Bifid spinous process of axis
41 Superior oblique
42 Rectus capitis posterior major
43 Inferior oblique
44 Sternocleidomastoid
45 Splenius capitis
46 Levator scapulae
47 Longissimus capitis
48 Semispinalis capitis
49 Semispinalis cervicis
50 Transverse sinus

51 Small infarct (see notes)

■ Section level

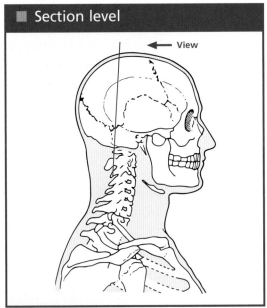

← View

■ Orientation

Superior

Right ← → Left

Inferior

■ Notes

This section passes through the posterior part of the opening in the tentorium cerebelli (**27**). Note the great cerebral vein (**26**), a short median vessel formed by the union of the two internal cerebral veins. It passes backwards to open into the anterior end of the straight sinus, which lies at the junction of the falx cerebri (**9**) with the tentorium cerebelli.

The dentate nucleus of the cerebellum (**34**) is the largest and most lateral of the four cerebellar nuclei. Fibres from this nucleus form the bulk of the superior cerebellar peduncle.

On the two T2-weighted images shown here, the extent of the cerebrospinal fluid is well demonstrated in image (A), especially in the subarachnoid space (**6**) around the gyri, but also in the cisterns around the base of the brain (**32**).

Also to be seen in image (A) is a small infarct (**51**); this is an area where there has been damage caused by interruption to the blood supply, most commonly due to a small embolus.

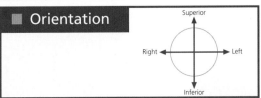

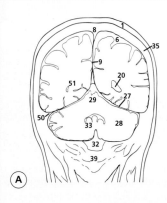

(A)

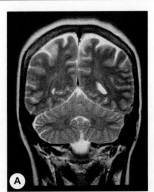

(A)

Coronal magnetic resonance image (MRI)

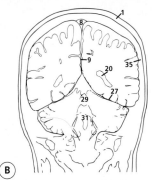

(B)

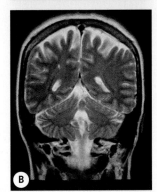

(B)

Coronal magnetic resonance image (MRI)

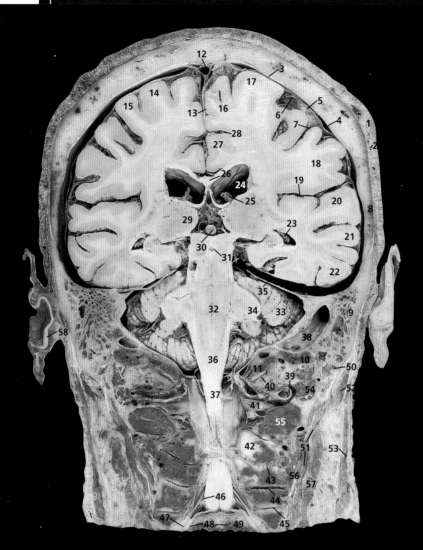

1 Skin and dense subcutaneous tissue	**18** Supramarginal gyrus	**33** Cerebellar hemisphere
2 Epicranial aponeurosis (galea aponeurotica)	**19** Lateral sulcus	**34** Middle cerebellar peduncle
3 Dura mater	**20** Superior temporal gyrus	**35** Tentorium cerebelli
4 Subdural space	**21** Middle temporal gyrus	**36** Termination of medulla oblongata
5 Arachnoid mater	**22** Inferior temporal gyrus	**37** Commencement of spinal cord
6 Subarachnoid space	**23** Choroid plexus within posterior horn of lateral ventricle (see 25)	**38** Sigmoid sinus
7 Pia mater		**39** Vertebral artery entering foramen magnum
8 Parietal bone	**24** Body of lateral ventricle	**40** Atlanto-occipital joint
9 Mastoid air cells within petrous part of temporal bone	**25** Choroid plexus within body of lateral ventricle (see 23)	**41** Posterior arch of atlas
10 Occipital bone	**26** Corpus callosum	**42** Lamina of axis
11 Margin of foramen magnum	**27** Cingulate gyrus	**43** Facet joint between C2/3 vertebrae
12 Superior sagittal sinus	**28** Cingulate sulcus	**44** Facet joint between C3/4 vertebrae
13 Falx cerebri	**29** Thalamus	**45** Facet joint between C4/5 vertebrae
14 Precentral gyrus	**30** Pineal gland	
15 Postcentral gyrus	**31** Aqueduct (of Sylvius)	
16 Para central lobule	**32** Pons	
17 Precentral gyrus		

46 Dorsal nerve root C5	**59** Occipital condyle
47 Dorsal root ganglion C5	**60** Dens of axis (odontoid peg of second cervical vertebra)
48 Ventral nerve root C5	
49 Body of fifth cervical vertebra	
50 Posterior belly of digastric	
51 Longissimus capitis	
52 Splenius capitis	
53 Sternocleidomastoid	
54 Superior oblique	
55 Inferior oblique	
56 Semispinalis capitis	
57 Levator scapulae	
58 Auricular cartilage of ear	

Section level

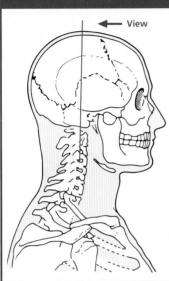

← View

Notes

This section provides an excellent view of the foramen magnum (**11**) in the coronal section. It can be appreciated that the medulla oblongata (**36**) terminates at its superior margin and the spinal cord (**37**) commences at its inferior margin.

The vertebral artery (**39**) passes over the posterior arch of the atlas (**41**) to enter the skull through the foramen magnum. The first cervical dorsal spinal ramus lies between the artery and posterior arch. Muscular branches of the artery supply the deep muscles of this region and anastomose with the occipital, ascending and deep cervical arteries.

Formation of the fifth cervical spinal nerve from its dorsal (**46**) and ventral (**48**) roots is seen clearly. Note that the dorsal root ganglion (**47**) lies within the intervertebral foramen between the fourth and fifth (**49**) cervical vertebrae.

The nerve roots in the cervical spine emerge cranial to their numbered vertebra (i.e. C5 roots emerge between C4 and C5; C8 emerges between C7 and T1).

In the thoracic, lumbar and sacral spine, roots emerge caudal to their numbered vertebra (i.e. L5 emerges between L5 and S1).

Note the close relationship between the pons (**32**), medulla oblongata (**36**) and the atlanto-occipital joints (**40**) and dens of the axis (odontoid peg) (**60**). This explains why injuries at the C1/C2 level are so serious and diseases that affect this region, e.g. rheumatoid arthritis eroding the dens of the axis (odontoid peg) and weakening ligaments, can be so disabling.

Orientation

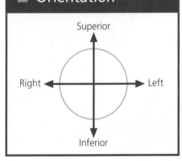

Superior

Right — Left

Inferior

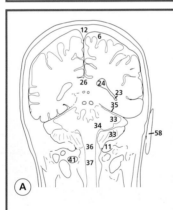

A

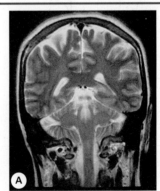

A

Coronal magnetic resonance image (MRI)

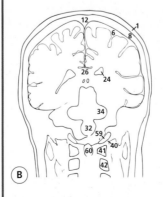

B

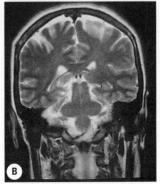

B

Coronal magnetic resonance image (MRI)

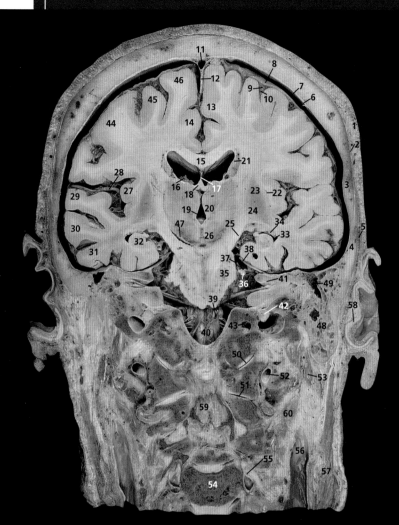

1 Skin and dense subcutaneous tissue	22 Claustrum	41 Facial nerve (VII) and vestibulocochlear nerve (VIII) entering internal auditory meatus within petrous part of temporal bone	49 Mastoid antrum within petrous part of temporal bone
2 Epicranial aponeurosis (galea aponeurotica)	23 Putamen		50 Atlanto-occipital joint
	24 Globus pallidus		51 Atlanto-axial joint
3 Parietal bone	25 Posterior limb of internal capsule		52 Vertebral artery within foramen transversarium of axis (see 39)
4 Temporal bone	26 Mamillary body	42 Glossopharyngeal nerve (IX), vagus nerve (X) and cranial part of accessory nerve (XI) entering jugular foramen within petrous part of temporal bone	53 Posterior belly of digastric
5 Temporalis	27 Insula		
6 Dura mater	28 Lateral cerebral fissure and branches of middle cerebral artery		54 Body of C4 vertebra
7 Subdural space			55 C4 dorsal root ganglion
8 Arachnoid mater			56 Internal jugular vein
9 Subarachnoid space	29 Superior temporal gyrus	43 Hypoglossal nerve (XII) entering hypoglossal canal within petrous part of temporal bone	57 Sternocleidomastoid
10 Pia mater	30 Middle temporal gyrus		58 Auricular cartilage of ear
11 Superior sagittal sinus	31 Inferior temporal gyrus		59 Dura of spinal canal
12 Falx cerebri	32 Hippocampus		60 Levator scapulae
13 Medial frontal gyrus	33 Inferior horn of lateral ventricle	44 Postcentral gyrus	
14 Cingulate gyrus	34 Tail of caudate nucleus	45 Precentral gyrus	61 Lateral ventricle
15 Body of corpus callosum	35 Pons	46 Superior frontal gyrus	62 Basilar artery
16 Choroid plexus within lateral ventricle	36 Trigeminal nerve (V)	47 Substantia nigra	63 Body of second cervical vertebra
	37 Trochlear nerve (IV)	48 Mastoid air cells within mastoid process of the petrous part of temporal bone	
17 Septum pellucidum	38 Free margin of tentorium cerebelli		
18 Fornix			
19 Third ventricle	39 Vertebral artery (see 52)		
20 Thalamus	40 Medulla oblongata		
21 Caudate nucleus			

Section level

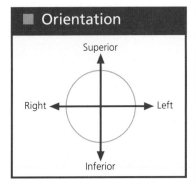

← View

Notes

The posterior limb of the internal capsule (**25**) is transected in this section and can be seen descending into the pons (**35**). Medial to the internal capsule can be seen the tail of the caudate nucleus (**21**) and the thalamus (**20**), while laterally lies the lentiform nucleus, made up of the putamen (**23**) and, more medially, the globus pallidus (**24**). Lateral to the lentiform nucleus lies the claustrum (**22**), sandwiching the narrow external capsule between the two.

The squamous part of the temporal bone (**4**) is the thinnest part of the calvarium. Contrast it with the densest part of the skull – the well-named petrous temporal bone (**49**).

The internal auditory meatus is cut along its length and demonstrates the facial nerve (VII) and vestibulocochlear, or auditory, nerve (VIII) lying within it (**41**).

MRI is an excellent method of demonstrating small acoustic neurinomata, which develop close to the internal auditory meatus. It is now possible to diagnose these benign tumours long before the bony meatus becomes enlarged.

These two magnetic resonance images, obtained at the same anatomical plane, graphically demonstrate the different information that can be obtained using different magnetic resonance parameters: image (A) is the proton-density image whereas image (B) is the T2-weighted image from a dual-echo acquisition.

Orientation

Superior

Right ← → Left

Inferior

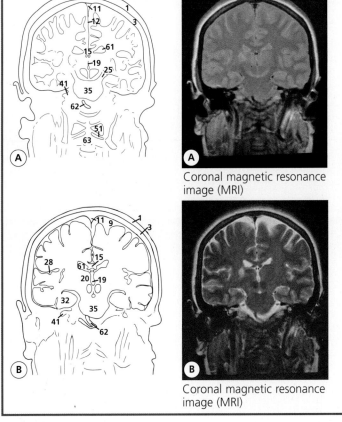

Coronal magnetic resonance image (MRI)

Coronal magnetic resonance image (MRI)

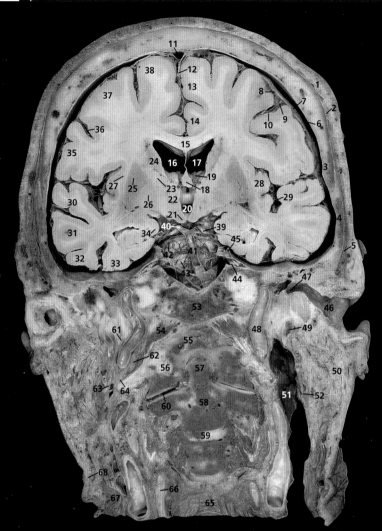

1 Skin and dense subcutaneous tissue
2 Epicranial aponeurosis (galea aponeurotica)
3 Parietal bone
4 Squamous part of temporal bone
5 Temporalis
6 Dura mater
7 Subdural space
8 Arachnoid mater
9 Subarachnoid space
10 Pia mater
11 Superior sagittal sinus
12 Falx cerebri
13 Medial frontal gyrus
14 Cingulate gyrus
15 Body of corpus callosum
16 Body of lateral ventricle
17 Septum pellucidum
18 Fornix

19 Choroid plexus with floor of lateral ventricle
20 Third ventricle
21 Mamillary body
22 Thalamus
23 Anterior limb of internal capsule
24 Caudate nucleus
25 Putamen
26 Globus pallidus
27 Claustrum
28 Insula
29 Lateral cerebral fissure and branches of middle cerebral artery
30 Superior temporal gyrus
31 Middle temporal gyrus
32 Inferior temporal gyrus
33 Lateral occipitotemporal gyrus
34 Parahippocampal gyrus adjacent (lateral) to hippocampus

35 Postcentral gyrus
36 Central sulcus
37 Precentral gyrus
38 Superior frontal gyrus
39 Oculomotor nerve (III)
40 Posterior cerebral artery
41 Basilar artery
42 Superior cerebral artery
43 Pons
44 Trigeminal nerve (V)
45 Free margin of tentorium cerebelli
46 External auditory meatus
47 Tympanic membrane
48 Internal carotid artery
49 Styloid process
50 Parotid gland
51 Internal jugular vein
52 Digastric
53 Base of occipital bone (clivus)

54 Rectus capitis anterior
55 Anterior atlanto-occipital membrane
56 Anterior arch of atlas
57 Dens of axis (odontoid peg of second cervical vertebra)
58 Body of axis
59 C2/3 intervertebral disc
60 Atlanto-axial joint
61 Glossopharyngeal nerve (IX)
62 Vagus nerve (X)
63 Spinal accessory nerve (XI)
64 Hypoglossal nerve (XII)
65 Posterior wall of pharynx
66 Thyroid cartilage
67 Sternocleidomastoid
68 Platysma

■ Section level

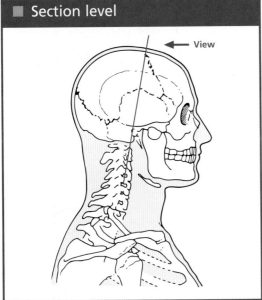

← View

■ Orientation

Superior

Right ← → Left

Inferior

■ Notes

This section passes through the external auditory meatus (**46**). This is about 37 mm long and has a peculiar S-shaped course, being directed first medially upwards and backwards, then medially and backwards, and finally medially forwards and downwards. The outer third of the canal is cartilaginous and somewhat wider than the medial osseous portion. It leads to the tympanic membrane, or eardrum (**47**), which faces laterally downwards and forwards.

This section provides a clear view of the dens (**57**) in coronal section and articulation with the anterior arch of the atlas (**56**). It also illustrates the importance of the transverse ligament of atlas keeping the dens of the axis (odontoid peg of second cervical vertebra) (**57**) in intimate contact with the atlas (first cervical vertebra).

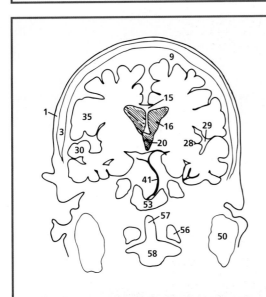

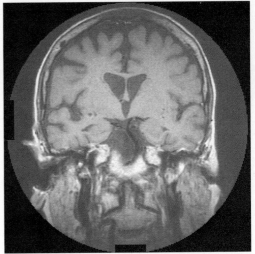

Coronal magnetic resonance image (MRI)

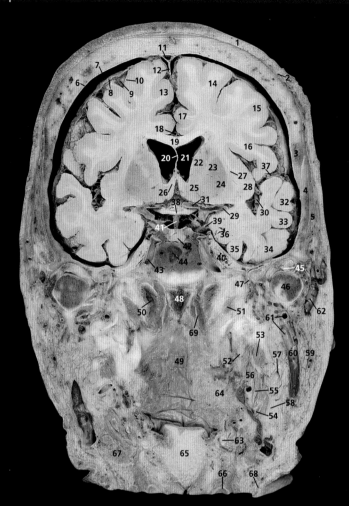

1	Skin and dense subcutaneous tissue	22	Head of caudate nucleus
2	Epicranial aponeurosis (galea aponeurotica)	23	Lentiform nucleus
3	Parietal bone	24	Putamen
4	Squamous part of temporal bone	25	Nucleus accumbens
5	Temporalis	26	Anterior column of fornix
6	Dura mater	27	Claustrum
7	Subdural space	28	Insula
8	Arachnoid mater	29	Origin of middle cerebral artery (see 30)
9	Subarachnoid space	30	Middle cerebral artery branches (see 29)
10	Pia mater	31	Origin of anterior cerebral artery (see 18)
11	Superior sagittal sinus	32	Superior temporal gyrus
12	Falx cerebri	33	Middle temporal gyrus
13	Medial frontal gyrus	34	Inferior temporal gyrus
14	Superior frontal gyrus	35	Lateral occipitotemporal gyrus
15	Middle frontal gyrus	36	Medial occipitotemporal gyrus
16	Inferior frontal gyrus	37	Lateral sulcus
17	Cingulate gyrus	38	Optic chiasma (II)
18	Pericallosal artery		
19	Body of corpus callosum		
20	Septum pellucidum		
21	Lateral ventricle		

39	Oculomotor nerve (III)	52	Internal carotid artery
40	Trigeminal ganglion	53	Styloglossus
41	Pituitary stalk	54	Tendon of digastric
42	Pituitary gland within pituitary fossa (sella turcica)	55	Stylohyoid
43	Internal carotid artery within cavernous sinus	56	Stylopharyngeus
44	Body of sphenoid bone and sphenoidal sinus	57	External carotid artery
45	Intra-articular disc of temporomandibular joint	58	Hypoglossal nerve (XII)
46	Head of mandible	59	Parotid gland
47	Middle meningeal artery within foramen spinosum of sphenoid bone	60	Retromandibular vein
48	Posterior wall of nasopharynx	61	Maxillary artery and vein
49	Posterior wall of oropharynx	62	Superficial temporal vein
50	Auditory (Eustachian) tube	63	Greater horn of hyoid bone
51	Levator veli palatini	64	Constrictor muscles of pharynx
		65	Cartilage of epiglottis
		66	Superior margin of lamina of thyroid cartilage
		67	Submandibular gland
		68	Platysma
		69	Longus capitis

Section level

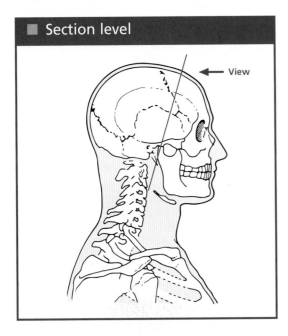

← View

Orientation

Superior

Right ← → Left

Inferior

Notes

The plane of this section passes through the head of the mandible (**46**) and the temporomandibular joint. The articular surfaces of the joint are covered with fibrocartilage (not hyaline cartilage as is usual in a synovial joint). The joint contains a prominent fibrocartilaginous intra-articular disc (**45**), which divides it into an upper and lower compartment.

The parotid gland (**59**) and the submandibular salivary gland (**67**) are in contact with each other, separated only by a sheet of fascia, the stylomandibular ligament.

The anterior limb of the internal capsule relates medially to the head of the caudate nucleus (**22**) and laterally to the putamen (**24**). See also the note on the posterior limb of the internal capsule in Coronal section 6.

The pituitary gland (**42**) can be seen lying within its fossa, in close relationship to the optic chiasma. An enlarging tumour of the pituitary gland classically produces the visual disturbance of bitemporal hemianopia because of pressure on the medial aspect of the chiasma. The modern pernasal trans-sphenoidal fibre-optic approach for pituitary surgery via the sphenoid sinus (**44**) can be appreciated in this section.

On this T1-weighted magnetic resonance image, the sphenoid (**44**) is very bright because there is virtually no sinus aeration; this is very variable. The bright signal reflects a high narrow content of bone.

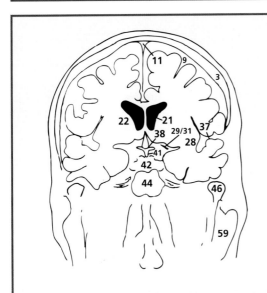

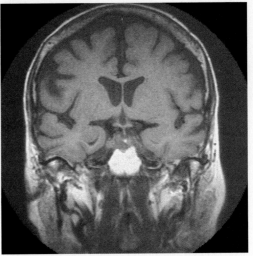

Coronal magnetic resonance image (MRI)

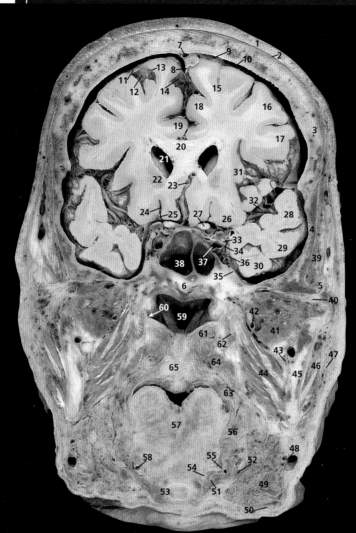

1 Skin and dense subcutaneous tissue
2 Epicranial aponeurosis (galea aponeurotica)
3 Parietal bone
4 Squamous part of temporal bone
5 Zygomatic process of temporal bone
6 Body of sphenoid bone
7 Superior sagittal sinus
8 Falx cerebri
9 Dura mater
10 Subdural space
11 Arachnoid mater
12 Subarachnoid space
13 Pia mater
14 Callosomarginal branch of anterior cerebral artery in longitudinal fissure
15 Superior frontal gyrus
16 Middle frontal gyrus

17 Inferior frontal gyrus
18 Medial frontal gyrus
19 Cingulate gyrus
20 Body of corpus callosum
21 Anterior horn of lateral ventricle
22 Head of caudate nucleus
23 Anterior cerebral artery
24 Olfactory sulcus
25 Olfactory tract (I)
26 Orbital gyri
27 Optic nerve (II)
28 Superior temporal gyrus
29 Middle temporal gyrus
30 Inferior temporal gyrus
31 Insula
32 Middle cerebral artery
33 Oculomotor nerve (III)
34 Abducent nerve (VI)
35 Maxillary nerve (Vⁱⁱ)

36 Ophthalmic nerve (III) with trochlear nerve (IV)
37 Internal carotid artery in cavernous sinus
38 Sphenoidal sinus
39 Temporalis
40 Intra-articular disc of temporomandibular joint
41 Lateral pterygoid
42 Maxillary artery
43 Inferior alveolar nerve and artery
44 Medial pterygoid
45 Ramus of mandible
46 Masseter
47 Parotid gland
48 Facial artery and vein
49 Submandibular gland
50 Platysma
51 Hyoglossus
52 Tendon of digastric

53 Body of hyoid bone
54 Lesser horn of hyoid bone
55 Stylohyoid ligament
56 Styloglossus
57 Intrinsic muscle of tongue
58 Lingual artery
59 Nasopharynx
60 Opening of auditory (Eustachian) tube (arrowed)
61 Levator veli palatini
62 Tensor veli palatini
63 Palatoglossus
64 Superior constrictor of pharynx
65 Soft palate

66 Internal carotid artery
67 Anterior clinoid process of sphenoid bone
68 Temporal lobe

■ Section level

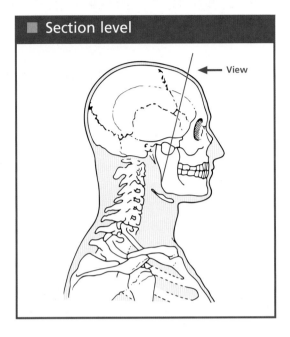

← View

■ Orientation

Superior

Right ← → Left

Inferior

■ Notes

The line of this section passes through the zygomatic process of the temporal bone (**5**), the posterior part of the tongue (**57**) and the body of the hyoid bone (**53**). We peer into the nasopharynx (**59**) with the termination of the auditory, or Eustachian, tube (**60**) just visible.

The oculomotor nerve (III) (**33**) passes through the sharp edge of the tentorium cerebelli to enter the cavernous sinus (**37**). The cerebral hemisphere, compressed by an extradural or subdural clot, presses upon the nerve at the tentorial edge and produces dilation of the pupil; hence, the neurosurgical aphorism, 'explore the side with the dilated pupil'. Damage to the internal carotid artery within the cavernous sinus (**37**), usually as a result of trauma, may produce a carotico-cavernous fistula and results in a pulsating exophthalmos.

The intrinsic muscles of the tongue (**57**) comprise longitudinal, transverse and vertical bands of muscle. These, acting alone or in combination, give the tongue its precise and highly variable mobility in speech and swallowing. Their nerve supply is the hypoglossal nerve (XII).

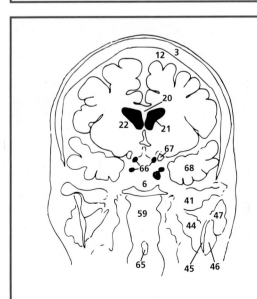

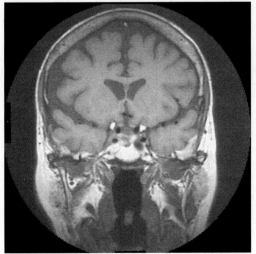

Coronal magnetic resonance image (MRI)

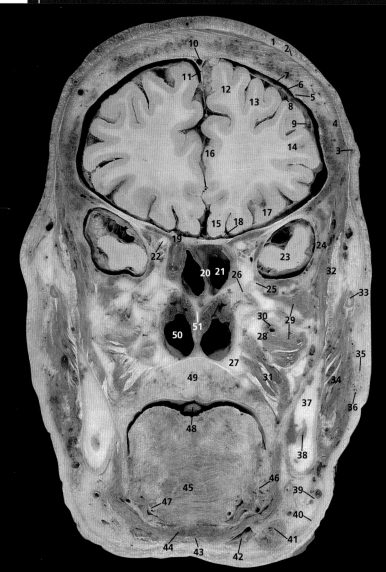

1 Skin and dense
  subcutaneous tissue
2 Epicranial aponeurosis
  (galea aponeurotica)
3 Branch of superficial
  temporal artery
4 Frontal bone
5 Dura mater
6 Subdural space
7 Arachnoid mater
8 Subarachnoid space
9 Pia mater
10 Superior sagittal sinus
11 Falx cerebri
12 Superior frontal gyrus
13 Middle frontal gyrus
14 Inferior frontal gyrus
15 Gyrus rectus
16 Cingulate gyrus
17 Medial orbital gyrus

18 Olfactory tract (I)
19 Lesser wing of
  sphenoid bone
20 Septum between
  sphenoidal sinuses
21 Sphenoidal sinus
22 Optic nerve (II)
23 Temporal lobe of brain
  within middle cranial
  fossa
24 Greater wing of
  sphenoid bone
25 Maxillary nerve within
  foramen rotundum of
  greater wing of
  sphenoid bone
26 Pterygopalatine
  ganglion
27 Medial pterygoid plate
  of sphenoid bone

28 Lateral pterygoid plate
  of sphenoid bone
29 Lateral pterygoid
30 Maxillary artery
31 Medial pterygoid
32 Temporalis
33 Zygomatic arch
34 Masseter
35 Accessory parotid
  gland
36 Parotid duct
37 Body of mandible
38 Inferior alveolar artery
  and nerve within
  mandibular canal
39 Facial artery and nerve
40 Platysma
41 Submandibular gland
42 Anterior belly of
  digastric

43 Mylohyoid
44 Geniohyoid
45 Transverse fibres of
  intrinsic muscle of
  tongue
46 Sublingual gland (deep
  part)
47 Lingual artery
48 Uvula
49 Palatine glands of soft
  palate
50 Nasal cavity
51 Nasal septum (vomer)

52 Anterior clinoid process
  (lesser wing of
  sphenoid bone)
53 Ramus of mandible
54 Nasopharynx

Section level

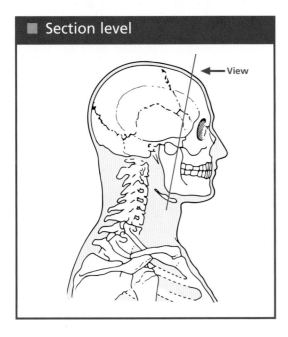

Orientation

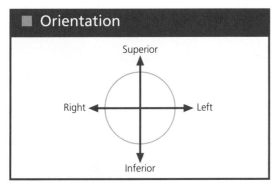

Notes

Do not be deceived! This section passes through the tip of the temporal lobe of the cerebrum (**23**), lying inferior to the lesser wing of the sphenoid (**19**) and not the orbit. Note that the plane of this section lies immediately anterior to the anterior horn of the lateral ventricle.

The parotid duct (**36**) can be palpated easily in the living subject by tensing the masseter muscle (**34**) and feeling along the upper part of the anterior border of this muscle just inferior to the zygomatic arch (**33**). The accessory parotid gland, or pars accessoria (**35**), is usually completely detached from the main gland and lies between the parotid duct and the zygomatic arch. It accounts for an occasionally very anteriorly placed parotid tumour.

The paired sphenoidal sinuses (**21**) lie within the body of the sphenoid bone and vary quite considerably in size and shape. They are rarely symmetrical, one often being much larger than the other and extending across the midline behind the other. Occasionally one overlaps the other sinus superiorly. Usually the septum (**20**) between the two sinuses is intact, although occasionally these communicate with each other.

As well as the main salivary glands, many other accessory salivary glands are found, some in the tongue, some between the crypts of the palatine tonsils and some on the inner aspects of the lip and cheeks. Large numbers are found in the posterior hard palate and the soft palate (**49**). They are mainly mucous in type and are occasional sites for the development of a pleomorphic salivary tumour.

The CT image is purposefully displayed at optimal setting for bony structure.

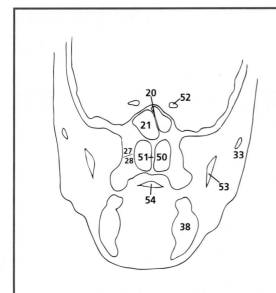

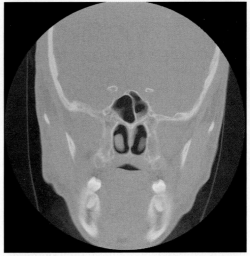

Coronal computed tomogram (CT)

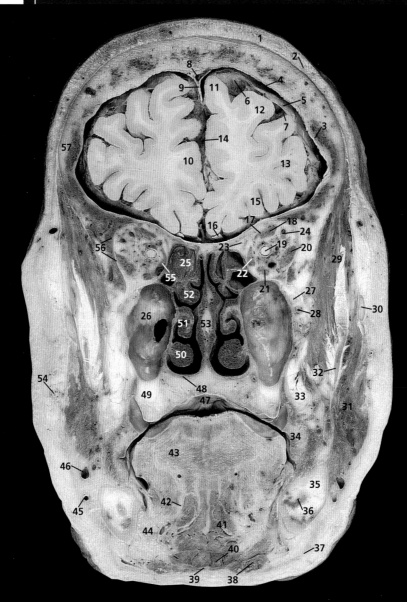

1 Skin and dense subcutaneous tissue
2 Epicranial aponeurosis (galea aponeurotica)
3 Dura mater
4 Subdural space
5 Arachnoid mater
6 Subarachnoid space
7 Pia mater
8 Superior sagittal sinus
9 Falx cerebri
10 Medial frontal gyrus

11 Superior frontal gyrus
12 Middle frontal gyrus
13 Inferior frontal gyrus
14 Longitudinal fissure
15 Orbital gyri
16 Olfactory tract (I)
17 Levator palpebrae superioris
18 Superior rectus
19 Optic nerve (II) in dural sheath
20 Lateral rectus
21 Inferior rectus
22 Medial rectus

23 Superior oblique
24 Branches of ophthalmic artery and vein
25 Ethmoidal air cells
26 Maxillary sinus
27 Maxillary nerve
28 Maxillary artery
29 Temporalis
30 Zygomatic arch
31 Masseter
32 Ramus of mandible
33 Buccal pad of fat
34 Buccinator
35 Body of mandible
36 Inferior alveolar nerve in mandibular canal

37 Platysma
38 Anterior belly of digastric
39 Mylohyoid
40 Geniohyoid
41 Genioglossus
42 Lingual artery
43 Transverse fibres of intrinsic muscle of tongue
44 Sublingual gland
45 Facial artery
46 Facial vein
47 Soft palate
48 Horizontal plate of palatine bone
49 Tuberosity of maxilla

50 Inferior nasal concha
51 Middle nasal concha
52 Superior nasal concha
53 Nasal septum
54 Parotid duct
55 Orbital part of ethmoid bone
56 Greater wing of sphenoid bone – orbital surface
57 Frontal bone

58 Zygoma
59 Dental artefacts (see notes)

Section level

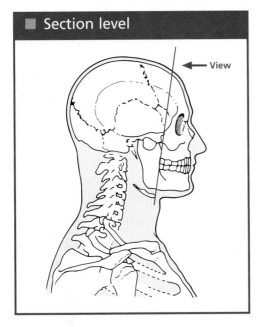

← View

Orientation

Superior

Right ← → Left

Inferior

Notes

This section does indeed pass through the posterior part of the cavity of the orbit and demonstrates the close packing of the extrinsic muscles (**17**, **18**, **20–23**) and blood vessels (**24**) with the orbital fat and optic (II) nerve (**19**). Note that the optic nerve is surrounded by an extension of the dura mater and is, therefore, bathed in cerebrospinal fluid. Raised intracranial pressure is thus transmitted in the cerebrospinal fluid along the sheath and results in the changes of papilloedema.

The ethmoidal air cells, or sinuses (**25**), are small, thin-walled cavities in the ethmoidal labyrinth. They range in number from three large to 18 small cells on either side and are separated from the orbit by the paper-thin orbital plate of the ethmoid. Orbital cellulitis can thus easily result from ethmoid sinusitis (see (**54**) in Coronal section 13).

The three nasal conchae (still often referred to by ear, nose and throat (ENT) surgeons as the turbinate bones) project downwards like three scrolls from the lateral wall of the nasal cavity. The lowest, the inferior (**50**), is the largest and broadest. It is a separate bone, unlike the middle (**51**) and superior (**52**), which are part of the ethmoid bone (**55**). The middle and superior conchae are joined anteriorly, but diverge away from each other posteriorly so that the superior concha can be visualized only at posterior rhinoscopy and is invisible on viewing through the anterior nares. Beneath each concha is a space, termed the superior, middle and inferior meatus, respectively.

Metallic material used in dental fillings creates substantial problems for coronal CT. Even with careful positioning and gantry angulation, problems may be unavoidable: On the image, note the distortion created by the presence of a metallic dental filling.

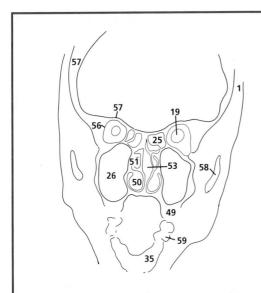

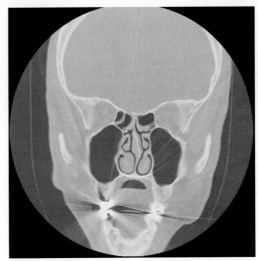

Coronal computed tomogram (CT)

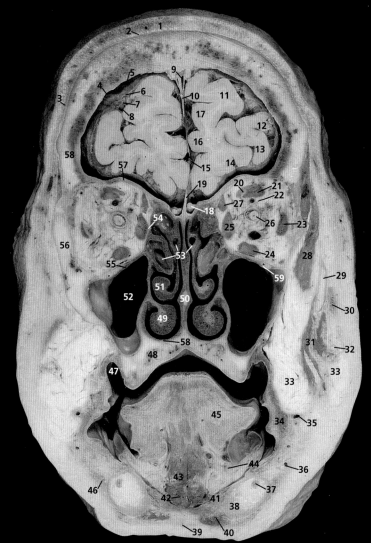

1 Skin and dense subcutaneous tissue
2 Epicranial aponeurosis (galea aponeurotica)
3 Frontal belly of occipitofrontalis
4 Dura mater
5 Subdural space
6 Arachnoid mater
7 Subarachnoid space
8 Pia mater
9 Superior sagittal sinus
10 Falx cerebri
11 Superior frontal gyrus
12 Middle frontal gyrus
13 Inferior frontal gyrus
14 Orbital gyri
15 Longitudinal fissure
16 Cingulate gyrus
17 Medial frontal gyrus
18 Posterior portion of olfactory bulb (I) lying on cribriform plate of ethmoid bone
19 Posterior part of crista galli
20 Levator palpebrae superioris
21 Superior rectus
22 Branches of ophthalmic artery and vein
23 Lateral rectus
24 Inferior rectus
25 Medial rectus
26 Optic nerve (II) in dural sheath
27 Superior oblique
28 Temporalis
29 Zygomatic arch
30 Zygomaticus major
31 Masseter
32 Parotid duct
33 Buccal fat
34 Buccinator
35 Facial vein
36 Facial artery
37 Inferior alveolar nerve in mandibular canal
38 Body of mandible
39 Platysma
40 Anterior belly of digastric
41 Mylohyoid
42 Geniohyoid
43 Genioglossus
44 Sublingual gland
45 Intrinsic muscle of tongue
46 Depressor anguli oris
47 Buccal vestibule
48 Palatine glands of soft palate
49 Inferior nasal concha
50 Nasal septum
51 Middle nasal concha
52 Maxillary sinus
53 Ethmoidal air cells
54 Orbital part of ethmoid bone
55 Orbital surface of maxilla
56 Zygomatic bone
57 Orbital part of frontal bone
58 Palatine process of maxilla
59 Infra-orbital artery and nerve within infra-orbital canal of maxilla

60 Teeth arising from mandible
61 Globe

Section level

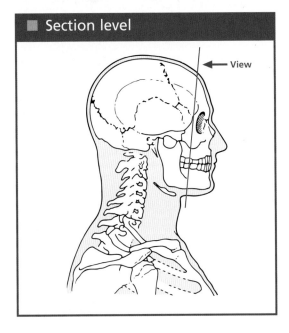

← View

Orientation

Superior

Right ←→ Left

Inferior

Notes

From the roof of the nasal cavity, some 20 olfactory nerve (I) filaments on each side perforate the dura and arachnoid over the cribriform plate and pass upwards through the subarachnoid space to enter the olfactory bulb (**18**). From here, the olfactory tract passes posteriorly on the inferior surface of the frontal lobe. Fractures crossing the anterior cranial fossa, with tearing of the overlying dura, may result in cerebrospinal rhinorrhoea, watery fluid draining into the nose. Untreated, this communication between the nasal cavity and the subarachnoid space inevitably results in meningitis.

The maxillary sinus, or antrum (**52**), occupying most of the body of the maxilla, is the largest of the nasal accessory sinuses. In dentulous subjects, conical elevations, which correspond to the roots of the first and second molar teeth, project into the floor of the sinus, which they occasionally perforate. Less commonly, the roots of the two premolars, the third molar and, rarely, the canine may also project into the sinus. Upper dental infection may thus involve the sinus, and dental extraction may result in an oromaxillary fistula. The sinus opens into the nasal cavity in the lowest part of the hiatus semilunaris below the middle concha (**51**). A second orifice is often present in or just below the hiatus.

CT in the coronal plane is used to demonstrate the anatomy of the maxillary sinus and its drainage into the nasal cavity. Some ENT surgeons now perform flexible endoscopic sinus surgery (FESS) to improve matters. This CT projection is also useful for assessing fractures of the floor of the orbit.

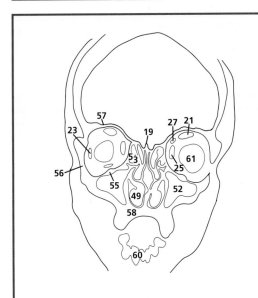

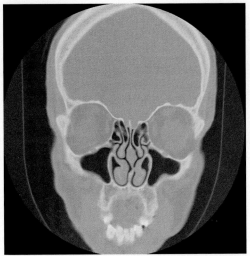

Coronal computed tomogram (CT)

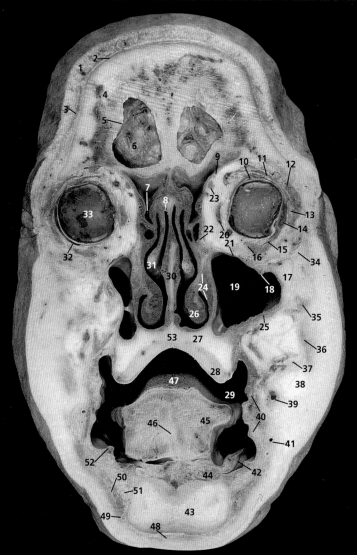

1 Skin and dense subcutaneous tissue
2 Epicranial aponeurosis (galea aponeurotica)
3 Occipital belly of occipitofrontalis
4 Frontal bone
5 Dura mater
6 Frontal lobe of brain covered with arachnoid mater and blood vessels within the anterior cranial fossa
7 Infundibulum draining frontal sinus
8 Roof of nasal cavity
9 Orbital part of frontal bone
10 Superior rectus
11 Levator palpebrae superioris
12 Lacrimal gland (orbital part)
13 Lacrimal gland (palpebral part)
14 Lateral rectus
15 Inferior oblique
16 Inferior rectus
17 Orbital margin of zygomatic bone
18 Infra-orbital artery and nerve within infra-orbital canal of maxilla
19 Maxillary sinus
20 Medial rectus
21 Orbital surface of maxilla
22 Lacrimal bone
23 Tendon of superior oblique
24 Nasolacrimal duct
25 Maxilla
26 Inferior nasal concha
27 Palatine process of maxilla
28 Alveolar process of maxilla
29 Vestibule of mouth
30 Nasal septum
31 Middle nasal concha
32 Scleral layer of orbit
33 Vitreous humour
34 Orbicularis oculi
35 Zygomaticus minor
36 Zygomaticus major
37 Parotid duct
38 Buccal fat pad
39 Facial vein
40 Buccinator
41 Facial artery
42 Mucous membrane of mouth
43 Mandible
44 Sublingual gland
45 Genioglossus
46 Median septum of tongue
47 Dorsum of tongue
48 Platysma
49 Depressor anguli oris
50 Depressor labii inferioris
51 Mental nerve
52 Sublingual papilla
53 Hard palate

54 Orbital margin of ethmoid bone
55 Crista galli of ethmoid bone

Section level

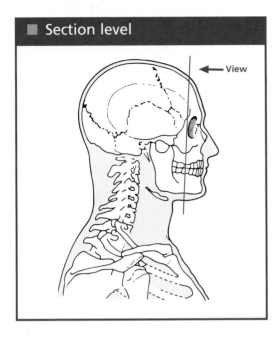

← View

Orientation

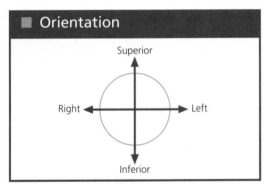

Superior

Right ← → Left

Inferior

Notes

The orbital part of the lacrimal gland (**12**) lies in the lacrimal fossa on the lateral part of the roof of the orbit supported by the lateral margin of levator palpebrae superioris (**11**). It projects around the lateral margin of this muscle and turns forward to form the palpebral part of the gland (**13**), which is visible through the superior fornix of the conjunctiva. Its dozen or so ducts drain into the superior fornix.

The nasolacrimal duct (**24**), about 2 cm in length, runs downwards and laterally to open into the inferior meatus below the inferior nasal concha (**26**), about 2 cm behind the nostril. Its mucosa is raised into several folds, which act as valves. These prevent air and nasal mucus being forced up the duct into the lacrimal sac when blowing the nose.

The buccal pad of fat (**38**) protrudes in front of the masseter to lie on the buccinator (**40**) immediately inferior to the parotid duct (**37**). Its estimated volume is 10 cm³. It is well developed in babies, where it forms a prominent elevation over the external surface of the face (the sucking pad). This helps to prevent collapse of the cheeks in vigorous sucking. It persists through life and is relatively 'protected', in that it does not decrease, even in emaciated subjects.

Note the paper-thin (lamina papyricea) orbital margin of the ethmoid bone (**54**). This portion and the relatively thin orbital margin of maxilla are liable to be damaged by a blow-out injury; the globe, being tougher, transmits injury to the walls of the orbit following trauma that is not absorbed by the bony margins. Squash balls are a particular culprit. The extrinsic eye muscles may get trapped between the fracture margins.

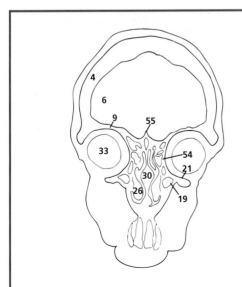

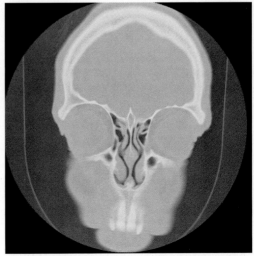

Coronal computed tomogram (CT)

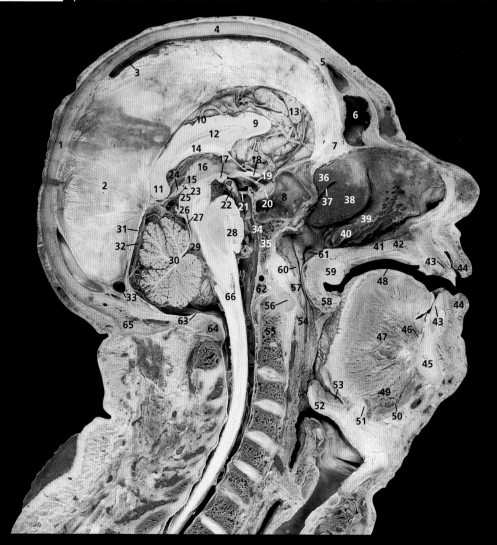

1 Occipital bone
2 Falx cerebri
3 Superior sagittal sinus
4 Parietal bone
5 Frontal bone
6 Frontal sinus
7 Crista galli of ethmoid
   bone
8 Sphenoidal sinus
9 Genu of corpus callosum
10 Body of corpus callosum
11 Splenium of corpus
   callosum
12 Septum pellucidum
13 Anterior lobe gyrus
14 Body of fornix
15 Third ventricle
16 Hypothalamus
17 Mamillary body
18 Optic chiasm
19 Pituitary stalk
20 Pituitary gland

21 Oculomotor nerve (III)
22 Posterior cerebral
   artery
23 Midbrain
24 Pineal body
25 Superior colliculus
26 Inferior colliculus
27 Aqueduct (of Sylvius)
   connecting third and
   fourth ventricles
28 Pons
29 Fourth ventricle
30 Cerebellum
31 Tentorium cerebelli
32 Straight sinus
33 Transverse sinus
34 Basilar artery
35 Clivus (basi-occipital
   and basi-sphenoid
   bones)
36 Superior nasal concha
37 Superior meatus

38 Middle nasal concha
39 Middle meatus
40 Inferior nasal concha
41 Inferior meatus
42 Hard palate
43 Central incisor (upper
   and lower)
44 Lip (upper and lower)
45 Body of mandible
46 Sublingual gland
47 Genioglossus
48 Dorsum of tongue
49 Geniohyoid
50 Mylohyoid
51 Body of hyoid bone
52 Epiglottis
53 Vallecula
54 Oral part of pharynx
   (oropharynx)
55 Dens of axis (odontoid
   peg of second cervical
   vertebra)

56 Anterior arch of atlas
   (first cervical vertebra)
57 Nasal part of pharynx
   (nasopharynx)
58 Uvula
59 Soft palate
60 Pharyngeal recess
61 Opening of auditory
   (Eustachian) tube
62 Anterior margin of
   foramen magnum
63 Posterior margin of
   foramen magnum
64 Posterior arch of atlas
65 External occipital
   protuberance
66 Medulla oblongata

67 Lateral ventricle

Section level

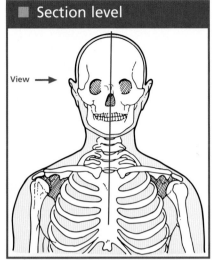

View →

Orientation

Superior

Posterior ← → Anterior

Inferior

Notes

Note that the nasal septum has been removed from this section in order to display the nasal conchae on the lateral wall.

The roof of the hard palate (**42**) lies at the level of the atlas (first cervical vertebra). Note that a clear anteroposterior view of the dens of the axis (second cervical vertebra) can be obtained on radiological examination by asking the patient to open the mouth widely.

This section illustrates the approach to the pituitary gland (**20**) via the transnasal trans-sphenoidal sinus (**8**) route at fibre-optic endoscopic surgery.

The frontal sinuses (**6**) vary considerably in size and are rarely symmetrical, the septum between the two usually being deviated to one or the other side. Each may be divided further by incomplete bony septa. Occasionally, one or both may be absent.

These two sagittal T1-weighted magnetic resonance images are very close to the median sagittal plane. Indeed, image (A) is so midline that the falx cerebri has been traversed. Image (B) is minimally lateral to the median sagittal plane and thus cerebral gyri and sulci are visible. The anatomy of the cerebral aqueduct and fourth ventricle is demonstrated well. So too is the important close relationship of the pituitary gland to the optic chiasm.

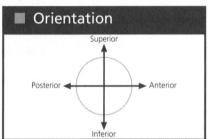

(A)

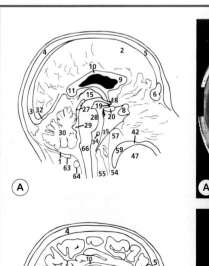

(B)

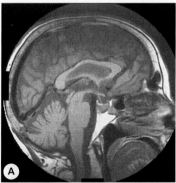

(A)

Sagittal magnetic resonance image (MRI)

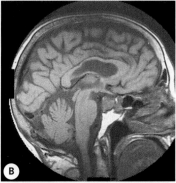

(B)

Sagittal magnetic resonance image (MRI)

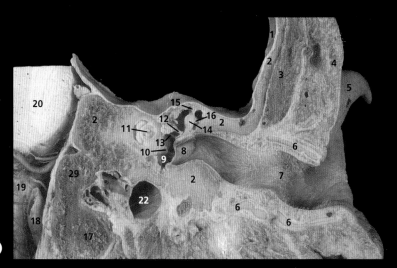

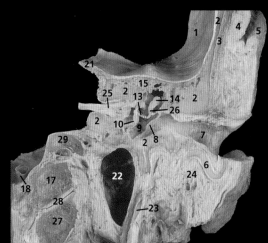

1 Dura mater	**12** Tendon of tensor tympani	**23** Styloid process
2 Temporal bone	**13** Stapes	**24** Parotid gland
3 Temporalis	**14** Head of malleus	**25** Facial nerve (VII) and
4 Skin and dense subcutaneous	**15** Tegmen tympani	vestibulocochlear nerve (VIII)
tissue	**16** Body of malleus	within the internal acoustic
5 Helix of left ear	**17** Occipital condyle	meatus
6 Auricular cartilage of ear	**18** Vertebral artery	**26** Long limb of incus
7 External acoustic meatus	**19** Medulla oblongata	**27** Atlas (first cervical vertebra)
8 Tympanic membrane	**20** Pons	**28** Atlanto-occipital joint
9 Cavity of middle ear	**21** Free margin of tentorium	**29** Occipital bone
10 Promontory of middle ear	cerebelli	
11 Cochlea	22 Internal jugular vein	

■ Section level

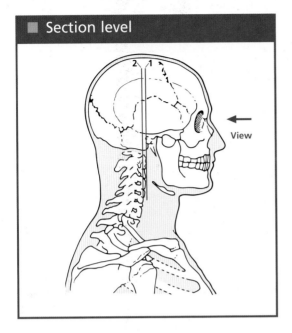

View

■ Orientation

Sections 1 and 2

- Superior
- Medial ←→ Left
- Inferior

CT images

- Superior
- Right ←→ Left
- Inferior

■ Notes

The external acoustic meatus (**7**) extends inwards to the tympanic membrane (**8**). The meatus is about 37 mm in length and has a peculiar S-shaped course, being directed first medially superiorly and anteriorly, then medially and backwards and then, at its termination, medially, anteriorly and inferiorly. The outer third of the canal is cartilaginous and somewhat wider than the inner osseous portion. The tympanic membrane (eardrum) separates the middle ear (**9**) from the external meatus. It is oval in outline and faces laterally, inferiorly and anteriorly. It is about 12 mm in its greatest (vertical) diameter and is slightly concave outwards. The middle ear, or tympanic cavity (**9**), is a slit-like cavity in the petrous temporal bone (**2**) and contains the three auditory ossicles. These are the malleus, whose body, or handle (**16**), is attached to the tympanic membrane, and a head (**14**) which articulates with the incus (**26**), which, in turn, articulates with the stapes (**13**). The base of the stapes is firmly adherent to the oval window, or fenestra vestibuli, of the inner ear. This comprises a complicated bony labyrinth that encloses the membranous labyrinth. This comprises the utricle and saccule, which communicate with the semicircular canals and the cochlea, respectively (**11**).

The intimate relationship of the facial nerve (VII) and the vestibulocochlear nerve (VIII) as they enter the internal auditory meatus (**25**) in the petrous part of the temporal bone (**2**) is demonstrated.

See also Coronal sections 5–7.

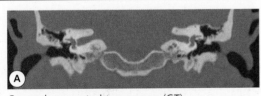

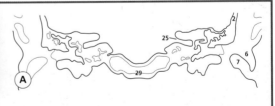

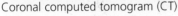
Coronal computed tomogram (CT)

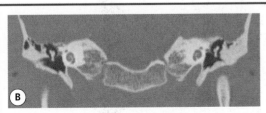

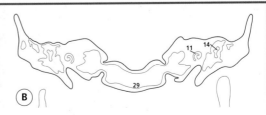

Coronal computed tomogram (CT)

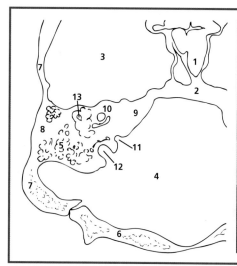
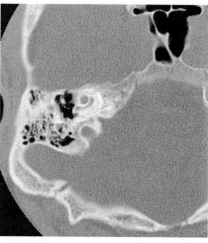

Axial computed tomogram (CT)

1 Sphenoidal sinus
2 Basi-spenoid joining basi-occiput (forming clivus)
3 Temporal lobe of brain (in middle cranial fossa)
4 Posterior cranial fossa
5 Mastoid air cells (within temporal bone)
6 Occipital bone
7 Temporal bone (petromastoid part)

8 Temporal bone (mastoid part)
9 Temporal bone (apex of petrous part)
10 Cochlea
11 Internal auditory meatus
12 Superior aspect jugular bulb
13 Malleus

■ Section level

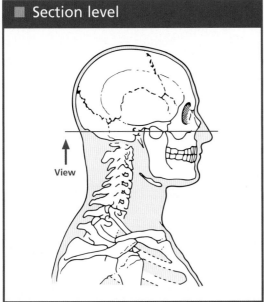

View

■ Orientation

Anterior

Right ← → Left

Posterior

■ Notes

This thin section CT image has been reconstructed using a bony algorithm and displayed at settings to demonstrate the bony structures. Hence the bone texture is well seen (and the detail of cerebral tissue absent). Such high resolution images are essential to study the anatomy of the inner ear before complex surgery.

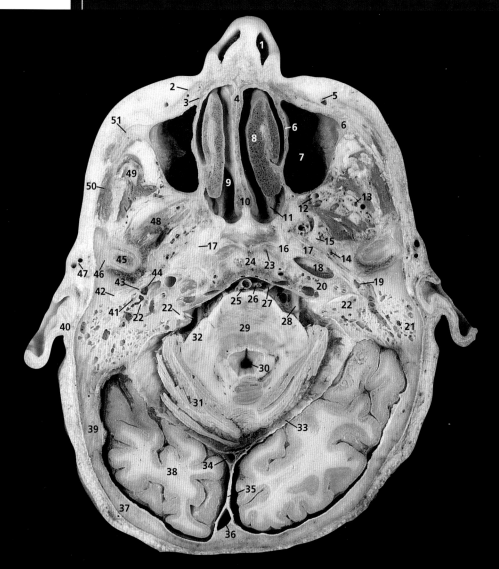

1 Vestibule of nose
2 Levator labii superioris alaeque nasi
3 Levator labii superioris
4 Cartilage of nasal septum
5 Facial vein
6 Maxilla
7 Maxillary sinus (antrum of Highmore)
8 Inferior nasal concha
9 Middle meatus
10 Vomer
11 Middle nasal concha
12 Maxillary artery
13 Pterygoid branch of maxillary artery
14 Middle meningeal artery
15 Mandibular nerve (V^{iii})

16 Greater wing of sphenoid
17 Cartilaginous roof of auditory (Eustachian) tube
18 Internal carotid artery
19 Junction of internal auditory tube and tympanic cavity
20 Petrous temporal bone
21 Mastoid air cells
22 Facial nerve (VII)
23 Longus capitis
24 Body of sphenoid
25 Basilar artery
26 Anterior inferior cerebellar artery
27 Abducent nerve (VI)
28 Trigeminal nerve (V)
29 Pons cerebri

30 Fourth ventricle
31 Cerebellum
32 Middle cerebellar peduncle
33 Tentorium cerebelli
34 Straight sinus
35 Falx cerebri
36 Superior sagittal sinus
37 Occipital bone (squamous part)
38 Occipital lobe of cerebrum
39 Squamous part of temporal bone
40 Pinna of ear
41 Malleus and incus
42 External auditory meatus
43 Tympanic membrane
44 Cavity of middle ear
45 Head of mandible

46 Temporomandibular joint
47 Superficial temporal artery and vein
48 Lateral pterygoid
49 Temporalis and tendon
50 Masseter
51 Zygomatic process of maxilla

52 Internal jugular vein (at origin)
53 Occipital bone (basilar part)
54 Postnasal space
55 Coronoid process of mandible
56 Medulla oblongata

Section level

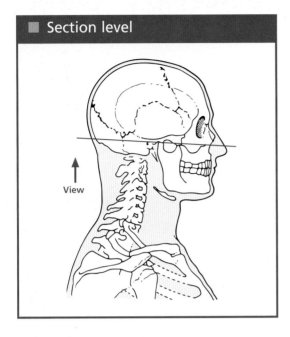

View

Orientation

Anterior

Right ← → Left

Posterior

Notes

This section passes through the vestibule of the nose (**1**), the inferior nasal concha (**8**), the temporomandibular joint (**46**), the pons (**29**) and the occipital lobe of the cerebrum (**38**).

The angulation of this magnetic resonance image does not tally exactly with this section; some of the anatomical features of the neck on this and subsequent sections are therefore better seen on other images.

The maxillary sinus (the antrum of Highmore) within the maxilla (**7**) is demonstrated well. Its orifice lies at a higher plane and drains into the middle meatus (**9**) below the bulla ethmoidalis. The fact that the opening of this antrum is situated at this high level accounts for the poor drainage and consequent frequency of infection.

Note that the lateral pterygoid muscle (**48**) inserts not only into a depression on the front of the neck of the mandible but also into the articular capsule of the temporomandibular joint (**46**) and its articular disc.

The postnasal space (**54**) lies between the nasopharynx and the basi-occiput (**53**) together with the anterior arch of the atlas. As well as containing the prevertebral muscles, this space contains variable quantities of lymphoid tissue (the pharyngeal tonsil, or adenoids). The size of the space is assessed readily on a lateral radiograph of the region. It is usually very narrow in adults (see Section 4, page 88) but can be very prominent in young children, whose adenoids are often very large.

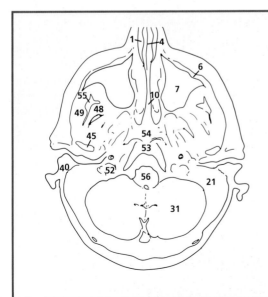

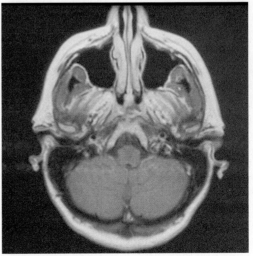

Axial magnetic resonance image (MRI)

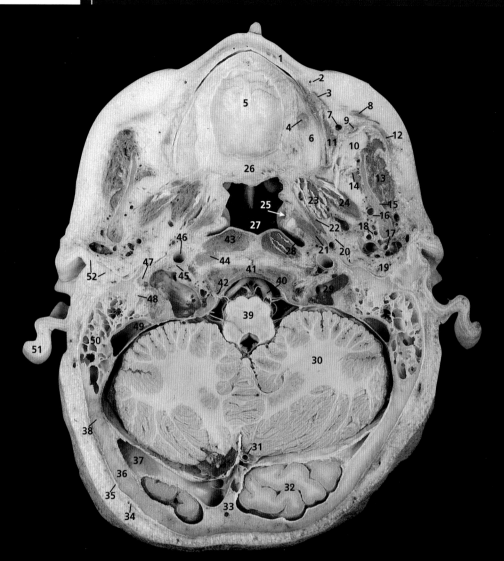

1 Orbicularis oris
2 Facial artery
3 Levator labii superioris
4 Mucosa of maxillary antrum
5 Hard palate
6 Alveolar process of maxilla
7 Facial vein
8 Zygomaticus major
9 Parotid duct
10 Buccal fat pad
11 Buccinator
12 Accessory parotid gland
13 Masseter
14 Temporalis and tendon
15 Ramus of mandible
16 Inferior alveolar artery and vein
17 Superficial temporal artery and vein

18 Maxillary artery and vein
19 Parotid gland
20 Lingual nerve, inferior alveolar nerve and nerve to mylohyoid (V^{iii})
21 Levator veli palatini
22 Tensor veli palatini
23 Medial pterygoid
24 Lateral pterygoid
25 Orifice of auditory tube (Eustachian tube) arrowed
26 Soft palate
27 Nasopharynx
28 Pharyngeal recess (fossa of Rosenmuller)
29 Internal jugular vein at origin
30 Cerebellum

31 Straight sinus at junction of tentorium cerebelli, falx cerebri and falx cerebelli
32 Occipital lobe of cerebrum
33 Internal occipital crest
34 Occipital artery and vein
35 Occipitofrontalis
36 Squamous part of occipital bone
37 Transverse sinus
38 Occipitomastoid suture
39 Medulla oblongata
40 Vertebral artery
41 Clivus of the basilar part of the occipital bone
42 Hypoglossal nerve (XII)
43 Longus capitis

44 Rectus capitis anterior
45 Glossopharyngeal nerve (IX), vagus nerve (X) and accessory nerve (XI)
46 Internal carotid artery
47 Styloid process
48 Facial nerve (VII)
49 Sigmoid sinus
50 Mastoid air cells of the temporal bone
51 Pinna of ear
52 Cartilage of external auditory meatus

53 Tonsil of cerebellum
54 Occipital bone (condyle)

■ Section level

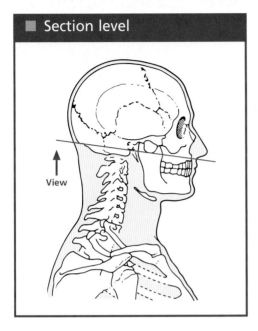

View

■ Orientation

Anterior

Right ◄─────► Left

Posterior

■ Notes

This section passes through the alveolar process of the maxilla (**6**) to reveal the hard palate (**5**) in its entirety. It then traverses the upper part of the ramus of the mandible (**15**), the mastoid air cells (**50**), the medulla oblongata (**39**), the cerebellum (**30**) and the posterior tip of the occipital lobe (**32**).

The floor of the maxillary sinus is formed by the alveolar process of the maxilla; several conical elevations, corresponding to the roots of the first and second molar teeth, project into the floor. An example of this is demonstrated here (**4**). Indeed, the floor is sometimes perforated by one or more of these molar roots.

This section gives a good view of the parotid duct (**9**) as it arches medially to penetrate the buccinator (**11**) and to enter the mouth at the level of the second upper molar tooth. The parotid duct is accompanied by a small, more or less detached, part of the gland that lies above the duct as it crosses the masseter; this is named the accessory part of the gland (**12**).

This section passes through the junctional zone between the falx cerebri, separating the occipital lobes of the brain (**32**), the falx cerebelli, separating the lobes of the cerebellum (**30**) and the tentorium cerebelli, which roofs the cerebellum. The straight sinus (**31**) is seen in section as it lies in the line of the junction of the falx cerebri and the tentorium cerebelli. The transverse sinus (**37**) lies in the attached margin of the tentorium cerebelli.

The facial nerve (**48**) (within the stylomastoid foramen) is demonstrated well in its immediate lateral relationship to the root of the styloid process (**47**).

Note that the orifice of the auditory tube (**25**) lies anterior to a depression – the pharyngeal recess (**28**). This helps to keep the orifice of the tube clear of secretions in the supine position.

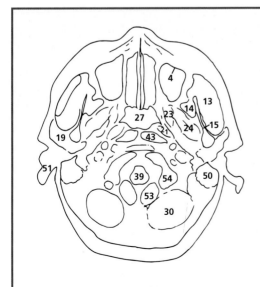

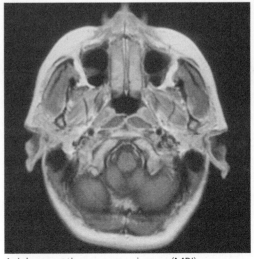

Axial magnetic resonance image (MRI)

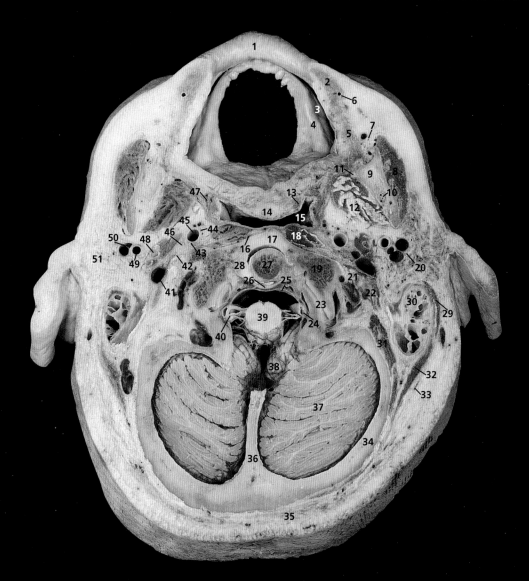

1 Upper lip
2 Orbicularis oris
3 Vestibule of mouth
4 Alveolus
5 Buccinator
6 Superior labial artery
7 Facial artery and vein
8 Masseter
9 Ramus of mandible
10 Inferior alveolar artery vein and nerve (V^{iii}) within mandibular canal
11 Lingual nerve (V^{iii})
12 Medial pterygoid
13 Tensor veli palatini
14 Soft palate
15 Nasopharynx
16 Anterior atlanto-occipital membrane

17 Anterior arch of atlas (first cervical vertebra)
18 Longus capitis
19 Lateral mass of atlas (first cervical vertebra)
20 Facial nerve (VII)
21 Roof of third part of vertebral artery
22 Rectus capitis lateralis
23 Atlanto-occipital joint
24 Fourth part of vertebral artery
25 Membrana tectoria
26 Superior longitudinal band of cruciform ligament
27 Dens of axis (odontoid process of second cervical vertebra)

28 Atlanto-axial joint
29 Sternocleidomastoid
30 Mastoid air cells of temporal bone
31 Posterior belly of digastric
32 Longissimus capitis
33 Splenius capitis
34 Squamous part of occipital bone
35 Trapezius
36 Internal occipital crest of occipital bone
37 Hemisphere of cerebellum
38 Tonsil of cerebellum
39 Spinal cord
40 Spinal root of accessory nerve

41 Internal jugular vein
42 Accessory nerve (XI) and hypoglossal nerve (XII)
43 Vagus nerve (X)
44 Sympathetic chain
45 Internal carotid artery
46 Glossopharyngeal nerve (IX)
47 Superior constrictor muscle of pharynx
48 Styloid process
49 External carotid artery
50 Retromandibular vein at bifurcation
51 Parotid gland

Section level

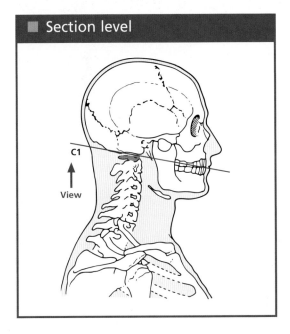

C1

View

Orientation

Anterior

Right — Left

Posterior

Notes

This section passes through the mouth at the level of the upper alveolus (**4**), the dens of the axis (**27**) at the articulation (**28**) with the anterior arch of the atlas (**17**) and posteriorly traverses the internal occipital crest of the occipital bone (**36**).

The radiographer obtains a clear anteroposterior view of the dens of the atlas (**27**) as it lies on the anterior arch of the axis (**17**) via the open mouth of the patient.

The third part of the vertebral artery (**21**) can be seen as it curves posterior to the lateral mass of the atlas (**19**) as it ascends to enter the vertebral canal by passing below the lower border of the posterior atlanto-occipital membrane. The fourth part (**24**) ascends anterior to the roots of the hypoglossal nerve.

Note how the last four cranial nerves (**42**, **43**, **46**) lie 'line astern' between the internal carotid artery (**45**) and the internal jugular vein (**41**) at the base of the skull.

The retromandibular vein (**50**) separates the parotid gland (**51**) into a superficial and deep lobe; it also demarcates the plane through which the facial nerve (**20**) and branches run.

The surgeon, in performing a subtotal superficial parotidectomy, establishes this plane, immediately superficial to the facial nerve.

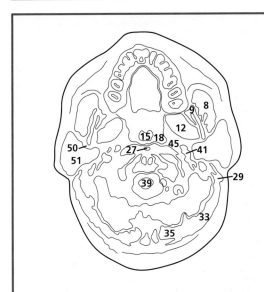

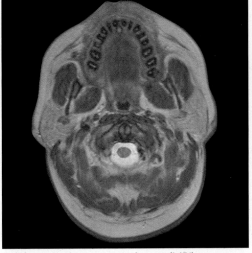

Axial magnetic resonance image (MRI)

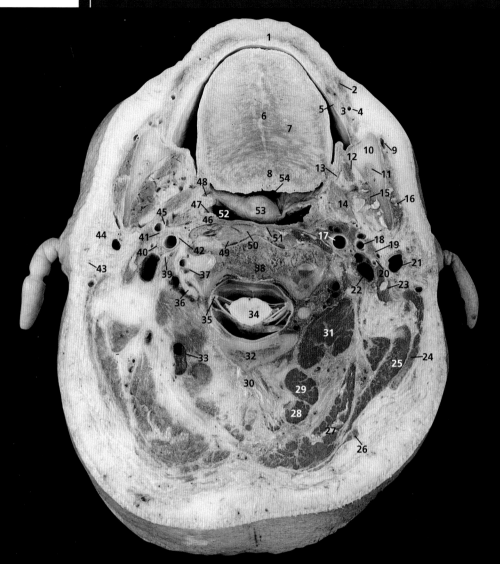

1 Orbicularis oris in lower lip
2 Depressor anguli oris
3 Buccinator
4 Anterior facial artery
5 Mucosa of lower lip
6 Median raphe of tongue
7 Intrinsic transverse muscle of tongue
8 Intrinsic superior longitudinal muscle of tongue
9 Facial vein
10 Ramus of mandible
11 Inferior alveolar artery vein and nerve (V^{iii}) within the mandibular canal
12 Mylohyoid
13 Lingual nerve (V^{iii})

14 Styloglossus
15 Medial pterygoid
16 Masseter
17 Internal carotid artery
18 External carotid artery
19 Stylohyoid
20 Posterior auricular artery and vein
21 External jugular vein
22 Internal jugular vein
23 Posterior belly of digastric
24 Sternocleidomastoid
25 Splenius capitis
26 Trapezius
27 Semispinalis capitis
28 Rectus capitis posterior minor
29 Rectus capitis posterior major

30 Ligamentum nuchae
31 Obliquus capitis inferior
32 Posterior arch of atlas (first cervical vertebra)
33 Occipital vein
34 Spinal cord within dural sheath
35 Dorsal root ganglion of second cervical nerve
36 Anterior primary ramus of second cervical nerve
37 Vertebral artery and vein within foramen transversarium
38 Body of axis (second cervical vertebra)
39 Sympathetic chain
40 Accessory nerve (XI)
41 Hypoglossal nerve (XII)

42 Vagus nerve (X)
43 Facial nerve (VII)
44 Parotid gland
45 Glossopharyngeal nerve (IX)
46 Palatopharyngeus
47 Tonsillar fossa
48 Palatoglossus
49 Longus capitis
50 Longus colli
51 Superior constrictor muscle of pharynx
52 Nasopharynx
53 Uvula
54 Oropharynx

55 Retromandibular vein

Section level

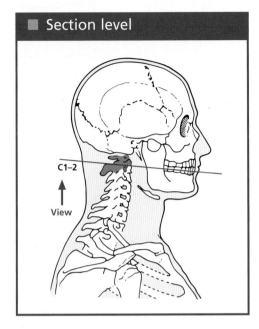

C1–2

↑
View

Orientation

Anterior

Right ← → Left

Posterior

Notes

This section passes through the tongue (**6**) and the body of the axis, the second cervical vertebra (**38**).

This section gives a useful appreciation of the inferior alveolar nerve and its accompanying vessels within the mandibular canal (**11**). An inferior alveolar nerve block, performed by injecting local anaesthetic at a point immediately medial to the anterior border of the ramus of the mandible and approximately 1 cm above the occlusal surface of the third molar tooth, will provide anaesthesia of all the teeth in that hemi-mandible as far as, and including, the first incisor. The skin and mucosa of the lower lip will also become numb (the mental branch of the nerve), and there is loss of sensation over the side of the tongue due to involvement of the adjacent, anteriorly placed, lingual nerve (see Axial Section 13, page 34). Note also the vertebral artery in its second part, together with its accompanying vein, within the foramen transversarium (**37**). The further course of this artery, in its third and fourth parts, can be seen in Axial section 3.

Note how close the posterior wall of the nasopharynx (**52**) lies to the body of the axis (**38**), and also to the anterior arch of the atlas in the previous section. The prevertebral space is thus normally very narrow on a lateral radiograph of the adult cervical spine (see Section 1, page 82).

This magnetic resonance image shows the parotid gland (**44**) very well. Note again how the retromandibular vein (**55**) separates the gland into superficial and deep portions.

The medial pterygoids are shown to good effect. The fat lying medially to these muscles in the parapharyngeal space shows up well on both MRI and CT imaging. Loss of this fat plane is an important sign when assessing the extent of tumours in this region.

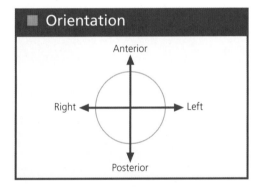

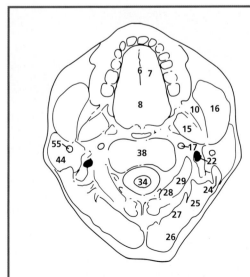

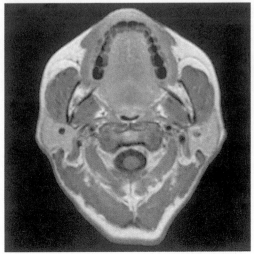

Axial magnetic resonance image (MRI)

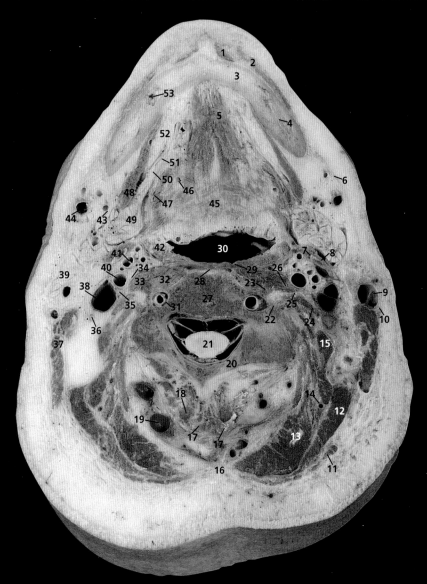

1 Mentalis
2 Orbicularis oris
3 Mandible
4 Inferior alveolar nerve (Vⁱⁱⁱ)
5 Genioglossus
6 Platysma
7 Posterior belly of digastric
8 Stylohyoid ligament
9 External jugular vein
10 Great auricular nerve
11 Trapezius
12 Splenius
13 Semispinalis capitis
14 Occipital artery
15 Levator scapulae
16 Ligamentum nuchae

17 Bifid spine of third cervical vertebra
18 Semispinalis cervicis
19 Occipital vein
20 Lamina of third cervical vertebra
21 Spinal cord within dural sheath
22 Posterior tubercle of transverse process of third cervical vertebra
23 Anterior tubercle of transverse process of third cervical vertebra
24 Scalenus medius
25 Anterior primary ramus of third cervical nerve
26 Scalenus anterior

27 Body of third cervical vertebra
28 Anterior longitudinal ligament
29 Superior constrictor muscle of pharynx
30 Oropharynx
31 Vertebral artery and vein within foramen transversarium
32 Longus colli
33 Longus capitis
34 Vagus nerve (X)
35 Sympathetic chain
36 Accessory nerve (XI)
37 Sternocleidomastoid
38 Internal jugular vein
39 Parotid gland

40 Internal carotid artery
41 External carotid artery
42 Palatine tonsil
43 Facial artery
44 Facial vein
45 Intrinsic transverse muscle of tongue
46 Lingual artery
47 Hyoglossus
48 Mylohyoid
49 Submandibular gland
50 Lingual nerve (Vⁱⁱⁱ)
51 Submandibular duct
52 Sublingual gland
53 Inferior alveolar artery, vein and nerve within mandibular canal

54 Hyoid

Section level

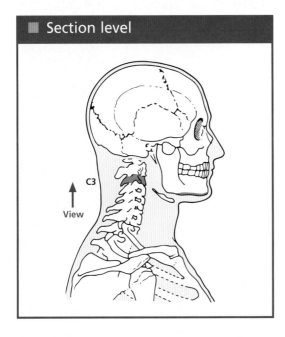

C3

View

Orientation

Anterior

Right ← → Left

Posterior

Notes

This section passes through the lower border of the body of the mandible (**3**), the oropharynx (**30**) and the third cervical vertebra (**27**).

It demonstrates how the parotid gland (**39**) projects deeply towards the side wall of the oropharynx (**30**). Indeed, a tumour of the deep portion of the gland may project into the tonsillar fossa and bulge the palatine tonsil (**42**) medially. An aneurysm of the internal carotid artery (**40**) similarly bulges into the tonsillar fossa medially and will give the unusual sign of visible pulsation of the palatine tonsil.

The vertebral vein (**31**) is smaller than the artery. Quite often it lies in its own compartment of the foramen transversarium. Sympathetic fibres from the superior cervical ganglion (C1,2,3,4) are conveyed as a plexus along the vertebral artery.

Genioglossus (**5**) is a triangular muscle placed close to, and parallel with, the median plane. It arises from the upper genial tubercle on the inner surface of the symphysis of the mandible (**3**) and spreads out in a fan-like form to enter the whole undersurface of the tongue from its root to its apex. It has the unique action of protruding the tongue, and this is used in the clinical testing of paralysis of the hypoglossal nerve (XII) (see Axial section 3, page 86).

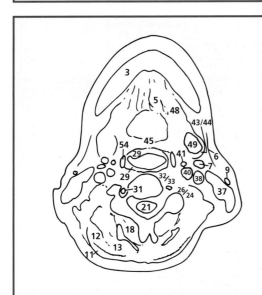

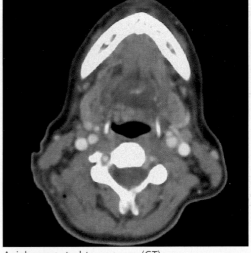

Axial computed tomogram (CT)

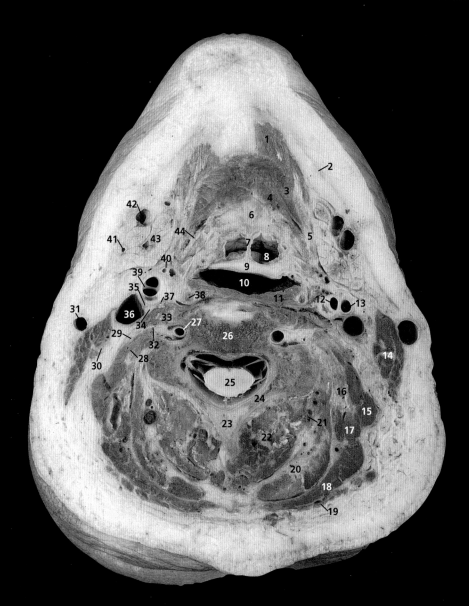

1 Anterior belly of digastric
2 Platysma
3 Mylohyoid
4 Hyoglossus
5 Tendon of digastric
6 Base of tongue
7 Glosso-epiglotic fold
8 Vallecula
9 Epiglottis
10 Laryngopharynx
11 Middle constrictor muscle of pharynx
12 Left internal carotid artery
13 Left external carotid artery

14 Sternocleidomastoid
15 Levator scapulae
16 Longissimus capitis and cervicis
17 Splenius cervicis
18 Splenius capitis
19 Trapezius
20 Semispinalis capitis
21 Deep cervical artery and vein
22 Semispinalis cervicis
23 Spine of fourth cervical vertebra
24 Lamina of fourth cervical vertebra
25 Spinal cord within dural sheath

26 Body of fourth cervical vertebra
27 Vertebral artery and vein within foramen transversarium
28 Scalenus medius
29 Anterior primary ramus of third cervical nerve
30 Accessory nerve (XI)
31 External jugular vein
32 Anterior primary ramus fourth cervical nerve
33 Scalenus anterior
34 Phrenic nerve
35 Vagus nerve (X)
36 Internal jugular vein
37 Sympathetic chain

38 Hyoid
39 Right common carotid artery at bifurcation
40 Superior thyroid artery
41 Facial artery
42 Facial vein
43 Submandibular salivary gland
44 Lingual artery

45 Mandible
46 Common carotid artery
47 Pre-epiglottic space
48 Superior cornu of thyroid cartilage
49 Aryepiglottic fold
50 Piriform fossa

Section level

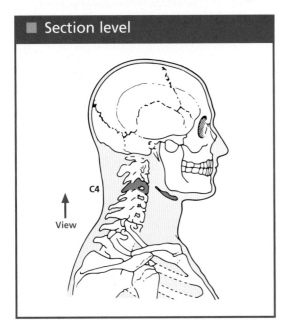

C4

View

Orientation

Anterior

Right ← → Left

Posterior

Notes

This section passes through the body of the fourth cervical vertebra (**26**), just shaving the inferior margin of the hyoid bone (**38**).

The fourth cervical vertebra marks the level of bifurcation of the common carotid artery. On the right side this is just occurring (**39**), and on the left it has already taken place (**12**, **13**). Note the marked atheromatous thickening of the internal carotid artery. On the CT image the plane passes through the common carotid arteries.

The external jugular vein (**31**) is the only structure of prominence lying in the superficial fascia of the posterior triangle of the neck. Immediately above the clavicle it pierces the deep fascia to enter the subclavian vein, as the only tributary of this vessel. Occasionally it is double (see **39**, Thorax, Axial section 1, page 102).

The way in which the lingual artery (**44**) passes deep to the hyoglossus muscle (**4**) to supply the tongue is demonstrated. On CT imaging, precise definition of the various intrinsic muscles of the tongue is difficult unless the fat planes are very pronounced.

The precise shape of the laryngopharynx (**10**), and indeed the whole airway system of the head and neck, depends on the phase of respiration, phonation etc. In practice, gentle inspiration is the most appropriate phase for routine CT imaging, but attempts at phonation and the Valsalva manoeuvre may be helpful.

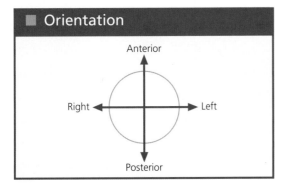

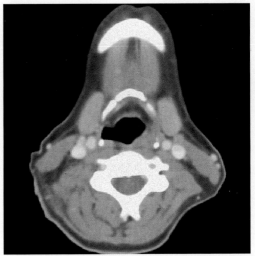

Axial computed tomogram (CT)

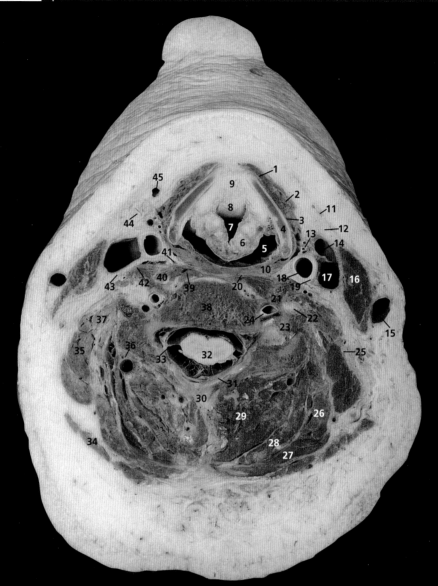

1 Sternohyoid
2 Omohyoid
3 Thyrohyoid
4 Lamina of thyroid cartilage
5 Laryngopharynx
6 Corniculate cartilage
7 Vestibule of larynx
8 Epiglottis
9 Pre-epiglottic space (fat filled)
10 Inferior constrictor muscle of pharynx
11 Platysma
12 Investing fascia of neck
13 Superior thyroid artery and vein
14 Common facial vein

15 External jugular vein
16 Sternocleidomastoid
17 Internal jugular vein
18 Common carotid artery
19 Vagus nerve (X)
20 Prevertebral fascia
21 Anterior tubercle of fifth cervical vertebra
22 Ventral ramus of fifth cervical nerve
23 Posterior tubercle of fifth cervical vertebra
24 Vertebral artery and vein within foramen transversarium
25 Accessory nerve (XI)
26 Splenius cervicis
27 Splenius capitis

28 Semispinalis capitis
29 Erector spinae
30 Spine of fifth cervical vertebra
31 Lamina of fifth cervical vertebra
32 Spinal cord within dural sheath
33 Ligamentum denticulatum
34 Trapezius
35 Levator scapulae
36 Deep cervical artery and vein
37 Scalenus medius
38 Body of fifth cervical vertebra
39 Longus colli
40 Longus capitis

41 Sympathetic chain
42 Scalenus anterior
43 Phrenic nerve
44 Submandibular salivary gland
45 Anterior jugular vein

46 Inferior horn of thyroid cartilage
47 Arytenoid cartilage
48 Cricoid cartilage
49 Vocal fold
50 Anterior border of thyroid cartilage

■ Section level

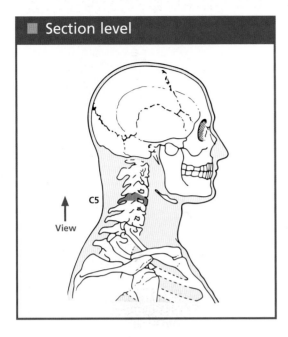

C5

↑
View

■ Orientation

Anterior

Right ← → Left

Posterior

■ Notes

This section passes through the body of the fifth cervical vertebra (**38**) and the lamina of the thyroid cartilage (**4**).

The attachment of the stem of the cartilage of the epiglottis (**8**) to the angle formed by the two laminae of the thyroid cartilage (**4**) is demonstrated at this level. Apart from the apices of the arytenoids, the epiglottis (**8**) is the only laryngeal cartilage made of yellow elastic cartilage. On either side of the epiglottis can be seen the groove of the vallecula. In deglutition, the epiglottis acts like a stone jutting into a waterfall: it deviates the food bolus to pass either side along the vallecula, thus keeping it away from the laryngeal orifice. The vallecula is a common site for impaction of a sharp swallowed object, such as a fish bone.

This section gives an excellent demonstration of the ligamentum denticulatum (**33**). This is a narrow fibrous sheet situated on each side of the spinal cord. Its medial border is continuous with the pia mater at the side of the spinal cord, while its lateral border presents a series of triangular tooth-like processes whose points are fixed at intervals to the dura mater. There are 21 such processes on each side; the last lies between the exits of the twelfth thoracic and first lumbar nerves.

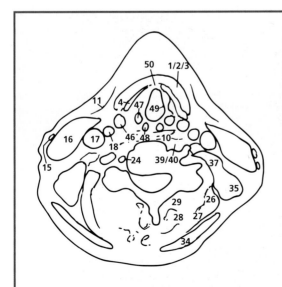

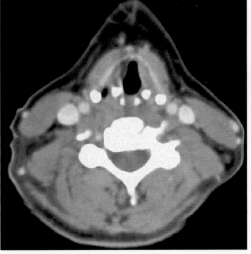

Axial computed tomogram (CT)

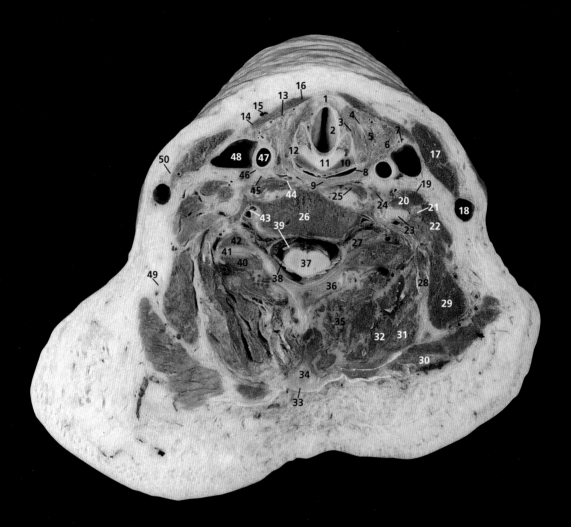

1 Anterior border of thyroid cartilage
2 Vocal fold
3 Lateral cricoarytenoid
4 Lamina of thyroid cartilage
5 Cricothyroid
6 Lateral lobe of thyroid gland
7 Superior thyroid artery and vein
8 Laryngopharynx
9 Inferior constrictor muscle of pharynx
10 Posterior cricoarytenoid
11 Cricoid cartilage
12 Inferior cornu of thyroid cartilage
13 Sternothyroid
14 Omohyoid

15 Anterior jugular vein
16 Sternohyoid
17 Sternocleidomastoid
18 External jugular vein
19 Phrenic nerve
20 Scalenus anterior
21 Ventral ramus of fifth cervical nerve
22 Scalenus medius
23 Ventral ramus of sixth cervical nerve
24 Longus capitis
25 Longus colli
26 Body of sixth cervical vertebra
27 Dorsal root ganglion of seventh cervical nerve
28 Splenius cervicis
29 Levator scapulae
30 Trapezius

31 Splenius capitis
32 Semispinalis
33 Ligamentum nuchae
34 Tip of spinous process of seventh cervical vertebra
35 Erector spinae
36 Lamina of sixth cervical vertebra
37 Spinal cord within dural sheath
38 Dorsal nerve root of seventh cervical nerve
39 Ventral nerve root of seventh cervical nerve
40 Inferior articular facet of sixth cervical vertebra
41 Interarticular facet joint between sixth

and seventh cervical vertebrae
42 Superior articular facet of seventh cervical vertebra
43 Vertebral artery and vein within foramen transversarium
44 Prevertebral fascia
45 Sympathetic trunk
46 Vagus nerve (X)
47 Common carotid artery
48 Internal jugular vein
49 Accessory nerve (XI)
50 Platysma

51 Outline of subglottic space

Section level

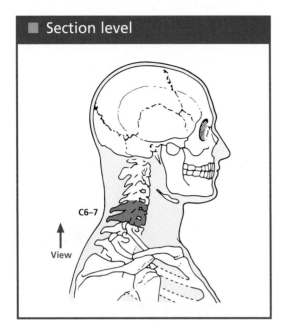

C6–7

↑
View

Notes

This section passes through the body of the sixth cervical vertebra (**26**) and traverses the cricoid cartilage (**11**). The cricoid is the only complete ring of cartilage throughout the respiratory system, but the plane of this section is above the narrow arch of the cricoid and only passes through its posterior lamina.

This section, together with the following section, provides a good appreciation of the relationships of the lateral lobe of the thyroid gland (**6**). Here, it is seen to be overlapped superficially by the strap muscles – the sternohyoid (**16**), omohyoid (**14**) and, on a deeper plane, the sternothyroid (**13**). Medially it lies against the larynx and laryngopharynx (**8**), and posteriorly it lies against the common carotid artery (**47**) and internal jugular vein (**48**). (See also CT image in Axial section 9.)

Note the demonstration of the relationship of the phrenic nerve (**19**) to the anterior aspect of scalenus anterior (**20**). The nerve is bound down to the underlying muscle by the overlying prevertebral fascia (**44**). Scalenus anterior (**20**) is thus an important landmark muscle to the surgeon. It sandwiches the subclavian artery and the brachial plexus roots between it and scalenus medius (**22**) and defines the phrenic nerve (**19**) on its anterior surface.

The ventral rami (**21**, **23**) of C5 and C6, together with C7, C8 and T1, form the brachial plexus; those of C1–4 form the cervical plexus.

The inferior surfaces of the vocal folds (**2**) can be seen within the larynx (see CT image in Axial section 7). The vestibular folds (false cords), which lie cranial to the vestibule of the larynx, are situated more cranially to this section.

Orientation

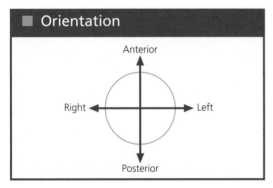

Anterior

Right ←→ Left

Posterior

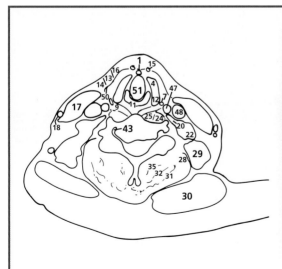

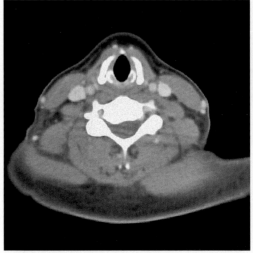

Axial computed tomogram (CT)

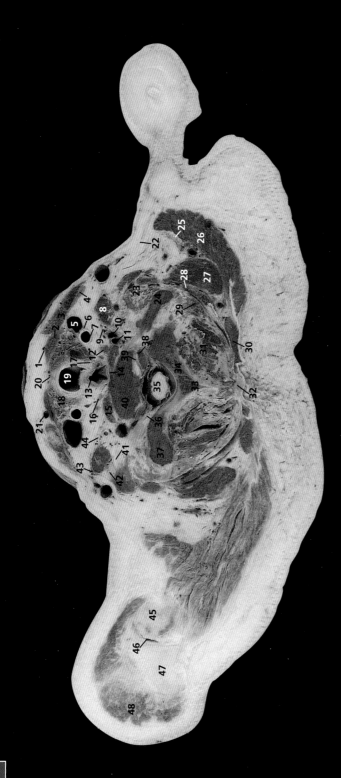

1 Sternohyoid
2 Sternothyroid
3 Sternocleidomastoid
4 Omohyoid
5 Internal jugular vein
6 Vagus nerve (X)
7 Common carotid artery
8 Scalenus anterior
9 Inferior thyroid artery
10 Vertebral vein
11 Vertebral artery
12 Deep cervical lymph node
13 Oesophagus
14 Prevertebral fascia
15 Longus colli

16 Parathyroid gland
17 Recurrent laryngeal nerve
18 Lateral lobe of thyroid gland
19 Trachea
20 Isthmus of thyroid gland
21 Anterior jugular vein
22 Investing (deep) fascia of the neck
23 Scalenus medius and posterior
24 Left first rib
25 Accessory nerve (XI)
26 Trapezius
27 Levator scapulae
28 Splenius
29 Semispinalis
30 Rhomboideus minor

31 Erector spinae
32 Ligamentum nuchae
33 Spinous process of first thoracic vertebra
34 Lamina of first thoracic vertebra
35 Spinal cord within dural sheath
36 Dorsal root ganglion of eighth cervical nerve
37 Transverse process of first thoracic vertebra
38 Part of body of first thoracic vertebra
39 Uncovertebral synovial joint between lip of T1 body and inferior aspect of C7

40 Body of seventh cervical vertebra
41 Ventral ramus of seventh cervical nerve
42 Ventral ramus of sixth cervical nerve
43 Phrenic nerve
44 Cervical sympathetic chain
45 Clavicle
46 Acromioclavicular joint
47 Acromion
48 Deltoid

49 External jugular vein

Section level

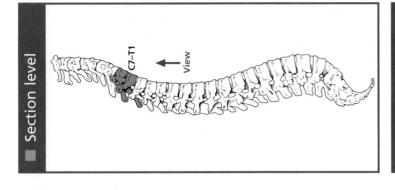

C7–T1

← View

Orientation

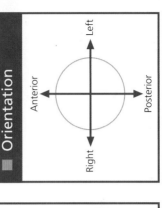

Left

Anterior

Posterior

Right

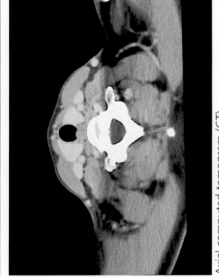

Axial computed tomogram (CT)

Notes

This section passes through the body of the seventh cervical vertebra (**40**) and through the tip of the shoulder, so that a sliver of the clavicle (**45**) and adjacent acromioclavicular joint (**46**) are shown.

Taken in conjunction with the previous section, the relationships of the lateral lobe of the thyroid gland (**18**) are demonstrated. In this section, it is overlapped by the strap muscles (**1**, **2**, **4**) and sternocleidomastoid (**3**). Medially it lies against the trachea (**19**) and oesophagus (**13**), while posteriorly it rests against the common carotid artery (**7**) and internal jugular vein (**5**). The inferior thyroid artery (**9**) passes transversely behind the common carotid artery to reach the thyroid gland. Note also the important posterior relationship of the lobe of the thyroid gland to the recurrent laryngeal nerve (**17**), lying in the tracheo-oesophageal groove.

The parathyroid glands (**16**) are usually four in number but vary from two to six. The superior glands are fairly constant in position, at the middle of the posterior border of the thyroid lobe above the level at which the inferior thyroid artery crosses the recurrent laryngeal nerve. The inferior glands are most usually situated near the lower pole of the thyroid gland below the inferior thyroid artery, but aberrant glands may be found in front of the trachea, behind the oesophagus, buried in the thyroid gland or descended into the superior mediastinum in company with thymic tissue.

On the CT image, the vertebral artery (**11**) is seen as it passes towards the gap between the foramina transversarium of the sixth and seventh cervical vertebrae. The bodies of the cervical vertebrae and the superior aspect of T1 have raised lips (uncinate processes) on each lateral margin of their superior surfaces. These processes enclose the intervertebral disc and articulate (**39**) with the inferior aspect of the adjacent vertebral body; they are prone to degenerative disease, which can lead to neurological problems.

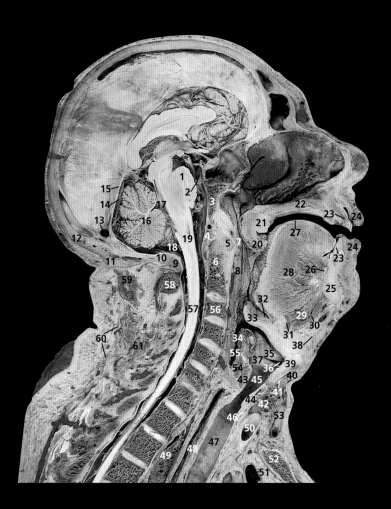

1	Pons	11	External occipital	29	Geniohyoid	46	Second tracheal ring
2	Basilar artery		protuberance	30	Mylohyoid	47	Trachea
3	Clivus (basi-occipital	12	Occipital bone	31	Body of hyoid bone	48	Oesophagus
	and basi-sphenoid	13	Transverse sinus	32	Vallecula	49	Superior lobe of left lung
	bones)	14	Straight sinus	33	Epiglottis	50	Brachiocephalic trunk
4	Anterior margin of	15	Tentorium cerebelli	34	Laryngeal part of	51	Brachiocephalic vein
	foramen magnum	16	Cerebellum		pharynx	52	Manubrium of sternum
5	Anterior arch of atlas	17	Fourth ventricle	35	Vestibular fold	53	Anterior jugular vein
	(first cervical vertebra)	18	Cisterna magna	36	Ventricle of larynx	54	Posterior cricoarytenoid
6	Dens of axis (odontoid	19	Medulla oblongata	37	Vocal fold (vocal cord)	55	Arytenoid cartilage
	peg of second cervical	20	Uvula	38	Platysma	56	Body of third cervical
	vertebra)	21	Soft palate	39	Lamina of thyroid		vertebra
7	Nasal part of pharynx	22	Hard palate		cartilage	57	Spinal cord
	(nasopharynx)	23	Central incisor (upper	40	Sternohyoid	58	Spinous process of
8	Oral part of pharynx		and lower)	41	Sternothyroid		second vertebra
	(oropharynx)	24	Lip (upper and lower)	42	Isthmus of thyroid gland	59	Semispinalis capitis
9	Posterior arch of atlas	25	Body of mandible	43	Lamina of cricoid	60	Trapezius
	(first cervical vertebra)	26	Sublingual gland		cartilage	61	Semispinalis cervicis
10	Posterior margin of	27	Dorsum of tongue	44	Arch of cricoid cartilage		
	foramen magnum	28	Genioglossus	45	Lower part of larynx	62	Occipital lobe of brain

■ Section level

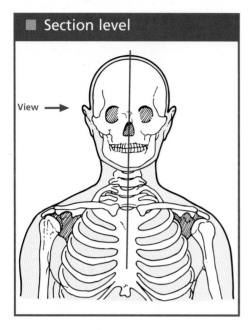

View →

■ Orientation

Superior

Posterior ←——→ Anterior

Inferior

■ Notes

The nasal septum has been removed from this section in order to display the nasal conchae on the lateral wall.

Cricothyroid puncture is performed between the thyroid cartilage (**39**) and the isthmus of the cricoid cartilage (**44**). Note that a tube inserted at this site will lie below the vocal folds (**37**),which are therefore free of danger.

Note that the junction of the larynx and trachea (**46**) lies at the level of the sixth cervical vertebra. This level also marks the junction of the pharynx (**34**) and the oesophagus (**48**).

These midline sagittal magnetic resonance images – (A) T1-weighted and (B) T2-weighted – demonstrate clearly the normal relationship of the pons, medulla and cervical spinal cord to the base of the skull, foramen magnum, dens of the axis (odontoid peg) and cervical canal. The anterior and posterior margins of the foramen magnum, the tip of the basi-occipital part of the clivus and the anterior margin of the occipital bone can be well appreciated.

Note the size of the cervical cord in relation to the spinal canal compared with the ratio more caudally; of course, the cervical canal carries many more white matter fibres. On T2 weighting (image B), there is only a relatively small amount of cerebrospinal fluid surrounding the cord; hence, the diameter of the spinal canal in this region is of key importance. If the canal is too narrow, then the inevitable degenerative changes of middle/old age that occur in the vertebral column can affect nerve roots supplying the arms (brachalgia) or even affect the cord to cause upper motor neurone signs.

The relationship of the anterior arch of the atlas (first cervical vertebra) to the dens (odontoid peg) of the axis (the body of the first cervical vertebra assimilated on to the body of the second cervical vertebra – the axis) is shown well. This pivot synovial joint allows rotation of the head and C1 on C2 and the rest of the spinal column.

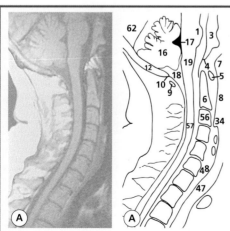

Sagittal magnetic resonance image (MRI)

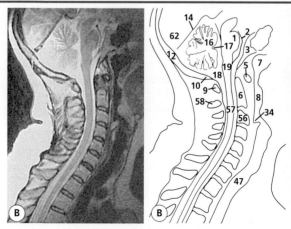

Sagittal magnetic resonance image (MRI)

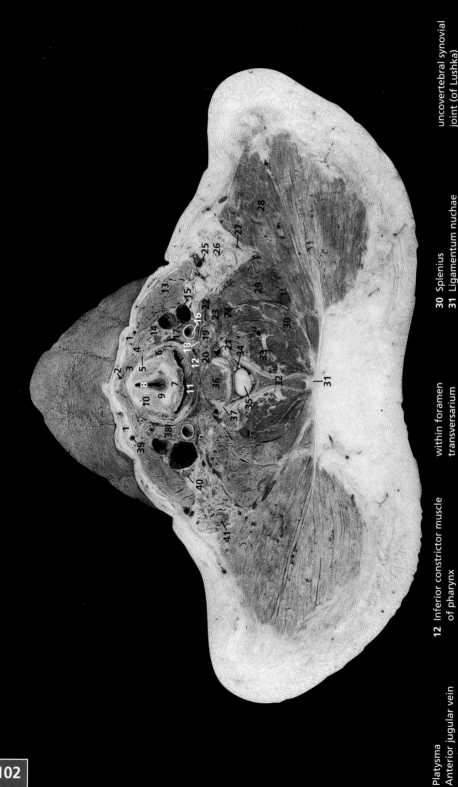

1 Platysma
2 Anterior jugular vein
3 Sternohyoid
4 Omohyoid
5 Sternothyroid
6 Thyroid cartilage
7 Cricoid cartilage
8 Rima glottidis
9 Arytenoid cartilage
10 Thyro-arytenoid
11 Pharynx

12 Inferior constrictor muscle of pharynx
13 Sternocleidomastoid
14 Common facial vein
15 Internal jugular vein
16 Common carotid artery
17 Vagus nerve (X)
18 Sympathetic chain
19 Longus capitis
20 Longus colli
21 Vertebral artery and vein

within foramen transversarium
22 Phrenic nerve
23 Scalenus anterior
24 Scalenus medius and posterior
25 External jugular vein
26 Fat of posterior triangle
27 Accessory nerve (XI)
28 Trapezius
29 Levator scapulae

30 Splenius
31 Ligamentum nuchae
32 Spine of fifth cervical vertebra
33 Erector spinae
34 Root of sixth cervical nerve
35 Spinal cord within dural sheath
36 Body of fifth cervical vertebra
37 Neurocentral or

uncovertebral synovial joint (of Lushka)
38 Lateral lobe of thyroid gland
39 Accessory anterior jugular vein
40 Lymph node of internal jugular chain
41 Cervical lymph node

■ Section level

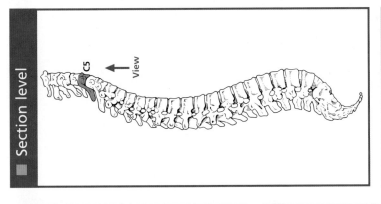

C5

← view

■ Orientation

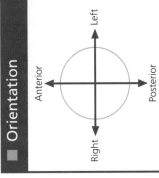

Left

Anterior — Posterior

Right

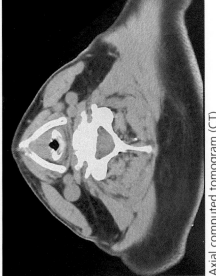

Axial computed tomogram (CT)

■ Notes

This section passes through the body of the fifth cervical vertebra (**36**), immediately above the level of the shoulder joint. Here the fibres of the trapezius (**28**) arch over the posterior extremity of the posterior triangle. Just below this level, at C6, lies the junction between the pharynx (**11**) and oesophagus, and the larynx (**6, 7, 9**) and the trachea. In both the section and the CT image, the pharynx (**11**) has a narrow anteroposterior diameter; it distends considerably during deglutition. On the CT image, the vocal cords of the rima glottidis (**8**) are adducted.

The posterior triangle of the neck has, at its boundaries, the posterior border of sternocleidomastoid (**13**) anteriorly, the anterior border of trapezius (**28**) posteriorly and the middle third of the clavicle below. Its floor comprises, from above downwards, splenius capitis (**30**), levator scapulae (**29**) and scalenus medius and posterior (**24**).

Not unusually, as in this case, the external jugular vein (**39**) is double.

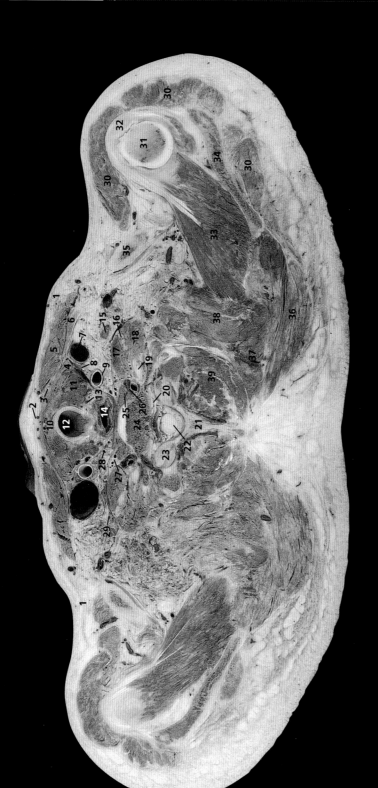

1 Platysma
2 Anterior jugular vein
3 Sternohyoid
4 Sternothyroid
5 Sternocleidomastoid
6 Omohyoid
7 Internal jugular vein
8 Vagus nerve (X)
9 Common carotid artery
10 Isthmus of thyroid gland
11 Lateral lobe of thyroid gland
12 Trachea

13 Recurrent laryngeal nerve
14 Oesophagus
15 Lymph node
16 Ventral ramus of sixth cervical
   nerve
17 Scalenus anterior
18 Scalenus medius
19 Ventral ramus of seventh cervical
   nerve
20 Dorsal root ganglion of eighth
   cervical nerve
21 Spine of seventh cervical vertebra –

vertebra prominens
22 Spinal cord within dural sheath
23 Inferior articular facet of seventh
   cervical vertebra
24 Body of seventh cervical vertebra
25 Longus colli
26 Vertebral artery and vein
27 Ascending cervical artery and vein
28 Inferior thyroid artery
29 Phrenic nerve
30 Deltoid
31 Head of humerus

32 Capsule of shoulder joint
33 Supraspinatus
34 Spine of scapula
35 Coracoid process of scapula
36 Trapezius
37 Rhomboideus minor
38 Levator scapulae
39 Erector spinae

40 External jugular vein

Section level

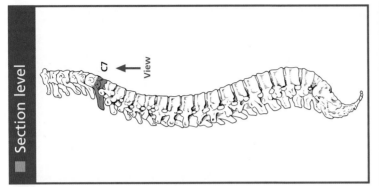

Orientation

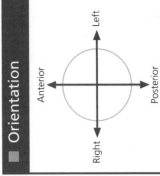

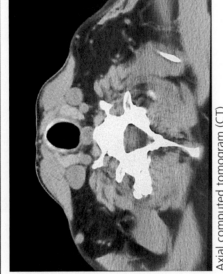

Axial computed tomogram (CT)

Notes

This section traverses the body of the seventh cervical vertebra, which bears the longest spine of the cervical series, the vertebra prominens (**21**). This is shorter, however, than the spine of T1, as can be ascertained easily by feeling the back of your own neck.

Three important relationships are demonstrated well. The recurrent laryngeal nerve (**13**) lies in the groove between the trachea (**12**) and the oesophagus (**14**). The phrenic nerve (**29**) hugs the anterior aspect of scalenus anterior (**17**) deep to the prevertebral fascia; three structures – the common carotid artery (**9**), the internal jugular vein (**7**) and the vagus nerve (**8**) – lie together within the fascial carotid sheath. The deep cervical chain of lymph nodes (**15**) lies lateral to the carotid sheath.

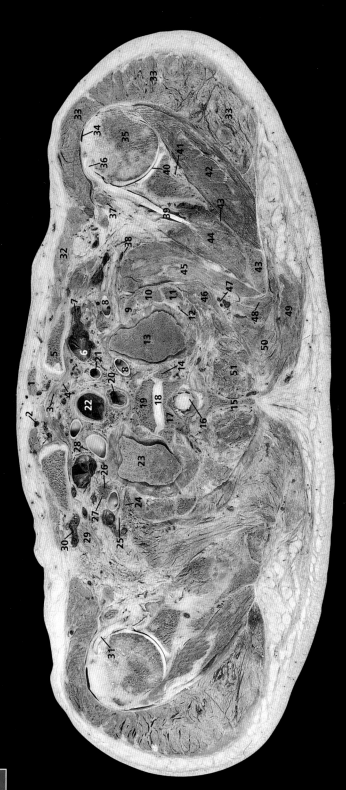

1 Sternocleidomastoid sternal head
2 Anterior jugular vein
3 Sternohyoid
4 Sternothyroid
5 Clavicle
6 Internal jugular vein – junction with left subclavian vein
7 Left subclavian vein
8 Subclavian artery
9 First rib
10 Intercostal muscles
11 Second rib
12 Intercostal neurovascular bundle
13 Apex of left lung
14 Head of second rib

15 Spine of first thoracic vertebra
16 Spinal cord within dural sheath
17 Part of body of second thoracic vertebra
18 Part of intervertebral disc between first and second thoracic vertebrae
19 Part of body of first thoracic vertebra
20 Oesophagus
21 Common carotid artery
22 Trachea
23 Right lung apex
24 Scalenus medius
25 Root of first thoracic nerve
26 Scalenus anterior

27 Phrenic nerve
28 Vagus nerve (X)
29 Subclavius
30 Right subclavian vein
31 Tendon of right biceps long head
32 Pectoralis major
33 Deltoid
34 Subdeltoid bursa
35 Head of humerus
36 Tendon of left biceps long head
37 Coracoid process of scapula
38 Nerve to serratus anterior
39 Tendon of subscapularis
40 Glenoid fossa of scapula
41 Suprascapular artery and vein

42 Infraspinatus
43 Scapula
44 Subscapularis
45 Serratus anterior
46 Serratus posterior superior
47 Superficial (transverse) cervical artery and vein
48 Rhomboideus minor
49 Trapezius
50 Rhomboideus major
51 Erector spinae
52 Supraspinatus
53 Pectoralis minor

Section level

T1–2

View

Orientation

Anterior

Left

Right

Posterior

B

Axial computed tomogram (CT)

A

Axial computed tomogram (CT)

Notes

This section, through the intervertebral disc between the first and second thoracic vertebrae (**18**), enters the apex of the thorax and traverses the apices of the upper lobes of the lungs (**13, 23**). There are considerable differences between the section and CT images at this level because the CT is performed with the arms elevated alongside the head in order to reduce artefacts from the humeri.

Here, posterior to the medial end of the clavicle (**5**), the internal jugular vein (**6**) joins with the subclavian vein (**7**) to form the brachiocephalic vein (see Axial section 4).

The intercostal neurovascular bundle (**12**) is seen well. Note that it comprises the intercostal vein, artery and nerve from above downwards; the nerve corresponds to the number of its

overlying rib and lies protected within the subcostal groove.

Only in transverse section is the extreme thinness of the blade of the scapula (**43**) appreciated fully.

One CT (A) is displayed at soft tissue settings (window level and width of grey scale), the other CT (B) at lung windows.

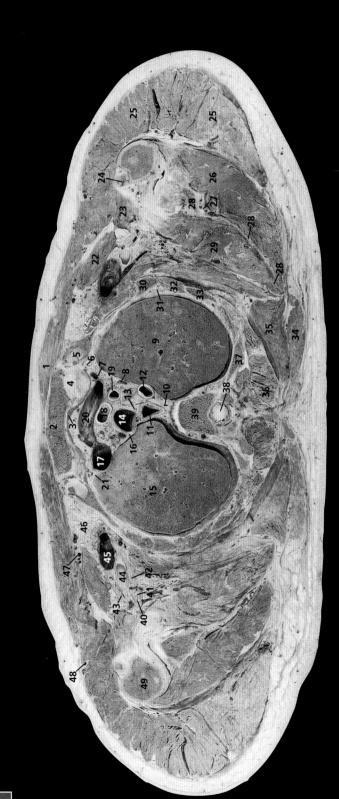

1 Pectoralis major
2 Manubrium of sternum
3 Sternothyroid
4 Sternoclavicular joint
5 First rib
6 Internal thoracic artery
7 Left phrenic nerve
8 Left vagus nerve (X)
9 Upper lobe of left lung
10 Thoracic duct
11 Oesophagus
12 Left subclavian artery
13 Left recurrent laryngeal nerve
14 Trachea

15 Upper lobe of right lung
16 Right vagus nerve (X)
17 Right brachiocephalic vein
18 Brachiocephalic artery
19 Left common carotid artery
20 Left brachiocephalic vein
21 Right phrenic nerve
22 Pectoralis minor
23 Coracobrachialis and biceps (short head)
24 Long head of biceps tendon
25 Deltoid
26 Infraspinatus
27 Suprascapular artery and vein

28 Scapula
29 Subscapularis
30 Second rib
31 Intercostal artery and vein and nerve
32 External and internal intercostal muscles
33 Third rib
34 Trapezius
35 Rhomboideus major
36 Erector spinae
37 Fourth rib with articulation of its head with body of third thoracic vertebra transverse process

38 Spinal cord within dural sheath
39 Body of third thoracic vertebra
40 Axillary nerve
41 Radial nerve
42 Ulnar nerve
43 Median nerve
44 Right axillary artery
45 Right axillary vein
46 Axillary fat
47 Pectoral branch of the acromiothoracic artery and vein
48 Cephalic vein
49 Shaft of humerus

Section level

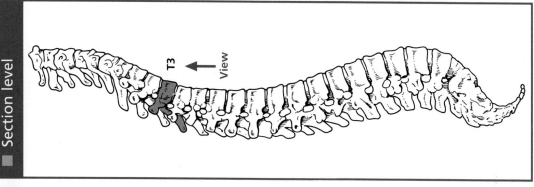

T3

← View

Orientation

Anterior

Left

Posterior

Right

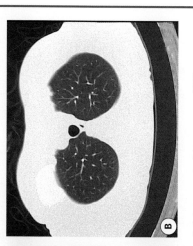

Axial computed tomogram (CT)

Ⓑ

Axial computed tomogram (CT)

Ⓐ

Notes

The contents of the upper mediastinum – including the oesophagus, trachea and great vessels – are demonstrated in this section, which traverses the manubrium and the third thoracic vertebra; these are also shown in Axial section 5.

This section also shows the walls and contents of the axilla. Note that the cephalic vein (**48**) runs in the deltopectoral groove between the medial edge of deltoid and the lateral edge of pectoralis major.

109

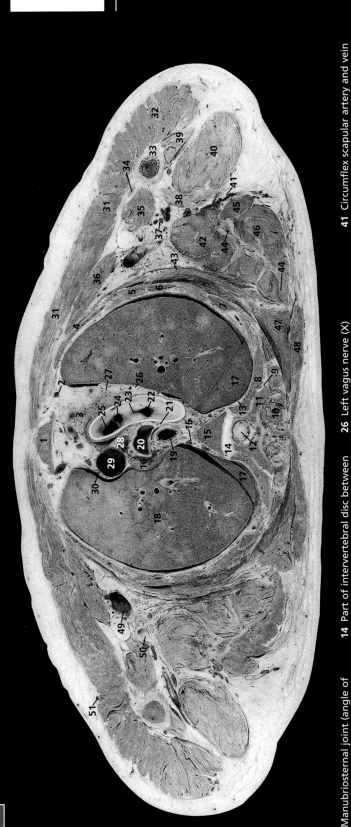

1 Manubriosternal joint (angle of Louis)
2 Internal thoracic artery and vein
3 Thymic residue within anterior mediastinal fat
4 Second rib
5 Intercostal
6 Third rib
7 Fourth rib
8 Fifth rib
9 Fifth costotransverse joint
10 Erector spinae
11 Transverse process of fifth thoracic vertebra
12 Spinal cord within dural sheath
13 Sympathetic chain

14 Part of intervertebral disc between fourth and fifth thoracic vertebrae
15 Part of body of fourth thoracic vertebra
16 Azygos vein
17 Apical segment lower lobe lung separated by oblique fissure from (18)
18 Upper lobe of lung
19 Oesophagus
20 Trachea at bifurcation
21 Recurrent laryngeal nerve
22 Left subclavian artery orifice
23 Aortic arch
24 Left common carotid artery orifice
25 Brachiocephalic artery orifice

26 Left vagus nerve (X)
27 Left phrenic nerve
28 Pretracheal lymph node
29 Superior vena cava
30 Right phrenic nerve
31 Pectoralis major
32 Deltoid
33 Shaft of humerus
34 Biceps – long head
35 Biceps – short head and coracobrachialis
36 Pectoralis minor
37 Subscapular artery vein and nerve
38 Latissimus dorsi
39 Triceps – lateral head
40 Triceps – long head

41 Circumflex scapular artery and vein
42 Subscapularis
43 Serratus anterior
44 Body of scapula
45 Teres minor
46 Infraspinatus
47 Rhomboideus
48 Trapezius
49 Axillary vein
50 Axillary artery
51 Cephalic vein
52 Oblique fissure

Section level

T4–5

View

Orientation

Anterior

Left

Posterior

Right

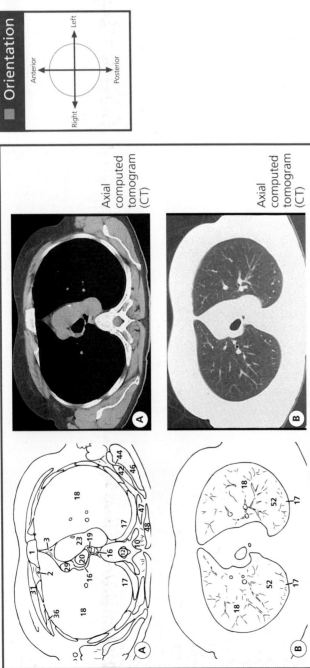

Axial computed tomogram (CT)

Axial computed tomogram (CT)

A

B

Notes

This section passes through the important anatomical level of the manubriosternal joint, the angle of Louis (**1**). At this joint articulate the second costal cartilage and rib (**4**), and it is from here that the ribs can be conveniently counted in clinical practice. Posteriorly this plane passes through the T4/5 intervertebral disc (**14**).

This plane demarcates the junction between the superior and the lower mediastinum, the latter of which is subdivided into the anterior mediastinum, in front of the pericardium, the middle mediastinum, occupied by the pericardium and its

contents, and the posterior mediastinum, behind the pericardium.

The trachea bifurcates at this level (**20**). In the living upright subject, however, the bifurcation may be as low as the level of T6, particularly in deep inspiration.

The cranial portions of the oblique fissures of the lungs (**17**, **52**) are traversed on this section. The normal oblique fissures are often not seen on conventional CT images of the lung parenchyma. The position can be inferred, however (see CT b) by the paucity of blood vessels; only small terminal vessels

are present in the lung parenchyma adjacent to a fissure.

Pretracheal nodes (**28**) may become enlarged due to a wide variety of disease processes. They are accessible for biopsy via mediastinoscopy.

Subscapularis (**42**) arises not only from the periosteum of the medial two-thirds of the subscapular fossa of the scapula but also from tendinous laminae in the muscle itself, which are attached to prominent transverse ridges on the subscapular fossa. This is shown clearly in this section.

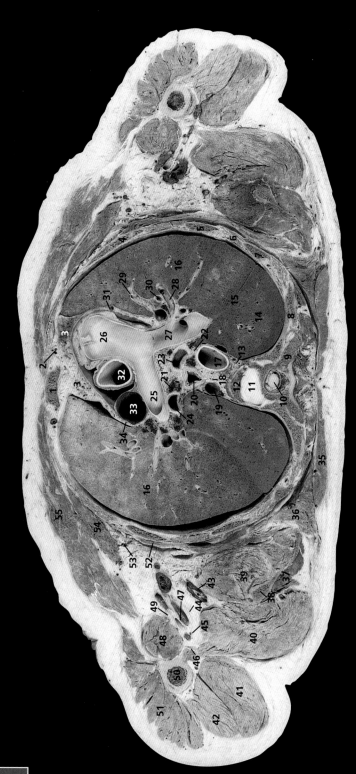

1 Body of sternum
2 Internal thoracic artery and vein
3 Thymic residue within anterior mediastinal fat
4 Third rib
5 Fouth rib
6 Intercostal muscle
7 Fifth rib
8 Sixth rib
9 Transverse process of sixth thoracic vertebra
10 Spinal cord within dural sheath
11 Part of intervertebral disc between fifth and sixth thoracic vertebrae
12 Part of body of fifth thoracic vertebra

13 Intercostal artery and vein
14 Lower lobe of lung
15 Oblique fissure
16 Upper lobe of lung
17 Descending aorta
18 Thoracic duct
19 Azygos vein
20 Oesophagus
21 Lymph node
22 Left vagus nerve (X)
23 Left main bronchus
24 Right intermediate bronchus
25 Right pulmonary artery
26 Pulmonary trunk
27 Left pulmonary artery
28 Pulmonary artery branch

29 Pulmonary vein tributary
30 Segmental bronchus
31 Left phrenic nerve with pericardiacophrenic artery
32 Ascending aorta
33 Superior vena cava
34 Right phrenic nerve
35 Trapezius
36 Rhomboideus major
37 Infraspinatus
38 Scapula
39 Subscapularis
40 Teres major
41 Triceps – long head
42 Triceps – lateral head
43 Subscapular artery and vein

44 Ulnar nerve
45 Radial nerve
46 Latissimus dorsi tendon
47 Axillary artery and vein
48 Biceps and coracobrachialis
49 Median nerve
50 Shaft of humerus
51 Deltoid
52 Serratus anterior
53 Lateral thoracic artery and vein
54 Pectoralis minor
55 Pectoralis major

56 Superior pulmonary vein
57 Left basal pulmonary artery
58 Breast

Section level

T5–6

View

Orientation

Anterior

Left

Posterior

Right

Axial computed tomogram (CT)

A

A

Axial computed tomogram (CT)

B

B

Notes

This section, traversing the upper body of the sternum (1) and the lower part of the body of the fifth thoracic vertebra (12), passes through the great arterial trunks as these emerge from the heart, the pulmonary trunk (26) and the ascending aorta (32).

On the CT image, the left main bronchus gives off its common upper lobe/lingular branch at this level. On the right, the upper lobe bronchus has already originated more cranially (on both CT images and section); hence, the term 'intermediate bronchus' (24) is applied to that portion of the right bronchus between its upper lobe and middle lobe branches.

At the left hilum, the superior pulmonary vein (56) lies anterior to the bronchus (23), which in turn lies anterior to the left basal pulmonary artery (57). On the right side, the vein (56) lies anterior to the right pulmonary artery, which lies anterior to the right intermediate bronchus (24).

In this subject, the right (25) and left (27) pulmonary arteries lie in the same axial plane. In most subjects, the left pulmonary artery is at a more cranial level than the right – hence the discrepancy between the section and CT image appearances. The branches of the pulmonary artery (28) that

accompany the segmental and subsegmental bronchi (30) usually lie dorsolaterally to these structures; each pulmonary segment receives an independent arterial supply. The bronchi usually separate the dorsolateral pulmonary artery branch from the ventromedially situated pulmonary vein tributary (29). Peripherally, many pulmonary venous tributaries run between, and drain adjacent, pulmonary segments. Thus, an individual bronchopulmonary segment will have its own bronchus and artery but not an individual pulmonary venous drainage.

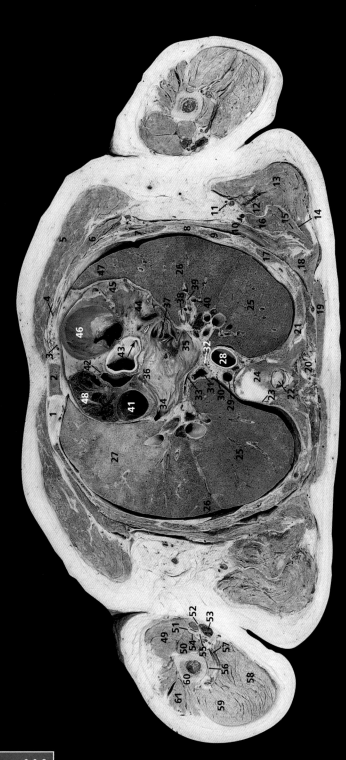

1 Third costal cartilage with adjacent sternocostal joint (see Notes)
2 Body of sternum
3 Internal thoracic artery and vein
4 Partially calcified third costal cartilage
5 Pectoralis major
6 Pectoralis minor
7 Third rib
8 Intercostal muscle
9 Fourth rib
10 Serratus anterior
11 Subscapular artery vein and nerve
12 Teres major
13 Latissimus dorsi
14 Infraspinatus

15 Scapula
16 Subscapularis
17 Fifth rib
18 Rhomboideus major
19 Trapezius
20 Erector spinae
21 Sixth rib, with adjacent costotransverse joint to transverse process of sixth thoracic vertebra
22 Spinal cord within dural sheath
23 Thoracic sympathetic chain
24 Body of sixth thoracic vertebra, with part of intervertebral disc between the sixth and seventh thoracic vertebrae
25 Lower lobe of lung

26 Upper lobe of lung
27 Middle lobe of right lung
28 Descending aorta
29 Azygos vein
30 Thoracic duct
31 Oesophagus
32 Left vagal plexus
33 Right vagal plexus
34 Right superior pulmonary vein
35 Left superior pulmonary vein
36 Left atrium
37 Left auricle (atrial appendage)
38 Left pulmonary vein tributary to lingula
39 Left bronchus segmental branch to lingula

40 Left pulmonary artery branch to lingula
41 Superior vena cava
42 Artefactual gap within the pericardial space
43 Ascending aorta, with orifice of left coronary artery (arrowed)
44 Left ventricle wall
45 Coronary artery (left anterior interventricular branch)
46 Infundibulum of right ventricle with pulmonary valves
47 Fibrous pericardium
48 Right auricle (atrial appendage)
49 Biceps

50 Coracobrachialis
51 Axillary artery and vein
52 Medial cutaneous nerves of arm and forearm
53 Basilic vein
54 Median nerve
55 Ulnar nerve
56 Triceps – medial head
57 Radial nerve with profunda brachii artery and vein
58 Triceps – long head
59 Triceps – lateral head
60 Shaft of humerus
61 Deltoid

62 Hemiazygos vein
63 Right coronary artery
64 Oblique fissure

Section level

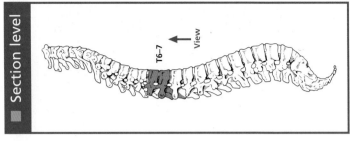

T6–7

← View

Orientation

Anterior

Posterior

Left

Right

Axial computed tomogram (CT)

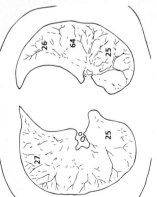

A

Axial computed tomogram (CT)

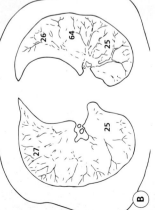

B

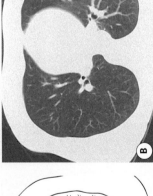

A

B

Notes

The plane of this section traverses the lower part of the body of the sixth thoracic vertebra (**24**). Anteriorly, it passes through the body of the sternum (**2**) at the level of the third costal cartilage (**1**). Note the adjacent sternocostal joint. These vary; the first lacks a synovial cavity, its costal cartilage being attached by fibrocartilage to the manubrium. The second to seventh joints are usually synovial (as in this subject), with the fibrocartilaginous articular surfaces on both the chondral and the sternal components of the joint. In some or all of these joints, however, an arrangement may be found similar to that of the first joint.

The presence of a pericardial effusion in this subject has produced an artefactual gap in the superior reflection of the pericardial space (**42**). The aorta at its origin (**43**) shows the orifice of the left coronary artery. The descending aorta (**28**) is normally more circular in outline than in this subject. Note that this section passes through the infundibulum of the right ventricle and demonstrates the pulmonary valves (**46**).

On the CT image, both the ascending aorta (**43**) and the region of the pulmonary valves (**46**) have indistinct outlines due to pulsation (compliance) of their walls during the 1-s data-acquisition time. (See also the ascending aorta on the left-hand image in Axial section 6.)

115

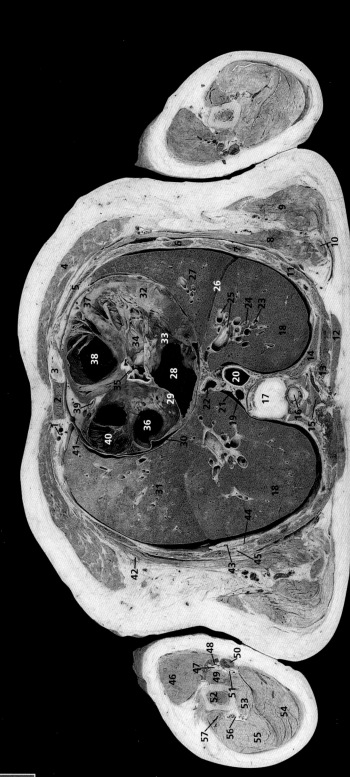

1 Internal thoracic artery and vein
2 Body of sternum
3 Fourth costal cartilage
4 Pectoralis major
5 Fourth rib
6 Fifth rib
7 Sixth rib
8 Serratus anterior
9 Latissimus dorsi
10 Scapula inferior angle
11 Seventh rib
12 Trapezius
13 Erector spinae
14 Eighth rib
15 Lamina of seventh thoracic vertebra

16 Spinal cord within dural sheath
17 Intervertebral disc between seventh and eighth thoracic vertebrae
18 Lower lobe of lung
19 Azygos vein
20 Descending aorta
21 Thoracic duct
22 Oesophagus
23 Pulmonary artery branch
24 Branches of left lower lobe bronchus
25 Pulmonary vein tributaries
26 Oblique fissure
27 Upper lobe of left lung
28 Left atrium

29 Interatrial septum
30 Phrenic nerve with pericardiacophrenic artery and vein
31 Middle lobe of right lung
32 Wall of left ventricle
33 Mitral valve
34 Vestibule of left ventricle (outflow tract) leading to root of aorta
35 Divided cusp of aortic valve
36 Right atrium
37 Anterior interventricular (descending) branch of left coronary artery
38 Right ventricle cavity

39 Right coronary artery
40 Right auricle (atrial appendage)
41 Fibrous pericardium
42 Nerve to serratus anterior
43 Intercostal neurovascular bundle
44 Innermost intercostal
45 External and internal intercostal muscles
46 Biceps
47 Median nerve with musculocutaneous nerve (lateral to it)
48 Brachial artery with two venae comitantes
49 Coracobrachialis

50 Basilic vein
51 Ulnar nerve
52 Shaft of humerus
53 Triceps – short head
54 Triceps – long head
55 Triceps – lateral head
56 Radial nerve with profunda brachii artery and vein
57 Deltoid

T7–8

View

Left

Anterior

Posterior

Right

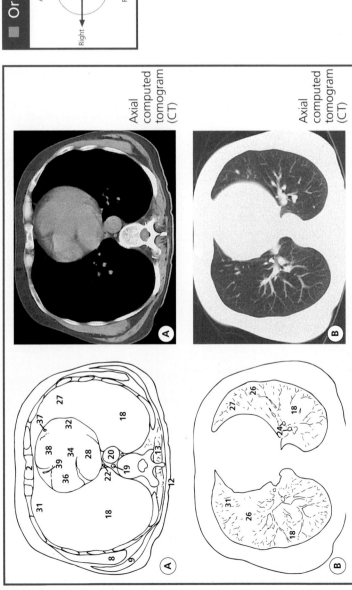

Axial computed tomogram (CT)

Axial computed tomogram (CT)

■ Notes

This section lies at the level of the intervertebral disc between the seventh and eighth thoracic vertebrae (17) and passes through the body of the sternum (2) at the level of the fourth costal cartilage (3). All four cardiac chambers can be seen and their relationships to each other appreciated. Note that the right atrium (36) forms the right border of the heart. The left atrium (28) is the major contribution to the base of the heart and lies immediately anterior to the

oesophagus (22), separated by the pericardium. The left ventricle (32) forms the bulk of the left border of the heart, and the right ventricle (38) constitutes the major component of the anterior cardiac surface.

In this subject, the left ventricular wall (32) becomes thinner in the region of the apex of the left ventricle, due to a previous myocardial infarction.

The interatrial septum (29) has a rather curious convexity. This has been caused by extensive post-

mortem thrombus in the right atrium (36). The septum is normally straighter.

The lower four or five digitations of serratus anterior (8) converge to insert on the costal aspect of the inferior angle of the scapula. This component of the muscle, together with the trapezius, powerfully pulls the inferior angle of the scapula forwards and upwards in raising the arm above the head.

117

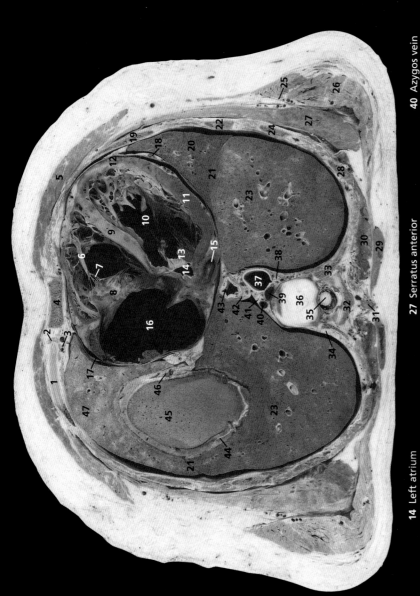

1 Fifth costal cartilage
2 Sternocostal joint
3 Internal thoracic artery and vein
4 Body of sternum
5 Pectoralis major
6 Papillary muscle
7 Chordae tendinae within right ventricular cavity
8 Triscupid valve
9 Interventricular septum
10 Left ventricular cavity
11 Normal left ventricular wall
12 Thinned left ventricular wall
13 Mitral valve

14 Left atrium
15 Coronary sinus
16 Right atrium
17 Fibrous pericardium
18 Left phrenic nerve, with pericardiacophrenic artery and vein
19 Fifth rib
20 Upper lobe of left lung (lingula)
21 Oblique fissure
22 Sixth rib
23 Lower lobe of lung
24 Seventh rib
25 Lateral thoracic artery and vein
26 Latissimus dorsi

27 Serratus anterior
28 Eighth rib
29 Trapezius
30 Erector spinae
31 Spine of eighth thoracic vertebra
32 Lamina of eighth thoracic vertebra
33 Ninth rib
34 Right sympathetic chain
35 Spinal cord within dural sheath
36 Intervertebral disc between eighth and ninth thoracic vertebrae
37 Aorta
38 Origin of eighth intercostal artery
39 Hemiazygos vein

40 Azygos vein
41 Thoracic duct
42 Oesophageal vagal plexus
43 Oesophagus
44 Dome of right hemidiaphragm
45 Apex of right lobe liver
46 Right phrenic nerve, with pericardiacophrenic artery and vein
47 Middle lobe of right lung

48 Inferior vena cava
49 Right ventricular cavity

Section level

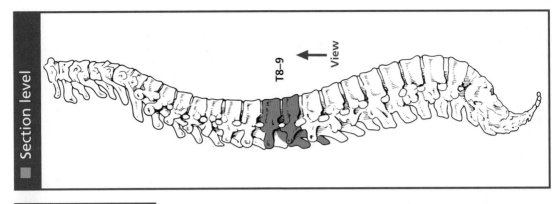

T8–9

← View

Orientation

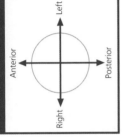

Anterior

Left

Right

Posterior

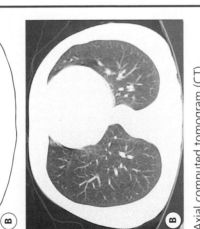

Axial computed tomogram (CT)

Axial computed tomogram (CT)

Notes

This section traverses the intervertebral disc between the eighth and ninth thoracic vertebrae (**36**) and slices through the dome of the right hemidiaphragm (**44**) and a sliver of the underlying right lobe of the liver (**45**).

In this section, there is considerable thinning and discoloration of the left ventricular wall at the apex (**12**), consistent with infarction associated with left anterior descending (interventricular) coronary arterial disease.

Note how only a tiny portion of the left atrium (**14**) is present on this section. This demonstrates that the left atrium is situated more cranially than the other three cardiac chambers.

The terminal fibres of the right phrenic nerve (**46**) usually pass through the vena caval opening in the diaphragm but may traverse the muscle itself.

119

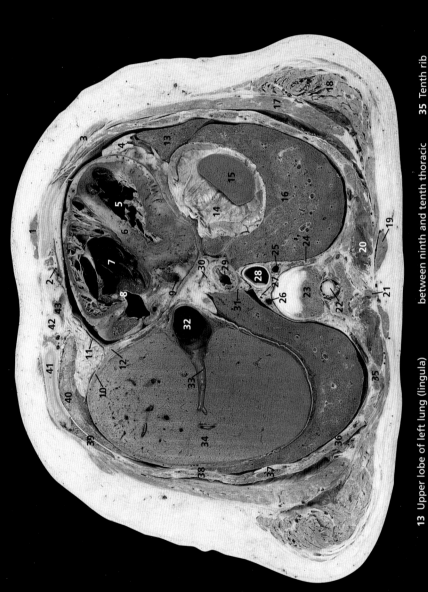

1 Pectoralis major
2 Internal thoracic artery and vein
3 External oblique
4 Extrapericardial pad of fat
5 Left ventricle
6 Interventricular septum
7 Right ventricle
8 Tricuspid valve
9 Coronary sinus
10 Diaphragm
11 Fibrous pericardium
12 Line of fusion of diaphragm and pericardium

13 Upper lobe of left lung (lingula)
14 Left dome of diaphragm
15 Spleen
16 Lower lobe of lung
17 Serratus anterior
18 Latissimus dorsi
19 Trapezius
20 Erector spinae
21 Tip of spine of eighth thoracic vertebra
22 Spinal cord within dural sheath
23 Body of ninth thoracic vertebra, with part of intervertebral disc

between ninth and tenth thoracic vertebrae
24 Left sympathetic chain
25 Hemiazygos vein
26 Azygos vein
27 Thoracic duct
28 Aorta
29 Oesophagus
30 Left vagus nerve (X)
31 Right vagus nerve (X)
32 Inferior vena cava
33 Right hepatic vein
34 Right lobe of liver

35 Tenth rib
36 Ninth rib
37 Eighth rib
38 Seventh rib
39 Sixth rib
40 Middle lobe of right lung
41 Sixth costal cartilage
42 Fifth costal cartilage
43 Sternum

44 Oblique fissure

Section level

T9–10

View

Orientation

Left

Anterior

Posterior

Right

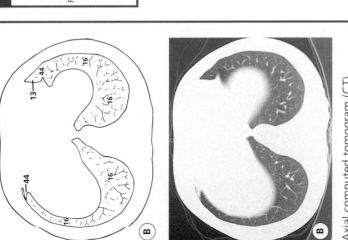

Axial computed tomogram (CT)

Axial computed tomogram (CT)

Notes

This section is at the level of the body of the ninth thoracic vertebra (**23**) and traverses the dome of the left diaphragm (**14**). The cranial portion of the spleen (**15**) is, therefore, revealed.

The fusion of the diaphragm (**10**) with the base of the fibrous pericardium (**11**) is shown clearly at this point.

The massive size of the hepatic veins as they drain into the inferior vena cava (**32**) is well demonstrated in this section, which passes through the right hepatic vein at its termination (**33**).

The aorta (**28**) at this level has become the immediate posterior relation of the oesophagus (**29**), just as it is about to pass through its hiatus in the diaphragm (**10**).

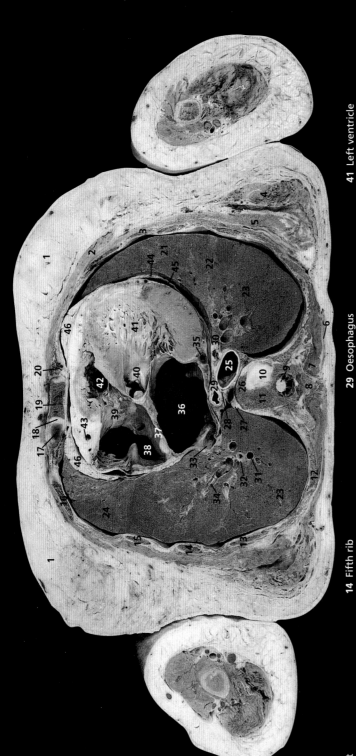

1 Breast
2 Pectoralis major
3 Intercostal muscles
4 Latissimus dorsi
5 Serratus anterior
6 Trapezius
7 Erector spinae
8 Spine of seventh thoracic vertebra
9 Spinal cord within dural sheath
10 Part of intervertebral disc between the seventh and eighth thoracic vertebrae
11 Body of seventh thoracic vertebra
12 Seventh rib
13 Sixth rib

14 Fifth rib
15 Fourth rib
16 Third rib
17 Third costal cartilage
18 Third sternocostal joint
19 Sternum
20 Internal thoracic artery and vein
21 Upper lobe of left lung (lingula)
22 Left oblique fissure
23 Lower lobe of lung
24 Middle lobe of right lung
25 Aorta
26 Azygos vein
27 Right sympathetic chain
28 Thoracic duct

29 Oesophagus
30 Mediastinal lymph node
31 Pulmonary arterial branch in lower lobe
32 Bronchus – segmental branch in lower lobe
33 Orifice of right inferior pulmonary vein
34 Right inferior pulmonary vein
35 Coronary sinus
36 Left atrium
37 Interatrial septum
38 Right atrium
39 Tricuspid valve
40 Aortic valve

41 Left ventricle
42 Right ventricle
43 Right coronary artery
44 Left phrenic nerve
45 Fibrous pericardium
46 Extrapericardial fat pad
47 Ascending aorta
48 Descending aorta
49 Pulmonary trunk
50 Right pulmonary artery
51 Superior vena cava
52 Left basal pulmonary artery
53 Upper lobe of right lung
54 Carcinoma right breast

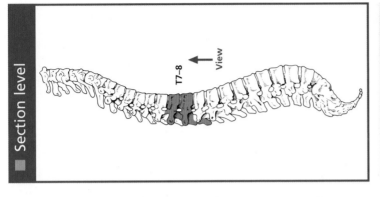

T7–8

View

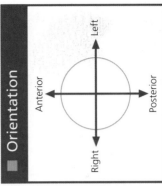

Anterior

Left

Right

Posterior

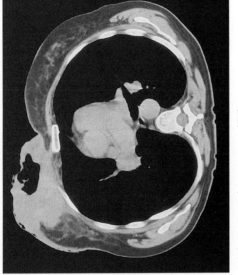

Axial computed tomogram (CT)

■ Notes

This section of a female subject passes through the body of the seventh thoracic vertebra (**11**) and through the third sternocostal joint (**18**). Note the general smaller configuration of the female thorax and the smaller, less bulky muscles.

The breast (**1**) contains the mammary gland. This extends vertically from the second to the sixth rib and transversely from the side of the sternum to near the mid-axillary line. The gland is situated within the superficial fascia and is separated from the fascia covering pectoralis major, serratus anterior and the external oblique muscle by loose areolar tissue. In old age, as in this subject, the glandular

tissue becomes atrophied. The inner wall of the left ventricle, immediately proximal to the aortic valve (**40**), is smooth-walled and termed the aortic vestibule.

This CT image shows a patient with a large carcinoma of the right breast, which has ulcerated and extended into, and infiltrated, a wide area of adjacent skin. The anatomical level is considerably more cranial than the cadaveric section; it corresponds closely to that shown in Axial section 6 of the male thorax.

Note that in this section, the margin of the mass of left ventricular muscle (**41**) has been cut across; there is infarction in the anterior free wall.

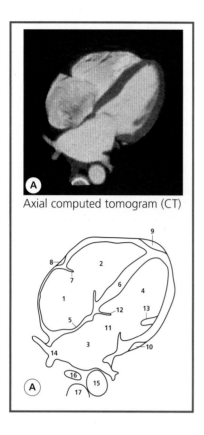

Axial computed tomogram (CT)

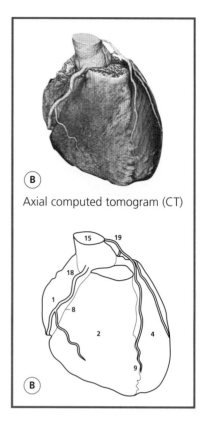

Axial computed tomogram (CT)

Images A–B

1 Right atrium
2 Right ventricle
3 Left atrium
4 Left ventricle
5 Interatrial septum
6 Interventricular septum
7 Tricuspid valve
8 Right atrioventricular groove for right coronary artery
9 Interventricular groove for anterior branch of left coronary artery
10 Left atrioventricular groove for circumflex branch of left coronary artery
11 Mitral valve
12 Anterior leaflet of mitral valve
13 Papillary muscle
14 Pulmonary vein
15 Aorta
16 Oesophagus
17 Thoracic vertebra
18 Right coronary artery
19 Left coronary artery

▪ Notes

Multidetector CT with rapid data acquisition has opened up huge opportunities for imaging the heart and great vessels. If the data for a whole revolution of the CT gantry can be acquired in less than 400 ms, then a considerable amount of information can be obtained in the relatively quiescent period of the cardiac cycle. If the patient's heart rate is slow and regular, then a succession of images can be obtained during one breath-hold at the same phase of the cardiac cycle; these can be combined and a three-dimensional dataset created. This can provide exceptional anatomical (and, increasingly, functional) information.

The four-chamber view (A) is a multiplanar two-dimensional reconstruction so that all four chambers can be seen on one oblique image. This is a standard view used in many imaging investigations, including CT, ultrasound and MRI. It allows direct comparison of the left and right sides of the heart. It elegantly shows the interventricular septum. The close relationship of the oesophagus to the posterior aspect of the left atrium explains the advantages of transoesophageal echocardiography.

The coloured three-dimensional surface rendered view of the ventricles and coronary arteries provides a good general overview but, in practice, the coronary arteries (B) are better displayed and analysed using more selective analysis tools.

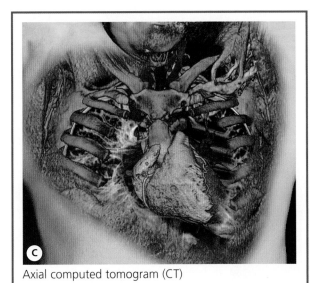

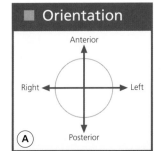

C

Axial computed tomogram (CT)

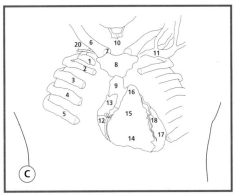

C

Image C

1 First rib (right)
2 Second rib
3 Third rib
4 Fourth rib
5 Fifth rib
6 Clavicle
7 Sternoclaviclar joint
8 Sternum – manubrium
9 Sternum – body
10 Hyoid bone
11 Left subclavian vein
12 Right atrium
13 Right atrial appendage
14 Right ventricle
15 Right ventricular outflow tract
16 Pulmonary trunk
17 Left ventricle
18 Left anterior descending – branch of left coronary artery
19 Right coronary artery
20 Right subclavian artery

■ Orientation

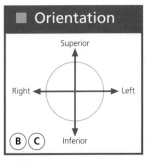

A

■ Orientation

B C

■ Notes

This edited 3D view of the chest (C) has been presented as a collage whereby the skin and subcutaneous tissues have been 'peeled away' to expose the internal structures of the chest. By using different window widths and colouring, it has been possible to demonstrate some lung detail in areas, which have not been obscured by overlying structures. These images were obtained during a long bolus injection of dilute iodinated contrast medium via the left arm. Hence the left subclavian vein (**11**) is well demonstrated but not the right. The heart, great vessels and coronary arteries are rendered opaque by the contrast medium and are well shown. It is just possible to see the right subclavian artery (**20**) between the right first rib (**1**) and the right clavicle (**6**). The coronary vessels are well shown with the left anterior descending artery (LAD, **18**) seen in the interventricular groove and the right coronary artery (**19**) seen in the right atrioventricular groove. Note the way that the 2nd rib (**2**) leads to the sterno-manubrial angle (of Louis). Of course the chondral part of the rib, which articulates with the sternomanubrial joint, is not sufficiently calcified to be seen at these settings.

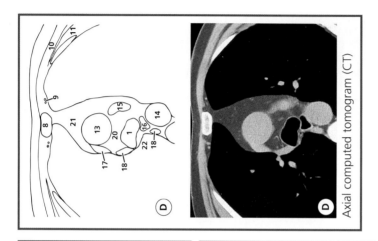

Axial computed tomogram (CT)

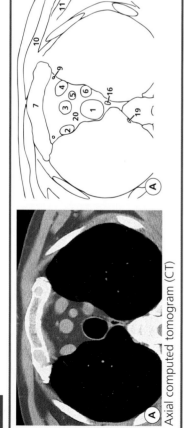

Axial computed tomogram (CT)

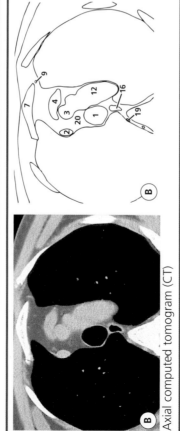

Axial computed tomogram (CT)

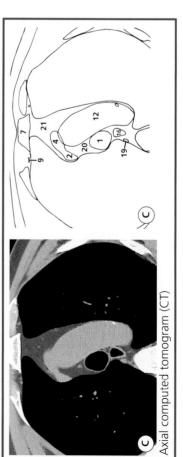

Axial computed tomogram (CT)

Images A–D

1 Trachea
2 Right brachiocephalic vein
3 Brachiocephalic artery
4 Left brachiocephalic vein
5 Left common carotid artery
6 Left subclavian artery
7 Manubrium of sternum
8 Body of sternum
9 Internal thoracic artery and vein
10 Pectoralis major
11 Pectoralis minor

12 Aortic arch (with fleck of calcification in wall in image C)
13 Ascending aorta
14 Descending aorta
15 Left pulmonary artery
16 Oesophagus
17 Superior vena cava
18 Azygos vein
19 Right superior intercostal vein
20 Fat in pretracheal space
21 Fat in anterior mediastinal space (with thymic remnant)
22 Azygos-oesophageal recess

■ Orientation

Anterior

Right — Posterior

Left

■ Section level

A
B
C
D

View

■ Notes

This patient has copious mediastinal fat, which makes the normal structures very conspicuous. Enlarged lymph nodes would show up well in such a patient (see Axial section 6). If such nodes lie in the pretracheal space (**20**), then biopsy material can be obtained via mediastinoscopy.

The trachea (**1**) is bifurcating on image D; this point is known as the carina. The left pulmonary artery (**15**) lies at a more cranial level than the right; it is just entering part of the section shown on image D. It appears indistinct because only part of the thickness of the slice is occupied by the

structure (partial volume effect). The space immediately caudal to the aortic arch and cranial to the bifurcation of the pulmonary artery is known as the subaortic fossa or aortopulmonary window. The ligamentum arteriosum (the obliterated ductus arteriosus passing from the left pulmonary artery to the aorta) runs through this space. This fossa may also contain enlarged lymph nodes.

The azygos vein (**18**) can be seen approaching the posterior aspect of the superior vena cava (**17**) on image D. This venous system, which developed at an early stage of embryological development of

the cardinal veins, is of immense importance when the vena cava becomes blocked for any reason (usually by a tumour). For example, in superior vena cava obstruction caused by mediastinal nodal enlargement secondary to carcinoma of the bronchus, the venous return from the head, neck and arms will go via collateral veins around the scapula and retrogradely in the intercostal veins into the azygos and thence back to the heart, bypassing the obstruction in the superior mediastinum.

127

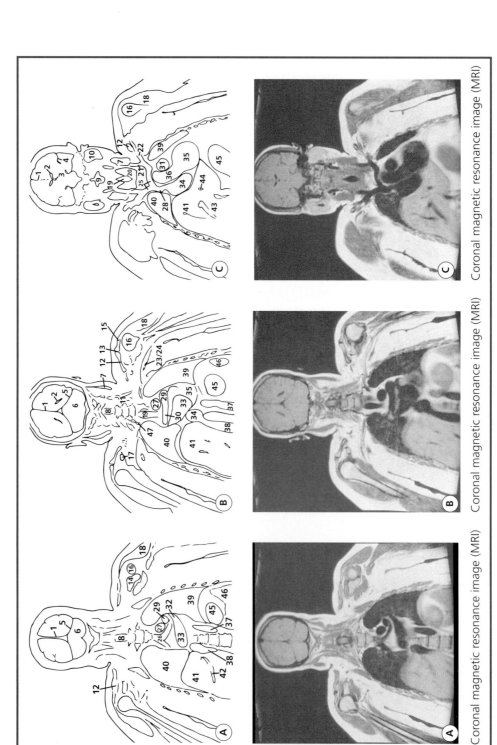

Coronal magnetic resonance image (MRI)

Coronal magnetic resonance image (MRI)

Coronal magnetic resonance image (MRI)

Section level

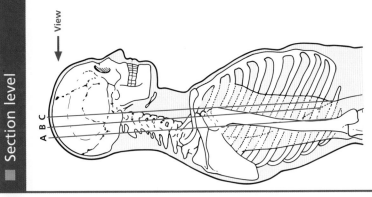

← View

A B C

Orientation

Superior

Left

Right

Inferior

1 Falx cerebri
2 Lateral ventricle
3 Third ventricle
4 Lateral sulcus (Sylvian fissure)
5 Tentorium cerebelli
6 Cerebellum
7 Sternocleidomastoid
8 Spinal cord
9 Second cervical vertebra (axis)
10 Parotid gland
11 Scalene muscles
12 Clavicle
13 Acromioclavicular joint
14 Glenoid fossa of scapula
15 Acromion process of scapula
16 Humeral head
17 Coracoid process of scapula
18 Deltoid
19 Trachea
20 Thyroid gland
21 Internal jugular vein
22 Subclavian vein
23 Axillary vessels
24 Brachial plexus and resulting nerves

25 Brachiocephalic vein
26 Carina (bifurcation of trachea into two main bronchi)
27 Aortic arch
28 Superior vena cava
29 Left pulmonary artery
30 Right pulmonary artery
31 Main pulmonary artery
32 Left superior pulmonary vein
33 Left atrium
34 Right atrium
35 Left ventricle
36 Ascending aorta
37 Descending aorta
38 Inferior vena cava
39 Left lung
40 Right lung
41 Liver
42 Right hepatic vein
43 Middle hepatic vein
44 Left hepatic vein
45 Stomach
46 Spleen
47 Vertebral artery

Notes

These three T1-weighted coronal magnetic resonance images are included to show the overall relations of the head, neck, thorax and upper abdomen. Only rarely would such a large field of view be used in clinical practice, as the anatomical spatial resolution is inevitably compromised. Of course, the exact relations on the coronal plane depend much on the degree of thoracic spine kyphosis, body habitus and degree of inspiration. The relations in this relatively obese subject are fairly representative.

A wide field of view is used when trying to compare structures on the two sides. The brachial plexus (image B, **24**) is a case in point. In breast cancer, the axilla may be affected both by nodal metastases and by the effects of radiotherapy. These can cause either neurological symptoms in the arm or lymphoedema. Coronal images of the two axillae together can be very helpful in this differentiation, which can be difficult on clinical grounds.

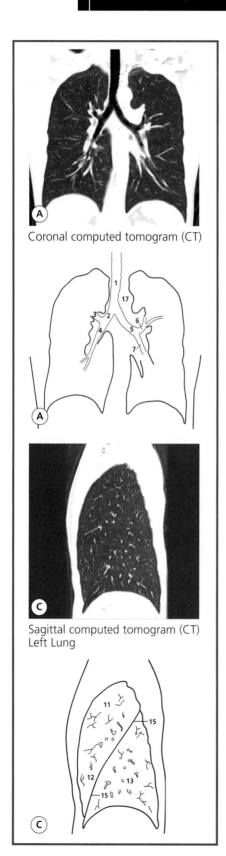

Coronal computed tomogram (CT)

Sagittal computed tomogram (CT)
Left Lung

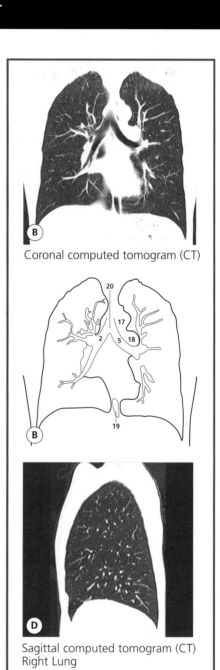

Coronal computed tomogram (CT)

Sagittal computed tomogram (CT)
Right Lung

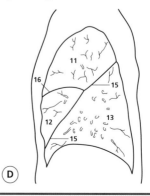

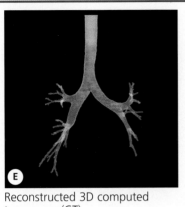

E

Reconstructed 3D computed
tomogram (CT)

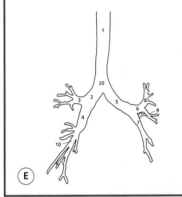

E

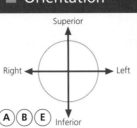

Orientation

Superior

Right ← → Left

(A)(B)(E) Inferior

Orientation

Superior

Anterior ← → Posterior

(C)(D) Inferior

1 Trachea	**12** Lingula (on the left)
2 Right main bronchus	**13** Lower lobe
3 Right upper lobe bronchus	**14** Middle lobe (on the right)
4 Bronchus intermedius	**15** Oblique fissure
5 Left main bronchus	**16** Horizontal fissure (on the
6 Left upper lobe/lingular	right)
bronchus	**17** Aortic knuckle
7 Left lower lobe bronchus	**18** Left pulmonary artery
8 Left upper lobe bronchus	**19** Oesophagus (containing
9 Left upper lobe lingular	some swallowed air)
bronchus	**20** Carina – the bifurcation of
10 Right lower lobe bronchus	the trachea
11 Upper lobe	

Notes

A spiral CT dataset of the chest at full inspiration has been obtained on a multidetector CT system. Next, the individual thin slices have been loaded together to form a three-dimensional volume with each voxel isometric so that the *x*, *y* and *z* resolutions of the resulting pixels are identical. This three-dimensional dataset can be analysed in a variety of ways.

The first two images show coronal multiplanar reconstructions viewed at lung settings to show the anatomy of the airways in this plane. The middle images shows sagittal reconstructions to demonstrate the lobes and fissures of the left and right lungs. The

lowest image is a three-dimensional reconstruction just extracting out the airways and accentuating the interface between air and soft tissue – this provides a graphic map of the anatomy of the trachea and main bronchi. These images elegantly show the more vertical nature of the right main bronchus (**2**) – hence the peanut and the endotracheal tube tend to enter the right side preferentially. They also show the greater length of the left main bronchus (**5**); on the right, the takeoff for the upper lobe bronchus can be very close to the carina (**20**, the point of bifurcation of the trachea into two main bronchi).

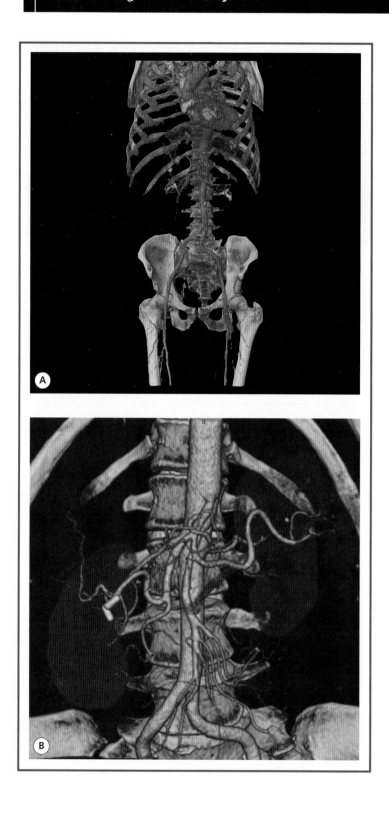

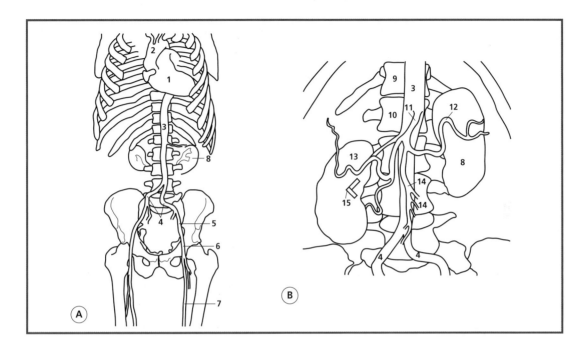

1 Heart	**9** Twelfth thoracic vertebra
2 Ascending aorta	**10** First lumbar vertebra
3 Abdominal aorta	**11** Coeliac artery
4 Common iliac artery	**12** Splenic artery
5 External iliac artery	**13** Hepatic artery
6 Common femoral artery	**14** Superior mesenteric artery
7 Superficial femoral artery	and arcade
8 Kidney and pelvicalyceal	**15** Cholecystectomy clips
system	

■ Orientation

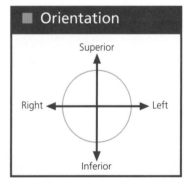

■ Notes

These two surface rendered 3D angiograms have been obtained on a modern CT system following the injection of standard iodinated contrast medium. The CT data were acquired during the aortic phase of the passage of contrast medium through the body and the images subsequently manipulated on the workstation.

On the left image the global view allows the relationship of the heart, aorta, iliac and femoral vessels to be appreciated in relation to the skeletal structures. A test dose of contrast medium has been given sometime before and this accounts for the dense iodine being excreted from the kidneys and pelvicalyceal system (**8**).

On the right image the patient has had a previous laproscopic cholecystectomy and the clips (**15**) can readily be identified as very dense structures overlying the right kidney and close to the hepatic artery (**13**). Note the way the aorta changes in calibre at the L1 level; it is smaller inferior to the coeliac artery, superior mensenteric artery and the two renal arteries. The superior mensenteric arcade is beautifully demonstrated (**14**). The tortuosity of the iliac vessels is normal in middle age and above. The renal and splenic parenchyma are only faintly seen in this early phase.

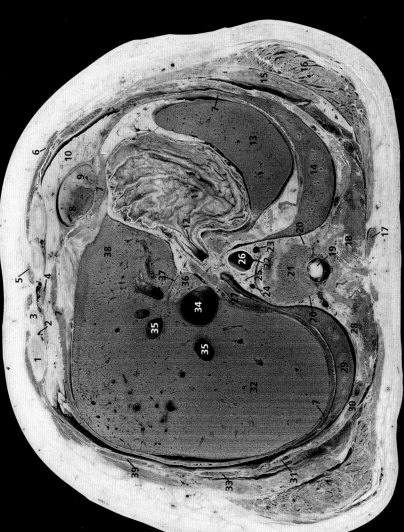

1 Sixth costal cartilage
2 Superior epigastric artery and vein
3 Seventh costal cartilage
4 Xiphoid
5 Rectus abdominis
6 External oblique
7 Diaphragm
8 Right ventricle

9 Left ventricle
10 Extrapericardial fat
11 Fundus of stomach
12 Oesophagogastric junction
13 Spleen
14 Lower lobe of left lung
15 Serratus anterior
16 Latissmus dorsi
17 Trapezius

18 Erector spinae
19 Spinal cord within dural sheath
20 Sympathetic chain
21 Body of tenth thoracic vertebra
22 Origin of intercostal artery
23 Hemiazygos vein
24 Azygos vein

25 Thoracic duct
26 Aorta
27 Right crus of diaphragm
28 Tenth rib
29 Lower lobe of right lung
30 Ninth rib
31 Eighth rib
32 Right lobe of liver
33 Seventh rib

34 Inferior vena cava
35 Hepatic vein
36 Caudate lobe of liver
37 Fissure for ligamentum venosum – lesser omentum
38 Left lobe of liver
39 Sixth rib
40 Oesophagus

Section level

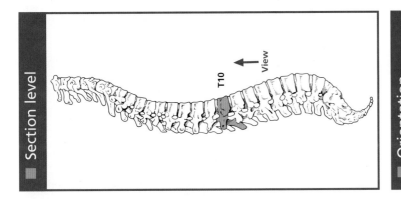

T10

View

Orientation

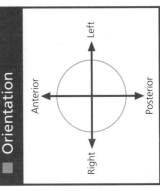

Anterior

Left

Right

Posterior

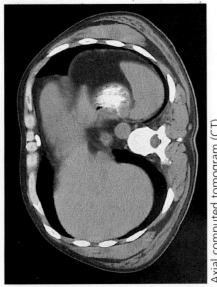

Axial computed tomogram (CT)

Notes

This section passes through the body of the tenth thoracic vertebra (**21**) and anteriorly transects the xiphoid (**4**).

The oesophagogastric junction (**12**) is seen in longitudinal section. This acts as a physiological sphincter in the prevention of reflux. The fundus of the stomach (**11**) contains air in the erect position but in the supine position is normally full of fluid. It is opaque in the CT image because of the ingested radio-opaque iodinated material.

The lesser omentum is the fold of peritoneum that extends to the liver from the lesser curvature of the stomach and the commencement of the duodenum. Superiorly it attaches to the porta hepatis and to the bottom of the fissure for the ligamentum venosum (**37**). At the cranial margin of this fissure, the lesser omentum reaches the diaphragm, where its two layers separate to surround the lower end of the oesophagus.

The ligamentum venosum is the thrombosed cord of the ductus venosus, which, in fetal life, connects the left portal vein to the anterior aspect of the inferior vena cava.

The spleen (**13**) lies against the diaphragm (**7**) opposite ribs 9 (**30**), 10 and 11. This section demonstrates clearly how a stab wound of the left lower chest posteriorly might traverse the pleural cavity, injure the lower lobe of the lung (**14**), traverse the diaphragm and lacerate the spleen. Similarly, a stab wound of the right chest at this level might injure the liver (**32**).

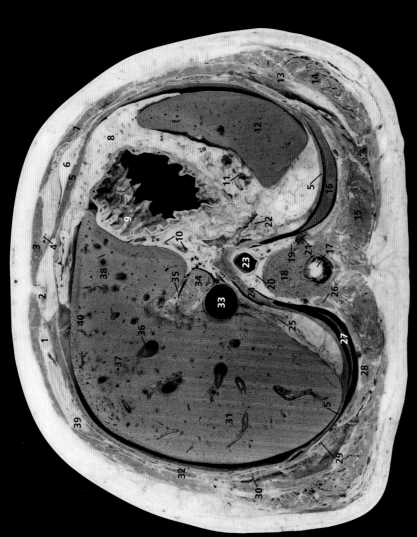

1 Seventh costal cartilage
2 Xiphoid
3 Rectus abdominis
4 Superior epigastric artery and vein
5 Diaphragm
6 Pericardial fat
7 External oblique
8 Greater omentum
9 Body of stomach
10 Left gastric artery branches

11 Splenic pedicle
12 Spleen
13 External oblique
14 Latissimus dorsi
15 Erector spinae
16 Lower lobe of left lung
17 Spinal cord within dural sheath
18 Body of eleventh thoracic vertebra
19 Intercostal artery

20 Thoracic duct
21 Intercostal vein
22 Left suprarenal gland
23 Aorta
24 Right crus of diaphragm
25 Right suprarenal gland
26 Head of eleventh rib
27 Lower lobe of right lung
28 Tenth rib
29 Ninth rib
30 Eighth rib

31 Right lobe of liver
32 Seventh rib
33 Inferior vena cava
34 Caudate lobe of liver
35 Lesser omentum in fissure for ligamentum venosum
36 Hepatic vein
37 Left lobe of liver medial segment
38 Left lobe of liver lateral segment

39 Sixth costal cartilage and rib
40 Falciform ligament
41 Portal vein
42 Pancreas
43 Left colic (splenic) flexure
44 Splenic vein
45 Left crus of diaphragm
46 Median arcuate ligament

Section level

T11

View

Orientation

Anterior — Left — Posterior — Right

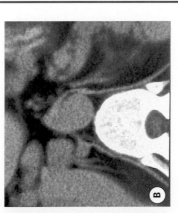

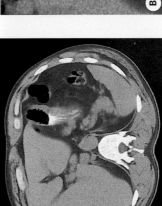

Axial computed tomograms (CTs)

Notes

This section passes through the body of the eleventh thoracic vertebra (**18**) and the xiphoid (**2**).

This is the most caudal section that transects intrathoracic viscera – note the pericardial fat (**6**) anteriorly and the lower lobe of the left lung (**16**).

The suprarenal glands (**22**, **25**) have a constant relationship to the diaphragmatic crura (**24**, **45**). Note on the CT images that the separate limbs of the suprarenal glands are demarcated.

The right crus of the diaphragm (**24**) on the CT image is often bulky. The crura change shape during respiration; normally they are bulkier on inspiration.

On the CT image, the pancreas (**42**) is just visible as it enters the plane of this section. It is seen better in more caudal sections. As the pancreas occupies only part of the section, its outlines are not demarcated sharply. This is another example of the 'partial volume' effect.

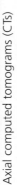

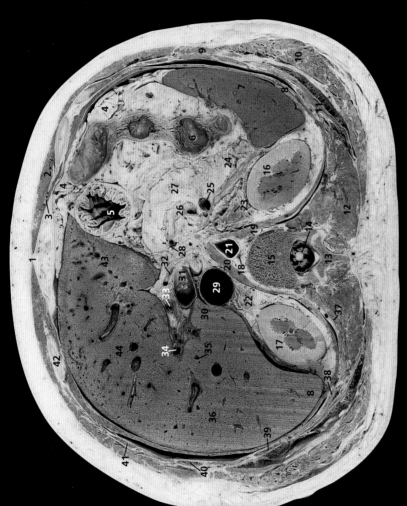

1 Linea alba
2 Rectus abdominis
3 Superior epigastric artery and vein
4 Greater omentum
5 Body of stomach
6 Left colic (splenic) flexure
7 Spleen
8 Diaphragm
9 External oblique
10 Latissimus dorsi

11 Serratus posterior inferior
12 Erector spinae
13 Spine of eleventh thoracic vertebra
14 Conus medullaris surrounded by cauda equina within dural sheath
15 Body of twelfth thoracic vertebra
16 Left kidney
17 Right kidney

18 Thoracic duct
19 Left crus of diaphragm
20 Right crus of diaphragm
21 Aorta
22 Right suprarenal gland
23 Left suprarenal gland
24 Tail of pancreas
25 Splenic vein
26 Splenic artery
27 Body of pancreas
28 Left gastric artery and vein

29 Inferior vena cava
30 Caudate lobe of liver
31 Portal vein
32 Hepatic artery
33 Common bile duct
34 Radicle of portal vein
35 Hepatic artery branch
36 Right lobe of liver
37 Twelfth rib
38 Eleventh rib
39 Tenth rib

40 Ninth rib
41 Eighth rib
42 Seventh costal cartilage
43 Left lobe of liver (lateral segment)
44 Left lobe of liver (medial segment)

45 Gall bladder
46 Ligamentum teres
47 Jejunum

Section level

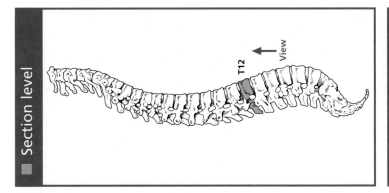

Orientation

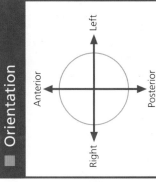

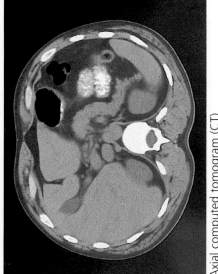

Axial computed tomogram (CT)

Notes

This section passes through the body of the twelfth thoracic vertebra (**15**). It demonstrates well the relationships of the structures at the porta hepatis – the common bile duct (**33**) anterior and to the right, the hepatic artery (**32**) anterior and to the left, and the portal vein (**31**) posterior to these structures. The inferior vena cava (**29**) lies immediately behind the portal vein; between the two is the epiploic foramen, or the aditus to the lesser sac (the foramen of Winslow). The division between the cortex (peripheral) and medulla (central) of the kidneys (**16, 17**) is shown well; in the plane of this division run the small arcuate vessels, which can just be identified in this section. Post-mortem changes account for the discrepancy in the differentiation between cortex and medulla in the left kidney.

Note on the lobes of the liver

The gross anatomical division of the liver is into right and left lobes, demarcated by the attachment of the falciform ligament on the anterior surface and by the fissures for the ligamentum teres and ligamentum venosum on its visceral surface. This is simply a gross anatomical descriptive term, with no morphological significance. Two subsidiary additional lobes are marked out on the visceral aspect of the liver – the quadrate lobe anteriorly, between the gall bladder fossa and the fissure for the ligamentum teres, and the caudate lobe posteriorly, between the groove for the inferior vena cava and the fissure for the ligamentum venosum. The transverse fissure for the porta hepatis separates the quadrate and caudate lobes. The distribution of the right and left branches of the hepatic artery and of the hepatic duct shows that the morphological division of the liver is into a right and left lobe demarcated by a plane that passes through the fossa of the gall bladder and the fossa of the inferior vena cava (the median plane of the liver). Morphologically, the quadrate lobe and the left half of the caudate lobe are part of the morphological left lobe of the liver. Further subdivision into hepatic segments is made by the Couinaud system (segments I–VIII).

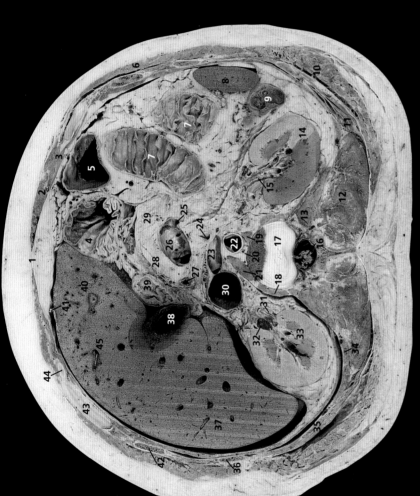

1 Linea alba
2 Rectus abdominis
3 Transversus abdominis
4 Stomach, body/antrum
5 Transverse colon
6 External oblique
7 Jejunum
8 Lower pole of spleen
9 Descending colon
10 Latissimus dorsi
11 Serratus posterior inferior
12 Erector spinae
13 Quadratus lumborum

14 Left kidney
15 Left renal vein (intrarenal portion); see also 23
16 Conus medullaris surrounded by cauda equina within dural sheath
17 Part of intervertebral disc between the twelfth thoracic and first lumbar vertebrae, with part of body of twelfth thoracic vertebra
18 Psoas major

19 Left crus of diaphragm
20 Thoracic duct
21 Right crus of diaphragm
22 Aorta
23 Left renal vein
24 Superior mesenteric artery
25 Splenic vein
26 Portal vein (commencement)
27 Common bile duct
28 Head of pancreas
29 Neck of pancreas
30 Inferior vena cava

31 Right renal artery
32 Right renal vein
33 Right kidney
34 Twelfth rib
35 Eleventh rib
36 Tenth rib
37 Right lobe of liver
38 Gall bladder
39 First part of duodenum (cap)
40 Left lobe of liver (lateral segment)
41 Falciform ligament

42 Ninth rib
43 Eighth costal cartilage
44 Ninth costal cartilage
45 Left lobe of liver (medial segment)
46 Right colic (hepatic) flexure

Section level

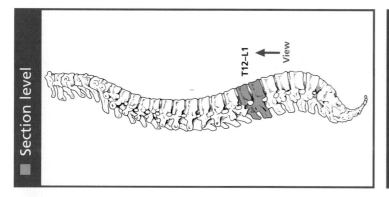

T12–L1

← View

Orientation

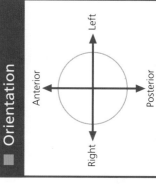

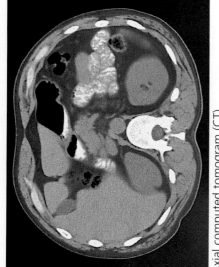

Axial computed tomogram (CT)

Notes

This section transects the intervertebral disc between the twelfth thoracic and the first lumbar vertebrae (**17**). The spinal cord tapers into the conus medullaris (**16**), which terminates, in this subject, at the level of the body of the first lumbar vertebra. The site of termination is variable, the range being from the disc between the twelfth thoracic and first lumbar vertebrae to the lower border of the second lumbar vertebra.

The plane of this section passes through the left renal vein (**23**) and demonstrates well the close relationship of this vein to the superior mesenteric artery (**24**), which passes forward from its aortic origin (**22**) immediately

superior to the vein. These features are demonstrated well on the CT image in Axial section 5. In exposure of the abdominal aorta (**22**), the surgeon can divide the left renal vein (**23**) in order to obtain additional access. The left kidney is not infarcted if this is done because the left renal vein receives the terminations of the left gonadal and left suprarenal veins, so that venous drainage of the left kidney can take place via collaterals from these vessels.

Note the circular folds of mucous membrane that project into the lumen of the small intestine transversely to its long axis (**7**). These are termed the *plicae circulares*. Radiologists and clinicians refer to these as *valvulae conniventes*.

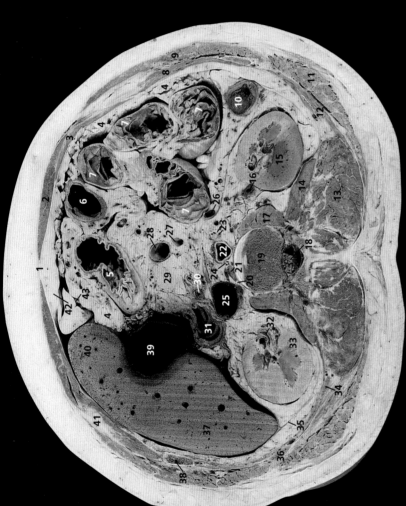

1 Linea alba
2 Rectus abdominis
3 Transversus abdominis
4 Greater omentum
5 Antrum of stomach
6 Transverse colon
7 Jejunum
8 Internal oblique
9 External oblique
10 Descending colon
11 Latissimus dorsi
12 Serratus posterior inferior

13 Erector spinae
14 Quadratus lumborum
15 Left kidney
16 Left ureter
17 Psoas major
18 Cauda equina within dural sheath
19 Body of first lumbar vertebra, with portion of intervertebral disc between the first and second lumbar vertebrae

20 Right sympathetic chain
21 Right crus of diaphragm
22 Aorta
23 Para-aortic lymph node
24 Cisterna chyli
25 Inferior vena cava
26 Inferior mesenteric vein
27 Superior mesenteric artery
28 Superior mesenteric vein
29 Head of pancreas
30 Common bile duct
31 Duodenum

32 Commencement of right ureter
33 Right kidney
34 Twelfth rib
35 Renal fascia
36 Eleventh rib
37 Right lobe of liver
38 Tenth rib
39 Gall bladder
40 Left lobe of liver (medial segment)
41 Ninth costal cartilage

42 Falciform ligament
43 Left lobe of liver (lateral segment)
44 Left renal vein
45 Renal cyst
46 Uncinate process pancreas

Section level

L1–2

View

Orientation

Anterior

Left

Posterior

Right

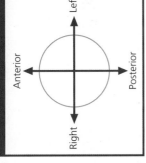

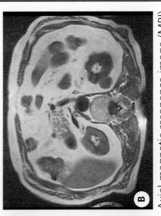

(A)

Axial computed tomogram (CT)

(B)

Axial magnetic resonance image (MRI)

Notes

This section passes through the body of the first lumbar vertebra (**19**), with a small portion of the intervertebral disc between the first and second lumbar vertebrae.

The kidneys (**15**, **33**) are embedded in a mass of fatty connective tissue termed the perirenal (perinephric) fat, which is thickest at their medial and lateral borders. The fibro-areolar tissue surrounding the kidney and perirenal fat condenses to form a sheath termed the renal fascia (**35**). At the lateral border of the kidney, the two layers of the renal fascia are fused. The anterior layer is carried medially anterior to the kidney and its vessels and merges with the connective tissue anterior to the aorta and inferior vena cava. The posterior layer extends medially in front of the fascia covering quadratus lumborum (**14**) and psoas major (**17**) and to the vertebrae and intervertebral discs. The perirenal fat and renal fascia (**35**) are surrounded by further retroperitoneal (pararenal) fatty connective tissue. The amount varies with the relative obesity of the subject.

In this section, a tiny portion of the lateral segment of the left lobe of the liver can be seen (**43**).

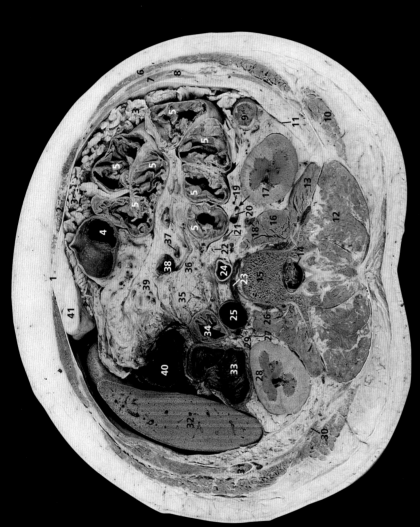

1 Linea alba
2 Rectus abdominis
3 Greater omentum
4 Transverse colon
5 Jejunum
6 External oblique
7 Internal oblique
8 Transversus abdominis
9 Descending colon
10 Latissimus dorsi
11 Renal fascia
12 Erector spinae

13 Quadratus lumborum
14 Cauda equina within dural
    sheath
15 Body of second lumbar
    vertebra
16 Psoas major
17 Left kidney
18 Left ureter
19 Left colic artery – ascending
    branch
20 Inferior mesenteric vein,
    with origin of left colic vein

    (arrowed)
21 Left testicular vein
22 Para-aortic lymph node
23 Left lumbar vein
24 Aorta
25 Inferior vena cava
26 Right lumbar vein
27 Right ureter
28 Right kidney
29 Right testicular vein
30 Twelfth rib
31 Eleventh rib

32 Right lobe of liver
33 Right colic (hepatic) flexure
34 Duodenum – second part
    (with ampulla marked with
    a white bristle)
35 Head of pancreas
36 Uncinate process of
    pancreas
37 Superior mesenteric artery
38 Superior mesenteric vein
39 Mesentery with mesenteric
    vessels

40 Gall bladder
41 Falciform ligament
42 Ascending colon
43 Right crus of diaphragm
44 Left renal vein
45 Left renal artery

Section level

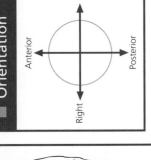

L2

View

Orientation

Anterior

Left

Posterior

Right

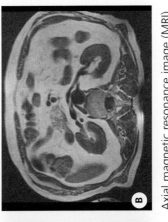

Axial computed tomogram (CT)

A

Axial magnetic resonance image (MRI)

B

Notes

This section passes through the body of the second lumbar vertebra (**15**). The plane of section passes through a prominent left lumbar vein (**23**) as it passes posterior to the aorta (**24**) to drain into the inferior vena cava (**25**). Occasionally, it may constitute the principal venous return from the left kidney, when it is termed a retro-aortic renal vein.

The right testicular vein (**29**) drains directly into the inferior vena cava, whereas the left testicular vein (**21**) (together with the left suprarenal vein) drains into the left renal vein.

This section passes through the second part of the duodenum (**34**). The orifice of the ampulla of Vater on its papilla is marked with a white bristle.

On both the section and the CT image, the uncinate process of the pancreas (**36**) is seen clearly. This lies posterior to the superior mesenteric artery (**37**) and vein (**38**) and is related closely to the entry point of the left renal vein (**44**) into the inferior vena cava (**25**).

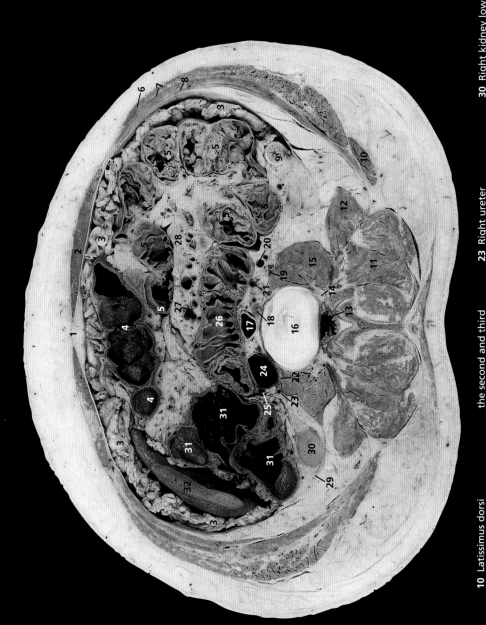

1 Linea alba
2 Rectus abdominis
3 Greater omentum
4 Transverse colon
5 Jejunum
6 External oblique
7 Internal oblique
8 Transversus abdominis
9 Descending colon

10 Latissimus dorsi
11 Erector spinae
12 Quadratus lumborum
13 Cauda equina within dural sheath
14 Root of second lumbar nerve
15 Psoas major
16 Intervertebral disc between the second and third lumbar vertebrae
17 Aorta
18 Para-aortic lymph node
19 Left ureter
20 Inferior mesenteric vein
21 Left testicular artery and vein
22 Right sympathetic chain

23 Right ureter
24 Inferior vena cava
25 Right testicular vein
26 Duodenum, third part
27 Superior mesenteric artery and vein
28 Mesentery with mesenteric vessels
29 Renal fascia

30 Right kidney lower pole
31 Ascending colon and right colic (hepatic) flexure
32 Right lobe liver

33 Ascending colon
34 Left kidney
35 Ileum

Section level

L2–3

← View

Orientation

Anterior

Left

Posterior

Right

Axial computed tomogram (CT)

Axial computed tomogram (CT)

■ Notes

This section passes through the intervertebral disc between the second and third lumbar vertebrae (16). It transects the most caudal part of the right lobe of the liver (32). The caudal extent of this lobe is variable and may project downwards in some subjects for a considerable distance as a broad tongue-like process (Riedel's lobe).

Note the third part of the duodenum (26) lying in the inverted V between the aorta (17) and the superior mesenteric vessels (27). Occasionally, this produces obstruction of the third part of the duodenum (duodenal ileus).

Seen clearly in this section are the three layers of muscles that constitute the lateral part of the anterior abdominal wall – the external oblique (6), internal oblique (7) and transversus abdominis (8). Medially, their aponeuroses form the sheath that surrounds the rectus abdominis (2). The anterior sheath comprises the aponeurosis of the external oblique together with the split anterior portion of the internal oblique; the posterior sheath is made up of the aponeurosis of the transversus abdominis reinforced by the posterior portion of the internal oblique. Below a line roughly halfway between the umbilicus and the pubis, the posterior sheath is deficient and all three aponeuroses pass in front of the rectus to form the anterior sheath. These muscles are demonstrated well on the CT image in Axial section 8.

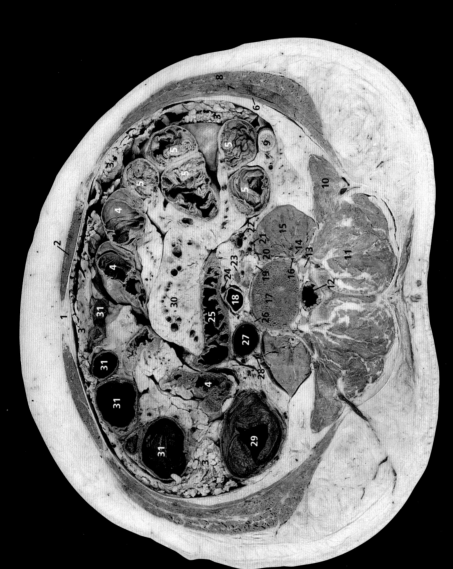

1 Linea alba
2 Rectus abdominis
3 Greater omentum
4 Ileum
5 Jejunum
6 Transversus abdominis
7 Internal oblique
8 External oblique
9 Descending colon

10 Quadratus lumborum
11 Erector spinae
12 Cauda equina within dural sheath
13 Dorsal root ganglion of third
   lumbar nerve
14 Ventral ramus of second lumbar
   nerve
15 Psoas major
16 Third lumbar artery

17 Body of third lumbar vertebra
18 Aorta
19 Left sympathetic chain
20 Left ureter
21 Left testicular artery and vein
22 Left colic artery and inferior
   mesenteric vein
23 Para-aortic lymph node
24 Inferior mesenteric artery

25 Duodenum, third part
26 Right sympathetic chain
27 Inferior vena cava
28 Right ureter
29 Ascending colon
30 Mesentery with mesenteric vessels
31 Transverse colon

Section level

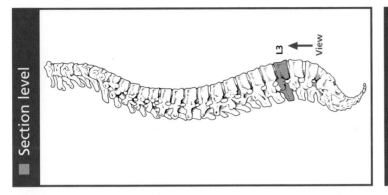

L3

View

Orientation

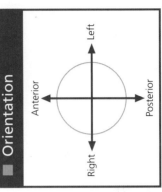

Left

Anterior

Posterior

Right

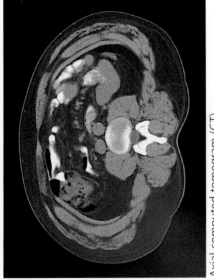

Axial computed tomogram (CT)

Notes

This section passes through the body of the third lumbar vertebra (**17**). This is just distal to the origin of the inferior mesenteric artery (**24**) from the anterior aspect of the aorta (**25**) posterior to the third part of the duodenum (**18**). This section is now caudal to the liver and the kidneys.

The ventral ramus of the second lumbar nerve (**14**) is seen in this section as it passes downwards and laterally into the psoas major (**15**). The first three lumbar nerves and the greater part of the fourth lumbar nerve form the lumbar plexus within the posterior part of the psoas major in front of the transverse processes of the lumbar vertebra.

The linea alba (**1**) is wide above the umbilicus and becomes quite narrow below this level (see page 164). This line marks the almost avascular blending of the rectus sheaths on either side and gives the surgeon rapid access to the abdominal cavity. The incision can, if necessary, be extended from the xiphoid to the pubic symphysis. The falciform ligament (see page 152) lies to the right-hand side of the incision.

Note the marked disparity between the patulous ascending colon (**29**) and the thick-walled, narrow descending colon (**9**).

149

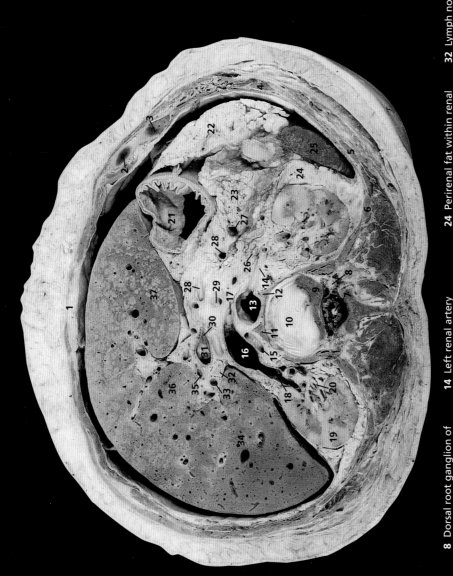

1 Linea alba
2 Eighth costal cartilage
3 Ninth rib/costal cartilage junction
4 Tenth rib
5 Eleventh rib
6 Twelfth rib
7 Cauda equina and termination of spinal cord within dural sheath

8 Dorsal root ganglion of first lumbar nerve
9 Part of body of first lumbar vertebra
10 Part of intervertebral disc between the first and second lumbar vertebrae
11 Right crus of diaphragm
12 Left crus of diaphragm
13 Aorta

14 Left renal artery
15 Right renal artery
16 Inferior vena cava
17 Left renal vein
18 Right renal vein
19 Kidney
20 Right ureter
21 Body of stomach
22 Greater omentum
23 Tail of pancreas

24 Perirenal fat within renal fascia
25 Spleen
26 Left suprarenal gland
27 Splenic vein
28 Splenic artery
29 Superior mesenteric artery
30 Termination of splenic vein
31 Commencement of portal vein

32 Lymph node in porta hepatis
33 Hepatic artery
34 Right lobe of liver
35 Common bile duct
36 Quadrate lobe of medial segment of left lobe of liver
37 Left lobe of liver, lateral segment

Section level

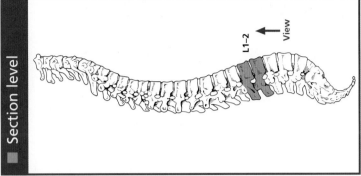

L1–2

← View

Orientation

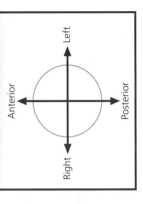

Left

Anterior

Posterior

Right

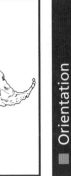

Axial computed tomogram (CT)

Notes

Axial sections 1 and 2 through the female abdomen should be compared with the male abdominal sections. There are wide individual variations in both the sexes, but a comparison of the 'typical' male and female abdomens reveals a greater accumulation of subcutaneous fat in the female in contrast to a higher proportion of intraperitoneal fat in the male subject.

This section passes through the intervertebral disc between the first and second lumbar vertebrae. This section shows well the quadrate lobe of the liver (**36**). Although the common bile duct (**35**) is usually the most anterolateral structure in the free (right) edge of the lesser omentum, variations are common. In this elderly female, the hepatic artery (**33**) is tortuous and thus is unusually

lateral. Anomalies of the hepatic artery are common. In 12 per cent of cases, the right hepatic artery derives from the superior mesenteric artery. The left hepatic artery or an accessory hepatic artery may originate from the left gastric, splenic or superior mesenteric artery. Occasionally, one or other of these vessels derives directly from the aorta.

Note the caudal tip of the left suprarenal gland (**26**), which may extend down to the left renal vein.

This section demonstrates the fascial layers that enclose the kidney (**19**). The kidney itself is enclosed in its renal capsule, which is readily stripped from the healthy organ. Surrounding this is the perirenal fat, contained within the renal fascia (**24**). A closed rupture of the kidney is usually contained and tamponaded by this fascial sheath.

151

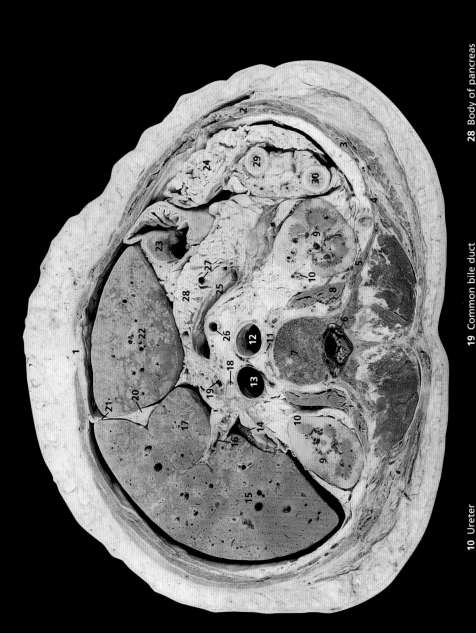

1 Linea alba
2 Tenth rib
3 Eleventh rib
4 Twelfth rib
5 Quadratus lumborum
6 Cauda equina within dural sheath
7 Body of second lumbar vertebra
8 Psoas major
9 Kidney

10 Ureter
11 Cisterna chyli
12 Aorta
13 Inferior vena cava
14 Caudate lobe of liver
15 Right lobe of liver
16 Neck of gall bladder
17 Left lobe of liver (medial segment)
18 Lymph node in porta hepatis

19 Common bile duct
20 Ligamentum teres
21 Falciform ligament
22 Left lobe of liver (lateral segment)
23 Body of stomach
24 Greater omentum
25 Splenic vein
26 Superior mesenteric artery
27 Splenic artery

28 Body of pancreas
29 Transverse colon
30 Descending colon

31 Spleen
32 Right suprarenal gland

Section level

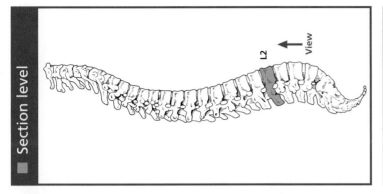

Orientation

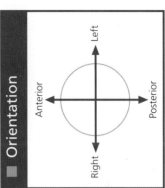

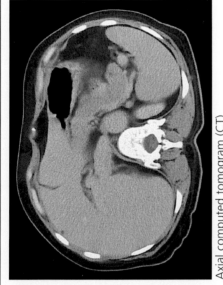

Axial computed tomogram (CT)

Notes

This section lies just caudal to the left colic (splenic) flexure, which joins the transverse colon (**29**) to the descending colon (**30**).

The tip of the papillary process of the caudate lobe of the liver (**14**) can be seen as a separate structure in the gap medial to the right lobe of the liver. The ligamentum teres (**20**) is the fibrotic remnant of the obliterated left umbilical vein. The falciform ligament divides the morphological left lobe of the liver into a lateral segment (**22**) and a medial

segment (**17**). The visceral aspect of this, between the falciform ligament and the gall-bladder bed (**16**), forms the anatomical quadrate lobe.

Although the left extremity of the transverse colon (**29**) and the upper extremity of the descending colon (**30**) are seen at this level, which is immediately inferior to the splenic flexure, this is above the level of the hepatic flexure of the right colon, which is displaced downwards by the right lobe of the liver.

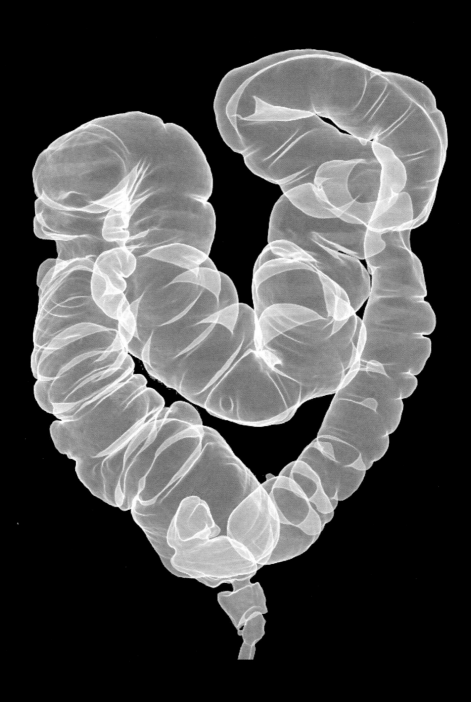

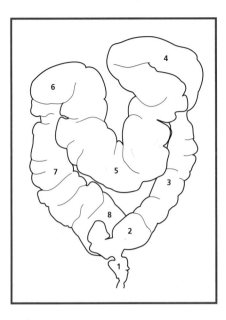

1   Tube in distal rectum
2   Sigmoid colon
3   Descending colon
4   Splenic flexure
5   Transverse colon
6   Hepatic flexure
7   Ascending colon
8   Caecum

◼ Orientation

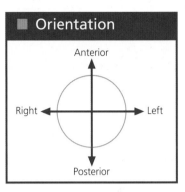

◼ Notes

This CT colonogram was obtained in the following way. First, the large bowel was cleaned by the oral administration of a standard purgative. The bowel was then distended by air via a small tube inserted by rectum. The wall of the bowel was enhanced by the use of a standard iodinated contrast agent administered intravenously. A spiral CT dataset was obtained on a multidetector CT system. Next, the individual thin slices were loaded together to form a three-dimensional volume, with each voxel isometric so that the x, y and z resolution of the resulting pixels was identical. This three-dimensional dataset can be analysed in a variety of ways – many people find software-generated virtual colonoscopy images helpful, where colour-rendered images allow a 'fly-through' approach that simulates what the endoscopist sees at standard colonoscopy. Others find standard multiplanar two-dimensional reconstructions helpful. For all such viewing, a roadmap of the whole colon is a valuable tool for orientation – hence this reconstructed image, which looks uncannily like the double-contrast barium enema of old.

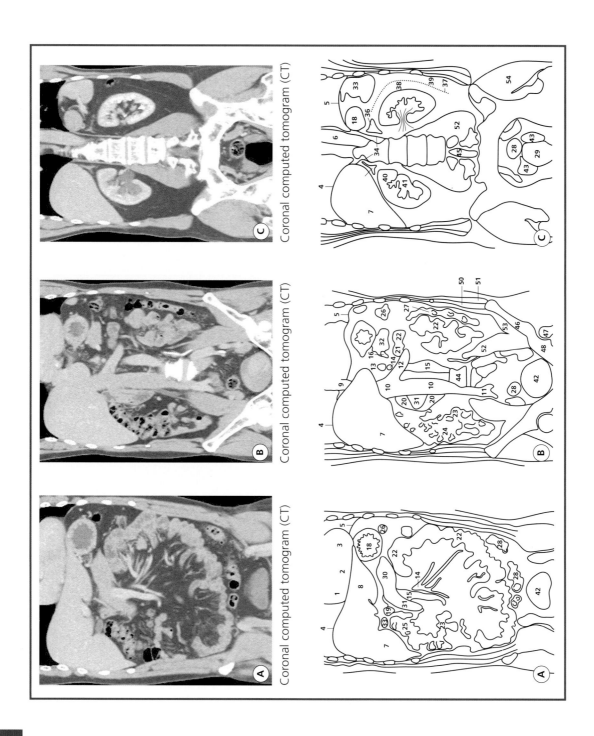

Coronal computed tomogram (CT)

Coronal computed tomogram (CT)

Coronal computed tomogram (CT)

Section level

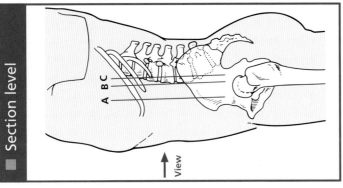

A B C

View

Orientation

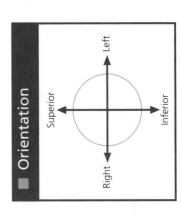

Left

Superior

Right

Inferior

1 Right atrium
2 Right ventricle
3 Left ventricle
4 Diaphragm (right side)
5 Diaphragm (left side)
6 Ascending aorta
7 Right lobe of liver
8 Left lobe of liver
9 Inferior vena cava – suprahepatic
10 Inferior vena cava – infrahepatic
11 Confluence of common iliac veins
12 Left renal vein
13 Coeliac trunk – hepatic, left gastric and splenic arteries
14 Superior mesenteric artery
15 Abdominal aorta
16 Splenic vein
17 Superior mesenteric vein
18 Fundus of stomach
19 Duodenum – cap (also known as D1)
20 Duodenum – second part (also known as D2)
21 Duodenum – fourth part (also known as D4) joining:
22 Jejunum
23 Ileum
24 Colon – ascending part
25 Colon – hepatic flexure
26 Colon – splenic flexure
27 Colon – descending part
28 Sigmoid colon
29 Rectum
30 Body of pancreas
31 Head of pancreas
32 Tail of pancreas
33 Gall bladder
34 Left and right crus of diaphragm
35 Right suprarenal (adrenal) gland
36 Left suprarenal (adrenal) gland
37 Renal (Gerota) fascia
38 Perirenal space
39 Pararenal space
40 Kidney
41 Renal pelvis (distended on right)
42 Bladder (urinary)
43 Seminal vesicle
44 Body of third lumbar vertebra
45 Thecal sac containing cauda equina
46 Ilium (and iliac crest)
47 Head of femur
48 Acetabulum
49 Transversus abdominis
50 Internal oblique
51 External oblique
52 Psoas major
53 Iliacus
54 Gluteus maximus

Notes

A spiral CT dataset of the abdomen was obtained on a multidetector CT system. The individual thin slices were loaded together to form a three-dimensional volume, with each voxel isometric, so that the x, y and z resolution of the resulting pixels is identical. This three-dimensional dataset can be analysed in a variety of ways – here in coronal multiplanar two-dimensional reformats.

Now that CT of the abdomen has become such a standard investigation for a wide range of abdominal conditions, the radiologist has to scroll through hundreds of axial images on a monitor. Some lesions are depicted better on coronal rather than axial images (e.g. asymmetry of the pelvicalyceal systems in the two kidneys in this case). To non-radiologists, such coronal views are a more intuitive method of looking at the abdomen than the source axial images.

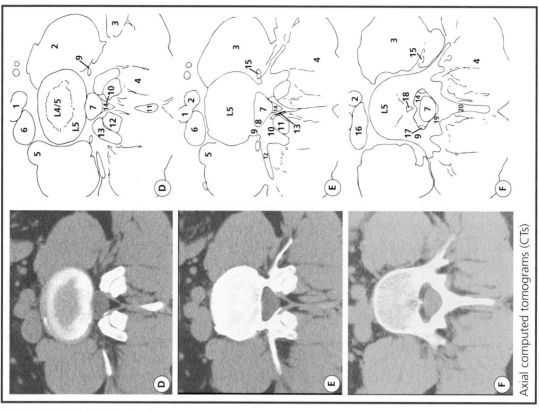

Axial computed tomograms (CTs)

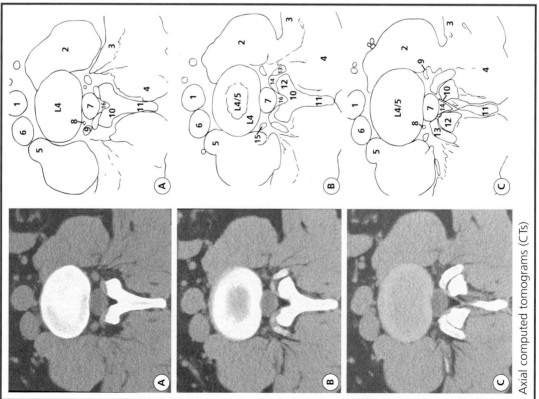

Axial computed tomograms (CTs)

Section level

Orientation

Images A–B

1 Aorta
2 Psoas major
3 Quadratus lumborum
4 Erector spinae
5 Psoas minor
6 Inferior vena cava
7 Dural sheath
8 Epidural vein
9 Dorsal root ganglion L4 in foramen between L4 and L5
10 Lamina L4
11 Spinous process L4
12 Inferior facet L4
13 Superior facet L5
14 Capsule L4/L5 facet joint
15 L4 nerve
16 Epidural fat

Images C–D

1 Aortic bifurcation
2 Psoas major
3 Quadratus lumborum
4 Erector spinae
5 Psoas minor
6 Inferior vena cava
7 Dural sheath
8 Epidural vein
9 Ventral ramus L4
10 Flaval ligament
11 Spinous process L4
12 Inferior facet L4
13 Superior facet L5
14 Epidural fat

Images E–F

1 Right common iliac artery
2 Left common iliac artery
3 Psoas major
4 Erector spinae
5 Psoas minor
6 Inferior vena cava
7 Dural sheath
8 Pouch for L5 root
9 Pedicle L5
10 Superior facet L5
11 Inferior facet L4
12 Transverse process of L5
13 Flaval ligament
14 Epidural fat
15 Ventral ramus L4
16 Confluence of common iliac veins
17 L5 nerve root sheath
18 Basi-vertebral vein
19 Lamina L5
20 Spinous process L5

Notes

This series of six computed tomograms (A–F) demonstrates the key anatomical features of a segment of the lumbar spine. Although all the features can also be demonstrated by magnetic resonance imaging (MRI), which is now the preferred test, computed tomography (CT) is perhaps easier to understand: bone appears white, soft tissues appear grey and fat appears black.

Images A–B

Image a traverses the slightly sclerotic endplate of L4. The dorsal root ganglion (**9**) lies in the foramen, immediately caudal to the L4 pedicle. Note how the dorsal root ganglion is demarcated clearly by normal epidural fat.

Images C–D

Image C traverses the L4/L5 disc. Note that the posterior aspect of the disc is concave with respect to the dural sheath (**7**). A normal disc at this anatomical level has either a concave or flat interface with the sheath. A convex disc here is indicative of an annular bulge. Note how the L4 ventral ramus (**9**) is now heading towards the psoas muscle

in which the lumbar plexus is formed. The dorsal ramus is too small to be resolved by CT; it would pass just lateral to the superior facet of L5.

Image D shows a portion of the L5 endplate surrounding the inferior aspect of the L4/L5 disc.

Images E–F

Image E transects the sclerotic endplate of L5. The flaval ligaments (**13**) running from the L4 to L5 laminae are shown well. Surgeons often operate through small openings in the flaval ligaments without the full laminectomy that used to be the standard approach for spinal surgery.

Image F passes through the body of the L5 vertebra – the normal bony architecture can be appreciated. The veins running through the body converge on the basi-vertebral vein (**18**), which has a small bony hood guarding its passage so that venous blood passes to the epidural veins (see **8** in image C). The right L5 root sheath (**17**) hugs the medial aspect of the pedicle (**9**).

Coronal magnetic resonance image (MRI)

Coronal magnetic resonance image (MRI)

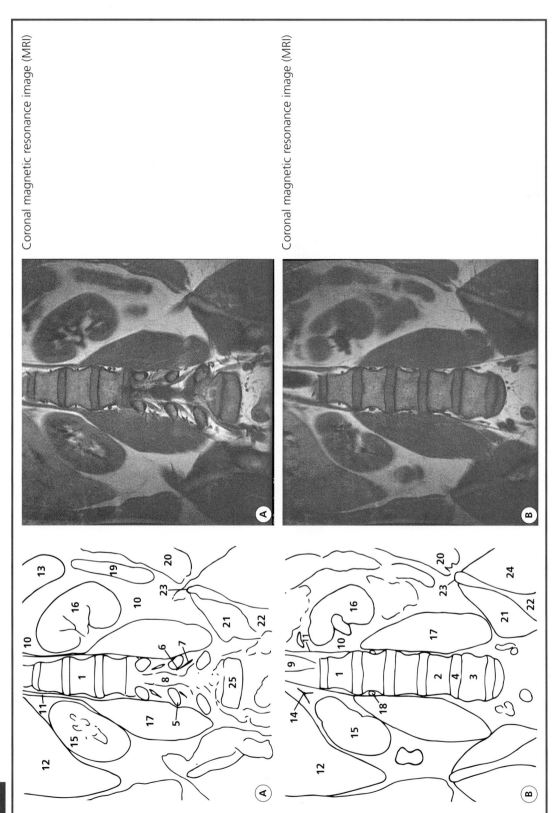

Section level

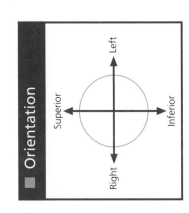

Orientation

Left

Superior

Right

Inferior

1 L1 vertebral body	8 Thecal sac
2 L4 vertebral body	9 Aorta
3 L5 vertebral body	10 Retroperitoneal fat
4 L4/L5 intervertebral disc	11 Crus of diaphragm
5 Pedicle	12 Liver
6 Nerve root sheath L4	13 Spleen
7 Dorsal root ganglion L4	14 Right adrenal gland

15 Right kidney	21 Iliacus
16 Left kidney	22 Ilium
17 Psoas	23 Iliac crest
18 Lumbar vein	24 Gluteal muscles
19 Descending colon	25 S1 vertebral body
20 Anterior abdominal-wall musculature	

Notes

Two coronal T1-weighted images elegantly show the relationship of the lumbar spine to the psoas muscles and kidneys (within retroperitoneal fat). Note that the kidneys lie in an oblique orientation, aligned to the lateral margins of the psoas muscles; thus, the upper poles lie in a more medial sagittal plane than the lower poles. Because of the lumbar lordosis, the upper poles lie in a more posterior coronal plane than the lower poles.

Because of the lumbar lordosis, the thecal sac and emerging nerve root sheaths can be seen in the L4 region, while vertebral bodies are demonstrated more superiorly and inferiorly. Note the way in which each nerve root sheath hugs the medial and inferior aspects of its associated pedicle (L4 root inferomedial to the L4 pedicle). The expansion for the dorsal root ganglion can just be appreciated. The fairly constant relationship of the L4/L5 disc space with the level of the superior iliac crest is shown

well; this is particularly useful in patients with lumbosacral anomalies (around 25 per cent of people).

Also apparent are the segmental lumbar veins, which drain blood from the epidural veins. These run anteriorly within a narrow, but important, fat plane alongside each vertebral body.

The psoas muscles (**17**) are particularly prominent in this individual. The superior attachment to the lateral aspects of the disc at the thoracolumbar junction is seen well. One can appreciate how a disc-space infection (often tuberculous) at this level could track inferiorly in and around the psoas muscle down to the iliacus and eventually present as a cold abscess in the inguinal region. The close relation of the adrenal to the right crus of the diaphragm (labelled **11** on the left) is apparent. The adrenal gland originates at this site, while the kidneys 'ascended' by differential growth during fetal life.

Sagittal T2-weighted magnetic resonance image (MRI)

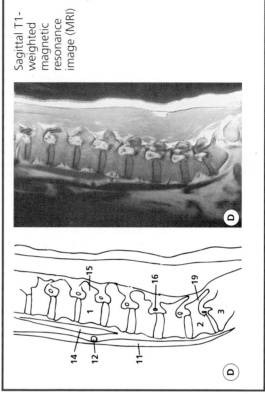

Sagittal T1-weighted magnetic resonance image (MRI)

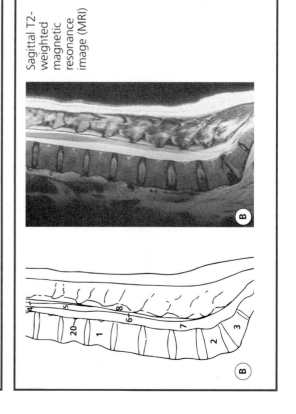

Sagittal T1-weighted magnetic resonance image (MRI)

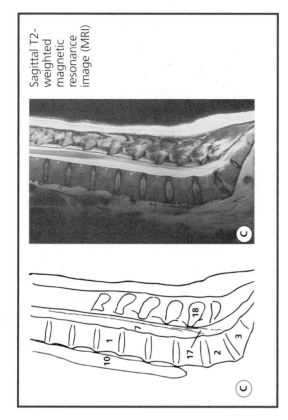

Sagittal T2-weighted magnetic resonance image (MRI)

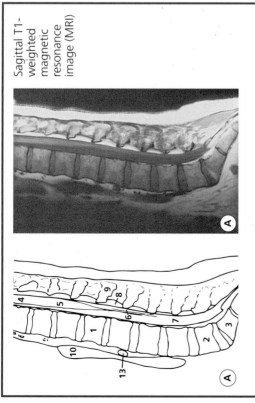

■ Section level

■ Orientation

1 L1 vertebral body	7 Cerebrospinal	11 Inferior vena cava	vertebra	18 Spinous process L4
2 L5 vertebral body	fluid within thecal	12 Right renal artery	16 L3 nerve root	19 Pars
3 S1 vertebral body	sac	13 Retro-aortic left	sheath/dorsal root	interarticularis L5
4 Spinal cord	8 Epidural fat	renal vein	ganglion	20 Basi-vertebral vein
5 Conus medullaris	9 Spinous process L1	14 Crus of diaphragm	17 Nerve roots within	
6 Cauda equina	10 Aorta	15 Pedicle of L1	cerebrospinal fluid	

■ Notes

Images A–B

These midline sagittal magnetic resonance images are of key importance in evaluating the lumbar spine (one of the commonest anatomical sites examined by MRI).

The anteroposterior diameter of the spinal canal can be assessed readily. This normally measures around 15 mm from the posterior aspect of the vertebral body to the anterior aspect of the laminar arch; values under 11.5 mm indicate a degree of spinal stenosis. The height of the disc spaces can be evaluated, as can the degree of hydration within. The normal disc space yields high signal intensity on T2 weighting (image B); a degenerate disc returns low signal intensity, and becomes narrower. In these images, the L5/S1 is slightly degenerate, as judged by the slight reduction of signal. There is a slight increase in fat content in the superior portion of S1 vertebral body, suggesting a longstanding disc abnormality.

These sagittal images also demonstrate clearly the slight expansion of the distal cord at the T12/L1 level (the conus medullaris). The collection of nerve roots that forms the cauda equina ('horse's tail') is seen well posteriorly within the canal when the patient lies supine (as during MRI). Because normal roots move freely within the cerebrospinal fluid, lumbar puncture is generally a very safe procedure at any level caudal to the conus medullaris.

Image C

A T2-weighted magnetic resonance image about 10 mm to the left of the median sagittal plane shown in the images A and B. Here, the segmental roots can be seen traversing the cerebrospinal fluid towards their respective nerve root sheaths and exit foramina. The aorta can just be seen anterior to the vertebral bodies.

Image D

A T1-weighted sagittal magnetic resonance image even more lateral than in image C. This is to the right of the midline, however, as the right renal artery can be seen passing anterior to the diaphragmatic crus and posterior to the inferior vena cava. This plane shows the exit foramina at several segmental levels. The classical shape has been said to resemble that of the human ear. The pedicles of two adjacent vertebral bodies form the superior and inferior boundaries of the foramen. The anterior margin is formed by the vertebral body superiorly and the posterolateral portion of the intervertebral disk inferiorly. Posteriorly lie the pars interarticularis, the flaval ligament and the facet joint. Narrowing of the disc space and degenerative changes in the facet joints will reduce the capacity of the foramen, and the flaval ligament gets thicker as the disc space narrows; all of these changes can contribute to nerve-root compression.

The nerve root sheaths, dorsal root ganglion and segmental nerve lie in the superior portion of the foramen. There are commonly two epidural veins in each foramen – a superior vein between the nerve root and the body/pedicle, and a second vein that usually lies much more caudally within the foramen. Remember that in the lumbar (and thoracic and sacral) spine, the segmental nerve root escapes caudal to its numbered vertebral body. For example, the L5 nerve root escapes caudal to the L5 pedicle through the L5/S1 foramen. Although the L5 root can be affected by a lateral L5/S1 disc herniation or facet joint degeneration, much more commonly it will be affected by a more central herniation at the L4/L5 level.

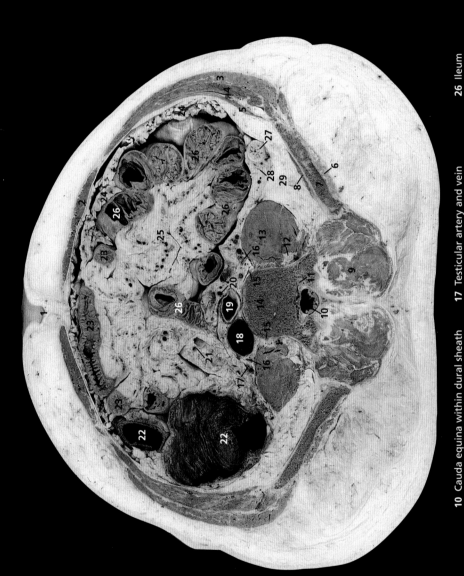

1 Umbilicus
2 Rectus abdominis
3 External oblique
4 Internal oblique
5 Transversus abdominis
6 Gluteus medius
7 Ilium
8 Iliacus
9 Erector spinae

10 Cauda equina within dural sheath
11 Dorsal root ganglion of fourth
    lumbar nerve
12 Ventral ramus of third lumbar
    nerve
13 Psoas major
14 Body of fourth lumbar vertebra
15 Lumbar sympathetic chain
16 Ureter

17 Testicular artery and vein
18 Inferior vena cava
19 Aorta
20 Inferior mesenteric artery and vein
21 Right colic artery and vein
22 Ascending colon
23 Jejunum
24 Greater omentum
25 Mesentery of small intestine

26 Ileum
27 Descending colon
28 Anterior pararenal fat of
    retroperitoneum
29 Posterior pararenal fat of
    retroperitoneum

30 Appendix vermiformis

Section level

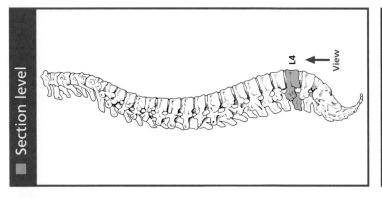

L4

← View

Orientation

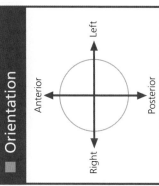

Left

Anterior

Posterior

Right

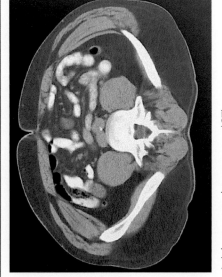

Axial computed tomogram (CT)

Notes

This section passes through the body of the fourth lumbar vertebra (**14**), the cranial portion of the iliac crests (**7**) and the umbilicus (**1**). There are wide individual variations in these landmarks, but the umbilicus is usually around the level of L4.

The inferior mesenteric artery (**20**) has just arisen from the aorta at the level of the third lumbar vertebra. More caudally, it will give rise to the superior rectal artery (see

Axial section 2, **24**). The accompanying inferior mesenteric vein (**20**) has a long ascending retroperitoneal course to enter the splenic vein.

The aorta (**19**) is commencing to bifurcate on both the section and the CT image. This level of bifurcation, anterior to the fourth lumbar vertebra, is surprisingly constant, even in subjects with gross arteriosclerosis or with aneurysmal dilation of the aorta.

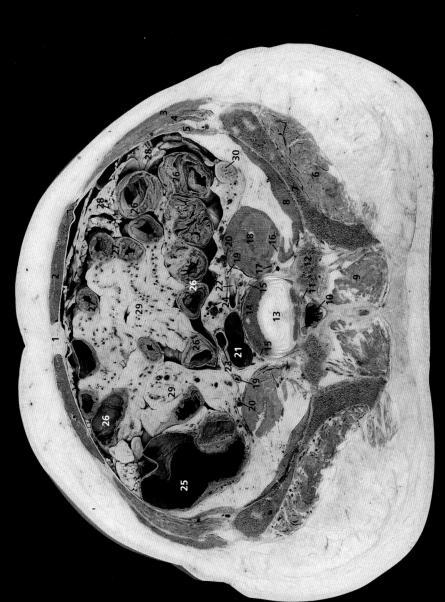

1 Linea alba
2 Rectus abdominis
3 External oblique
4 Internal oblique
5 Transversus abdominis
6 Gluteus medius
7 Ilium
8 Iliacus
9 Erector spinae

10 Cauda equina within dural sheath
11 Root of fifth lumbar nerve
12 Transverse process of fifth lumbar vertebra
13 Part of intervertebral disc between fourth and fifth lumbar vertebrae
14 Part of body of fourth lumbar vertebra
15 Lumbar sympathetic chain

16 Femoral nerve
17 Obturator nerve
18 Psoas major
19 Ureter
20 Testicular artery and vein
21 Inferior vena cava at origin
22 Left common iliac artery
23 Right common iliac artery
24 Superior rectal artery and vein

25 Ascending colon
26 Ileum
27 Jejunum
28 Greater omentum
29 Mesentery of small bowel
30 Descending colon

31 Appendix vermiformis

Section level

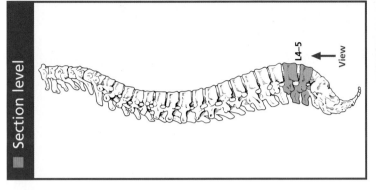

L4–5

← View

Orientation

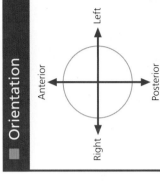

Left

Anterior — Posterior

Right

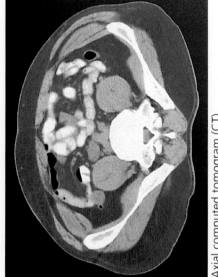

Axial computed tomogram (CT)

Notes

This section transects the intervertebral disc between the fourth and fifth lumbar vertebrae (**13**). The lumbar sympathetic chain (**15**) is visualized well as it lies on the fourth lumbar vertebral body (**14**); it is overlapped on the right by the inferior vena cava (**21**) and on the left by the common iliac artery (**22**). More cranially, it lies just lateral to the aorta.

The transverse processes of the fifth lumbar vertebra (**12**) are bulky and all but reach the sacrum, particularly (in this subject) on the left side. Reference to Axial section 3 shows partial sacralization of L5, a very common variation.

The superior rectal artery (**24**) is the continuation of the inferior mesenteric artery after this has given off its left colic branch (see Axial section 1).

The inferior vena cava (**21**) is seen at its commencement. Its oval shape in the section (more markedly oval in the CT image) is produced by the convergence of the two common iliac veins at this level.

The intervertebral discs (**13**) account for nearly 25 per cent of the total length of the spinal column. They are composed at their circumference of laminae of fibrous tissue, forming the annulus fibrosus. At their centre is the soft, pulpy, highly elastic nucleus pulposus, which is especially prominent in the lumbar region. This is considered to represent the remains of the fetal notochord. With increasing age, the nucleus becomes progressively less differentiated from the annulus and is gradually replaced with fibrocartilage.

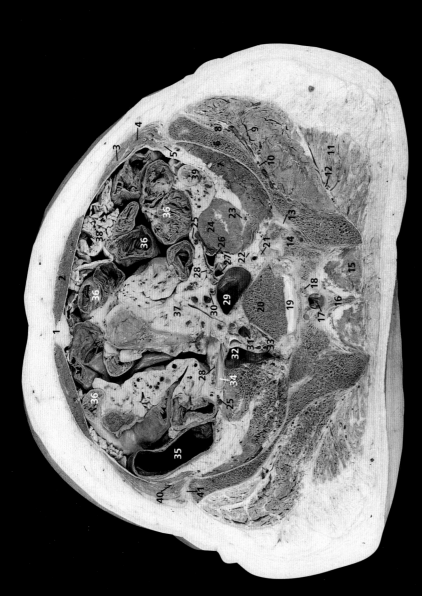

1 Linea alba
2 Rectus abdominis
3 External oblique
4 Internal oblique
5 Transversus abdominis
6 Ilium
7 Iliacus
8 Gluteus minimus
9 Gluteus medius
10 Superior gluteal artery vein and nerve

11 Gluteus maximus
12 Inferior gluteal artery vein and nerve
13 Sacroiliac joint
14 Lateral mass of sacrum
15 Erector spinae
16 Spine of first segment of sacrum
17 Cauda equina within dural sheath
18 Root of first sacral nerve

19 Part of lumbosacral disc
20 Part of body of fifth lumbar vertebra
21 Ventral ramus of fifth lumbar nerve
22 Obturator nerve
23 Femoral nerve
24 Psoas major
25 Testicular artery and vein
26 Left external iliac artery
27 Left internal iliac artery

28 Ureter
29 Left common iliac vein
30 Superior rectal artery and vein
31 Superior gluteal artery and vein within pelvis
32 Right common iliac vein
33 Right internal iliac vein
34 Right common iliac artery at bifurcation
35 Ascending colon

36 Ileum
37 Mesentery of small bowel
38 Greater omentum
39 Descending colon
40 Iliohypogastric nerve
41 Ilioinguinal nerve, with deep circumflex iliac artery and vein

42 Left external iliac vein
43 Left internal iliac vein

Section level

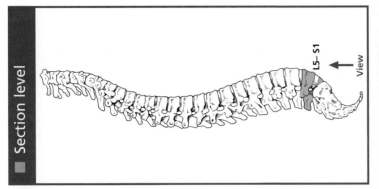

L5– S1

View

Orientation

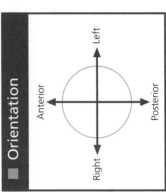

Left

Anterior

Posterior

Right

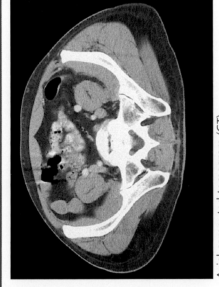

Axial computed tomogram (CT)

Notes

This section traverses the sacroiliac joint (**13**), the lumbosacral disc (**19**) and a lower part of the body of the fifth lumbar vertebra (**20**). There is some asymmetry of the lateral mass of the sacrum (**14**) in this subject, the left side being larger. This is because there is a small articulation (just visible) between the left sacral mass and the sacralized left L5 transverse process (see also Axial section 2). These variations are very common.

An intravenous injection of contrast medium was given before the CT image series, hence the opacification of the blood vessels.

The superior gluteal vessels (**31**) arise from the internal iliac vessels. Together with the superior gluteal nerve (**10**), they emerge from the pelvis through the greater sciatic foramen above piriformis and then run between and supply gluteus medius (**9**) and gluteus minimus (**8**). The inferior gluteal artery, vein and nerve (**12**) emerge below piriformis and supply gluteus maximus (**11**).

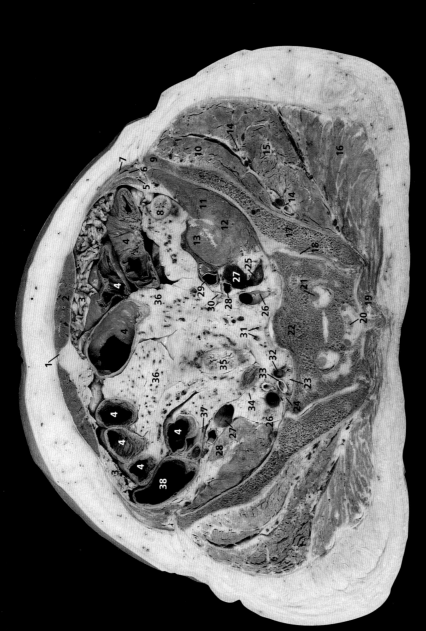

1 Linea alba
2 Rectus abdominis
3 Greater omentum
4 Ileum
5 Transversus abdominis
6 Internal oblique
7 External oblique aponeurosis
8 Descending colon
9 Anterior superior iliac spine
10 Gluteus minimus

11 Iliacus
12 Femoral nerve
13 Psoas major
14 Superior gluteal artery and vein
15 Gluteus medius
16 Gluteus maximus
17 Ilium
18 Sacroiliac joint
19 Erector spinae
20 Filum terminale within sacral canal

21 Second sacral nerve root
22 Sacrum, second segment
23 Lumbosacral trunk
24 Obturator nerve
25 Iliolumbar vein
26 Internal iliac vein
27 External iliac vein
28 Internal iliac artery
29 External iliac artery
30 Left ureter

31 Median sacral artery and vein
32 Superior gluteal vein
33 Superior gluteal artery
34 Right ureter
35 Sigmoid colon
36 Mesentery of ileum
37 Appendix vermiformis
38 Caecum

Section level

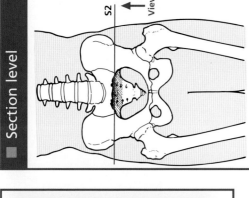

Orientation

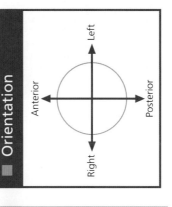

Axial computed tomogram (CT)

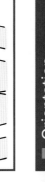

Notes

This section transects the second segment of the sacrum (**22**). Note that in this subject, the gluteal muscles on the right side are smaller and paler than those on the left (**10**, **15**, **16**). This subject had suffered a cerebrovascular accident that resulted in a right-sided paresis.

The sacroiliac joint (**18**) is a synovial joint. Since, as can be seen in this section, the sacral component is markedly wider anteriorly than posteriorly, the weight of the body tends to project it forward. This is resisted by the powerful posterior sacroiliac ligament on either side.

The appendix vermiformis (**37**) lies posterior to the ileum (**4**) in this section – the retro-ileal position. Much more commonly, the post-mortem appendix lies behind the caecum (65 per cent of cases) or descends into the pelvis (30 per cent of cases) (see the CT images in Axial sections 1 and 2).

The superior gluteal vessels in their pelvic (**32**, **33**) and gluteal (**14**) course are demonstrated clearly (see also Axial section 3).

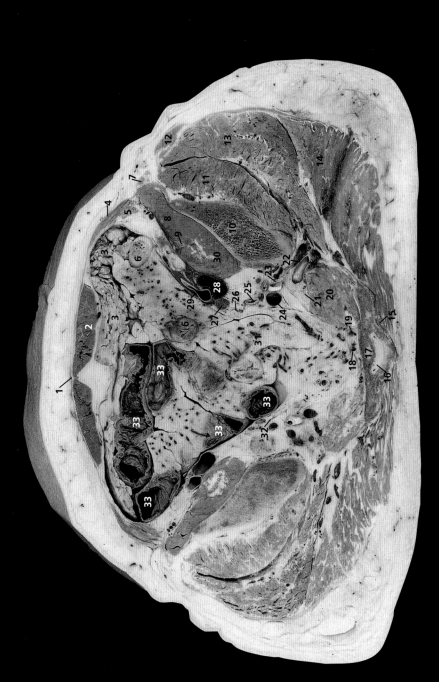

1 Linea alba
2 Rectus abdominis
3 Greater omentum
4 Internal oblique
5 Transversus abdominis
6 Sigmoid colon
7 Sartorius
8 Iliacus
9 Femoral nerve
10 Ilium

11 Gluteus minimus
12 Tensor fasciae latae
13 Gluteus medius
14 Gluteus maximus
15 Erector spinae
16 Sacral canal
17 Sacrum, third segment
18 Median sacral artery and vein
19 Lateral sacral artery and vein
20 Piriformis

21 Sciatic nerve
22 Superior gluteal artery and vein
23 Obturator artery and vein
24 Internal iliac vein
25 Internal iliac artery
26 Left ureter
27 Lymph node
28 External iliac vein
29 External iliac artery
30 Psoas major

31 Sigmoid mesocolon
32 Right ureter
33 Ileum

34 Bladder
35 Vas deferens
36 Inferior epigastric artery

Section level

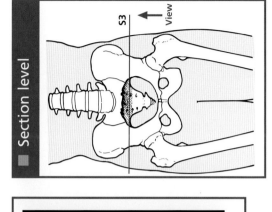

S3

View

Orientation

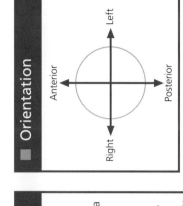

Left

Anterior

Posterior

Right

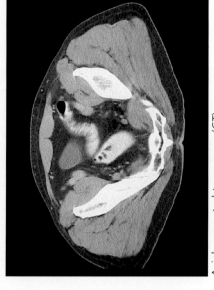

Axial computed tomogram (CT)

Notes

This section passes through the sacrum at its third segment (**17**). At this level, the sacral canal (**16**) lies below the termination of the dural sac, which ends at the second segment of the sacrum. The sacral canal now contains only the filum terminale and the lowermost sacral nerve roots, together with loose extradural fat. The sacral hiatus is, therefore, a useful portal of entry for the performance of an extradural nerve block.

Piriformis (**20**) arises from the front of the sacrum by three digitations, attached to the portions of bone between the pelvic sacral foramina and also to the grooves leading laterally from these foramina. The superior gluteal vessels (**22**), together with the superior gluteal nerve, pass above

piriformis through the greater sciatic foramen. In this subject, piriformis is paler and less bulky on the right side than on the left side as a result of a previous cerebrovascular accident (see Axial section 4). Piriformis is a bulky muscle that must be traversed when using the greater sciatic foramen as a route for percutaneous pelvic aspiration. On the CT image, there is asymmetry of the piriformis muscles due to a degree of scoliosis.

The ureter (**26**) descends into the pelvis characteristically immediately anterior to the internal iliac artery (**25**). It lies immediately deep to the pelvic peritoneum, crossed only by the vas deferens, which is seen in Axial section 6.

173

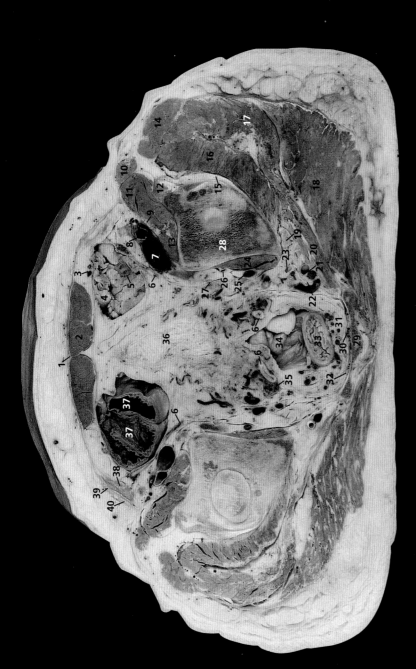

1 Linea alba
2 Rectus abdominis
3 Inferior epigastric artery and vein
4 Greater omentum
5 Sigmoid colon
6 Vas deferens
7 External iliac vein
8 External iliac artery
9 Femoral nerve
10 Sartorius
11 Iliacus
12 Rectus femoris straight head tendon

13 Psoas major and tendon
14 Tensor fasciae latae
15 Iliofemoral ligament
16 Gluteus minimus
17 Gluteus medius
18 Gluteus maximus
19 Sciatic nerve
20 Piriformis
21 Inferior gluteal artery and vein
22 Pudendal nerve
23 Internal pudendal artery
24 Obturator internus

25 Obturator vein
26 Obturator artery
27 Obturator nerve
28 Acetabulum (ilial portion)
29 Sacrum, fourth segment
30 Median sacral artery and vein
31 Superior rectal artery and vein
32 Lateral sacral artery and vein
33 Rectum
34 Rectosigmoid junction
35 Seminal vesicle
36 Fundus of bladder

37 Ileum
38 Transversus abdominis
39 Internal oblique
40 External oblique

41 Perirectal (mesorectal) fat
42 Pararectal fat (with branches of internal iliac artery and vein)
43 Perirectal (mesorectal) fascia

Section level

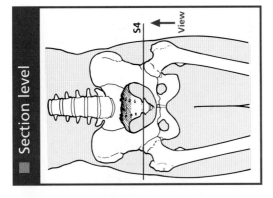

Orientation

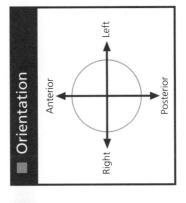

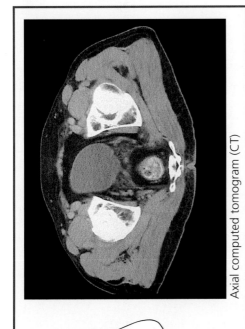

Axial computed tomogram (CT)

Notes

This section passes through the fourth segment of the sacrum (**28**), the superior portion of the acetabulum (**29**) and the fundus of the bladder (**36**). The rectum (**33**) lies immediately in front of the sacrum, separated by the median sacral vessels (**30**); it commences just cranial to this line of section on the third sacral segment. The rectosigmoid junction is also seen (**34**).

The vas deferens (**6**) is the most medial structure crossing the side wall of the pelvis immediately deep to the pelvic peritoneum. More caudally, it will join the seminal vesicle (**35**) to form the ejaculatory duct.

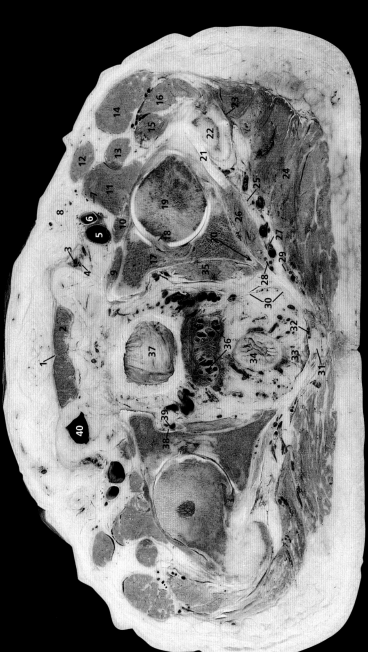

1 Linea alba
2 Rectus abdominis
3 Spermatic cord
4 Vas deferens
5 Femoral vein
6 Femoral artery
7 Femoral nerve
8 Lymph node
9 Pectineus
10 Psoas major and tendon
11 Iliacus
12 Sartorius

13 Rectus femoris
14 Tensor fasciae latae
15 Gluteus minimus
16 Gluteus medius
17 Acetabulum (pubic portion)
18 Ligamentum teres
19 Femoral head
20 Ischium, leading to ischial spine
   (arrowed)
21 Obturator internus tendon
22 Greater trochanter
23 Trochanteric bursa

24 Gluteus maximus
25 Sciatic nerve
26 Gemellus superior
27 Inferior gluteal artery and vein
28 Pudendal nerve and inferior
   pudendal artery and vein
29 Sacrospinous ligament
30 Perirectal (mesorectal) fascia
   separating perirectal fat from
   pararectal fat
31 Sacrum, fifth segment
32 Lateral sacral artery and vein

33 Superior rectal artery and vein in
   perirectal (mesorectal) fat
34 Rectum
35 Obturator internus
36 Seminal vesicle
37 Bladder
38 Obturator nerve
39 Obturator artery and vein
40 Patent processus vaginalis (indirect
   inguinal hernia sac)

Section level

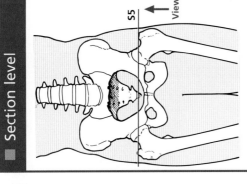

S5

View

Orientation

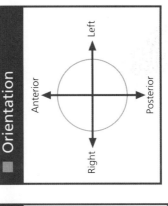

Anterior

Left

Right

Posterior

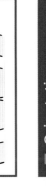

Axial computed tomogram (CT)

Notes

This section traverses the last (fifth) segment of the sacrum (**31**). The sacrospinous ligament (**29**) is transected as it passes forward to the ischial spine (**20**).

This section gives an excellent illustration of the hip joint at the level of the ligamentum teres (**18**). The ligamentum teres (**18**) transmits an artery, a branch of the obturator artery, to the femoral head, which is its sole source of blood in childhood. Damage to this vessel (Perthes' disease or slipped femoral epiphysis) may lead to avascular necrosis of the femoral head.

The superior rectal vessels (**33**) can be seen as they lie in the loose perirectal (mesorectal) fat, which also contains lymphatic vessels, lymph nodes and the pelvic plexuses lying on the rectal wall. The perirectal fat is separated from the pararectal fat by the perirectal (mesorectal) fascia (**30**).

Note that this subject has an indirect inguinal hernia sac on the right side (**40**).

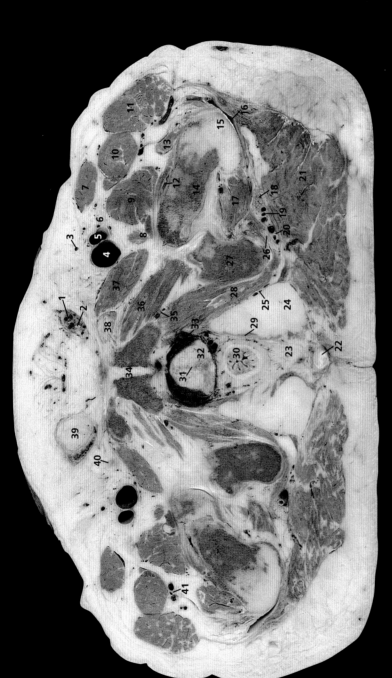

1 Spermatic cord
2 Vas deferens
3 Great saphenous vein
4 Femoral vein
5 Femoral artery
6 Femoral nerve
7 Sartorius
8 Psoas major and tendon
9 Iliacus
10 Rectus femoris
11 Tensor fasciae latae
12 Hip joint capsule

13 Vastus lateralis
14 Femoral neck
15 Greater trochanter
16 Trochanteric bursa
17 Quadratus femoris
18 Sciatic nerve
19 Inferior gluteal artery and vein
20 Internal pudendal artery and vein
   and pudendal nerve (see also 25)
21 Gluteus maximus
22 Coccyx
23 Mesorectum

24 Ischiorectal fossa
25 Pudendal (Alcock's) canal
26 Obturator internus tendon
27 Ischium
28 Obturator internus
29 Levator ani (puborectalis portion)
30 Rectum
31 Prostatic urethra
32 Prostate
33 Prostatic venous plexus
34 Symphysis pubis
35 Obturator artery and vein

36 Obturator externus
37 Pectineus
38 Superior ramus of pubis
39 Extraperitoneal fat related to
   hernia sac
40 Inguinal lymph node
41 Lateral circumflex femoral artery
   and vein

42 Inferior rectal artery
43 Body of penis

Section level

Orientation

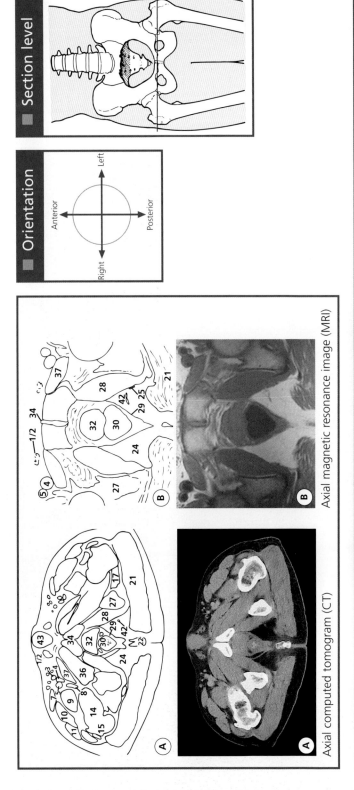

Axial computed tomogram (CT)

Axial magnetic resonance image (MRI)

Notes

This section passes through the coccyx (**22**) and the symphysis pubis (**34**). In the standing position, the horizontal plane that passes through the coccyx corresponds to the superior margin of the symphysis.

The ischiorectal fossa (**24**) is wedge-shaped; its base points to the surface of the perineum, while its apex is the junction of obturator internus (**28**) and levator ani (**29**), covered respectively by the obturator fascia and the inferior fascia of the pelvic diaphragm. Medially it is bounded by the external anal sphincter and levator ani, laterally by the

tuberosity of the ischium and the obturator fascia, and posteriorly by the lower border of gluteus maximus (**21**) and the sacrotuberous ligament. Anteriorly lies the urogenital diaphragm, but the fossa is prolonged as a narrow recess above this diaphragm, where it is limited by the fusion between the inferior fascia of the pelvic diaphragm and the superior fascia of the urogenital diaphragm.

The internal pudendal vessels and the pudendal nerve (**20**) enter the perineum through the lesser sciatic foramen and then traverse the pudendal canal of Alcock (**25**). This canal comprises a special

sheath of fascia fused with the lower part of the obturator fascia.

The left common femoral artery (**5**) is about to divide into the superficial femoral and profunda femoris on the section. On the CT image, this has already taken place.

The spermatic cord (**1**) and vas deferens (**2**) are seen clearly on the left-hand side. On the right, these are compressed by extraperitoneal fat related to this subject's indirect inguinal hernia (**39**). This hernia is seen well in Axial section 7.

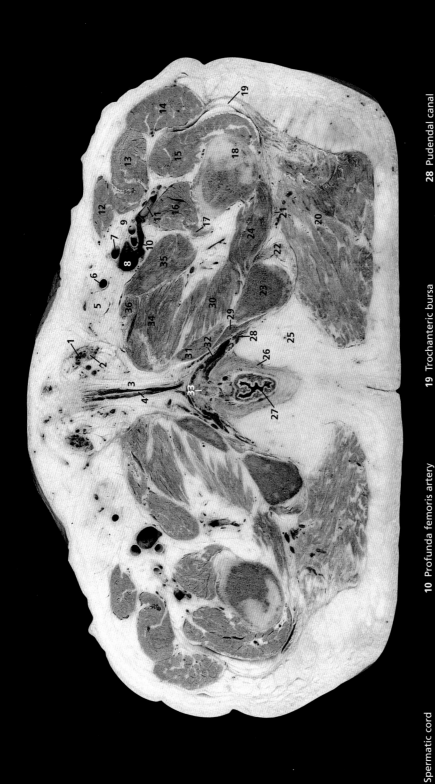

1 Spermatic cord
2 Vas deferens
3 Tunica albuginea of penis
4 Corpus cavernosum (body)
5 Inguinal lymph node
6 Great saphenous vein
7 Superficial femoral artery
8 Femoral vein
9 Femoral nerve
10 Profunda femoris artery
11 Lateral circumflex femoral vein
12 Sartorius
13 Rectus femoris
14 Tensor fasciae latae
15 Vastus lateralis
16 Iliacus
17 Tendon of psoas major
18 Greater trochanter
19 Trochanteric bursa
20 Gluteus maximus
21 Sciatic nerve
22 Biceps femoris tendon
23 Ischial tuberosity
24 Quadratus femoris
25 Ischiorectal fat
26 Levator ani
27 Anorectal junction
28 Pudendal canal
29 Obturator internus
30 Obturator externus
31 Pubis-inferior ramus
32 Corpus cavernosum (crus)
33 Urethra (in distal prostate)
34 Adductor brevis
35 Pectineus
36 Adductor longus

Section level

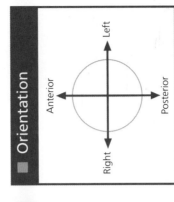

Orientation

Anterior

Left

Posterior

Right

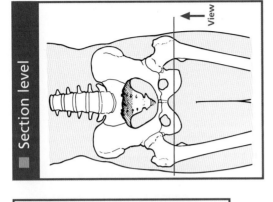

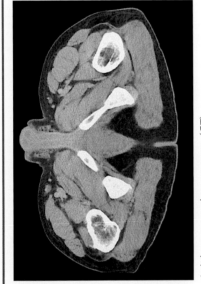

Axial computed tomogram (CT)

Notes

This section lies caudal to the coccyx and pubis but passes through the level of the ischial tuberosity (**23**). The plane of section cuts through the anorectal junction (**27**), around which lies levator ani (**26**).

The ischiorectal fossa, filled with fat (**25**), which is

described in Axial section 8, can be seen to communicate with the fossa on the other side, posterior to the anal canal. The inferior rectal artery is seen clearly in the centre of the fossa on the left-hand side.

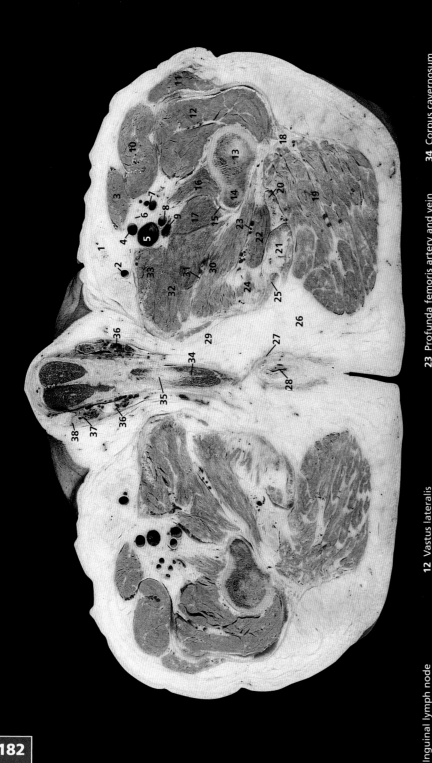

1 Inguinal lymph node
2 Great saphenous vein
3 Sartorius
4 Superficial femoral artery
5 Superficial femoral vein
6 Femoral nerve
7 Lateral circumflex femoral artery and vein
8 Profunda femoris artery
9 Profunda femoris vein
10 Rectus femoris
11 Tensor fasciae latae
12 Vastus lateralis
13 Femur
14 Lesser trochanter
15 Tendon of psoas major
16 Iliacus
17 Pectineus
18 Gluteus maximus tendon
19 Gluteus maximus
20 Sciatic nerve
21 Biceps femoris and semitendinosus tendons
22 Quadratus femoris
23 Profunda femoris artery and vein first perforating branches
24 Semimembranosus
25 Ischium
26 Ischiorectal fat
27 Levator ani
28 Anal canal
29 Gracilis
30 Adductor magnus
31 Obturator nerve, deep branch
32 Adductor brevis
33 Adductor longus
34 Corpus cavernosum
35 Urethra
36 Pampiniform plexus
37 Spermatic cord
38 Vas deferens
39 Corpus cavernosum (crus)
40 Obturator externus

Section level

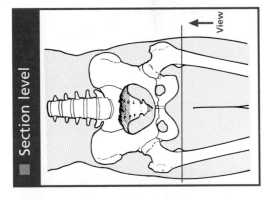

Orientation

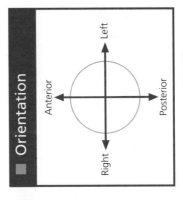

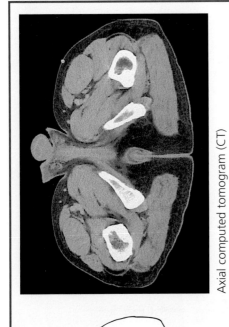

Axial computed tomogram (CT)

Notes

This section is completely below the pelvic girdle and transects the upper ends of the femoral shafts (**13**) at the level of the lesser trochanter (**14**). It transects the anal canal (**28**). The bulky gluteus maximus provides a good target for intramuscular injections of medications. It is worth considering the site of the sciatic nerve (**20**). Many patients have so much fat overlying the gluteal muscles that supposedly intramuscular injections are in fact placed in overlying adipose tissue!

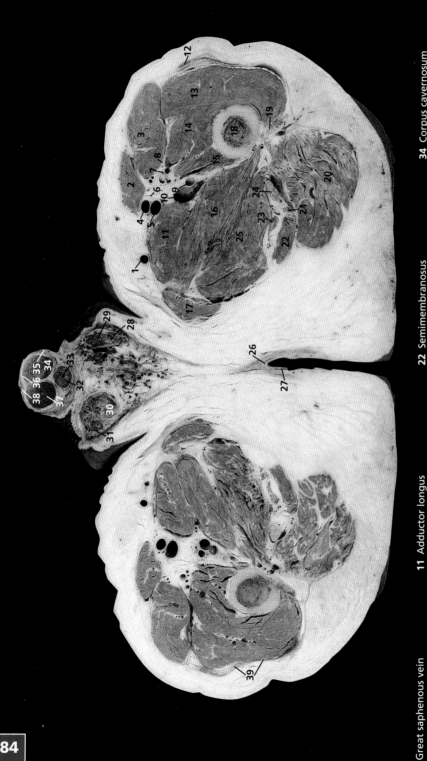

1 Great saphenous vein
2 Sartorius
3 Rectus femoris
4 Superficial femoral artery
5 Superficial femoral vein
6 Saphenous nerve
7 Lateral circumflex femoral artery and vein (inferior branch)
8 Femoral nerve (branch to quadriceps)
9 Profunda femoris artery
10 Profunda femoris vein

11 Adductor longus
12 Tensor fasciae latae
13 Vastus lateralis
14 Vastus intermedius
15 Vastus medialis
16 Adductor brevis
17 Gracilis
18 Femoral shaft
19 Gluteus maximus tendon
20 Gluteus maximus
21 Biceps femoris – tendon of long head

22 Semimembranosus
23 Semitendinosus tendon
24 Sciatic nerve
25 Adductor magnus
26 External anal sphincter
27 Anal verge
28 Vas deferens
29 Spermatic cord
30 Testis – upper pole
31 Pampiniform plexus
32 Corpus spongiosum
33 Urethra

34 Corpus cavernosum
35 Penile fascia
36 Tunica albuginea of penis
37 Deep artery of penis
38 Dorsal vein of penis
39 Investing fascia of thigh – fascia lata

40 Quadratus femoris

Section level

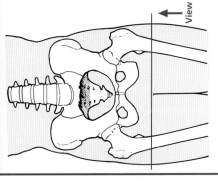

Orientation

Left

Anterior

Posterior

Right

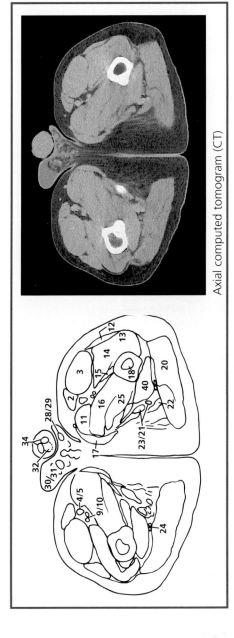

Axial computed tomogram (CT)

Notes

This section passes through the anal verge (**27**), surrounded by the external anal sphincter (**26**). It demonstrates well the structure of the penis in transverse section. The penile urethra (**33**) is surrounded by the corpus spongiosum (**32**). Above and lateral to this, on either side, are the corpora cavernosa (**34**). These structures are bound together within the penile fascia (**35**). The deep artery of the penis (**37**) is a branch of the internal pudendal artery, which ends in the deep perineal pouch by dividing into the deep and the dorsal arteries of the penis and the artery to the bulb. The deep artery supplies the corpus cavernosum, the dorsal artery supplies the prepuce and glans, and the artery to the bulb supplies the corpus spongiosum.

This section also demonstrates the upper pole of the testis (**30**), surrounded by its tunica albuginea, and also the vas deferens (**28**), surrounded by the pampiniform plexus (**31**).

The saphenous nerve (**6**), a branch of the femoral nerve, is seen here entering the adductor, or subsartorial, canal (Hunter's canal). This is an aponeurotic tunnel in the middle third of the thigh, formed posteriorly by adductor longus (**11**), more distally by adductor magnus (**25**), anterolaterally by vastus medialis (**15**) and anteromedially by sartorius (**2**). Its contents are the superficial femoral artery (**4**) and vein (**5**), the saphenous nerve (**6**) and the nerve to vastus medialis. (See also Lower limb – Thigh – Axial section 3.) The saphenous nerve (**6**) itself is of clinical interest. It is entirely sensory and is a branch of the femoral nerve just distal to the inguinal ligament. It becomes subcutaneous by emerging from the femoral canal at the posterior aspect of sartorius above the knee and descends, in company with the great saphenous vein, to the medial side of the foot as far as the base of the hallux. It is the longest cutaneous nerve in the body.

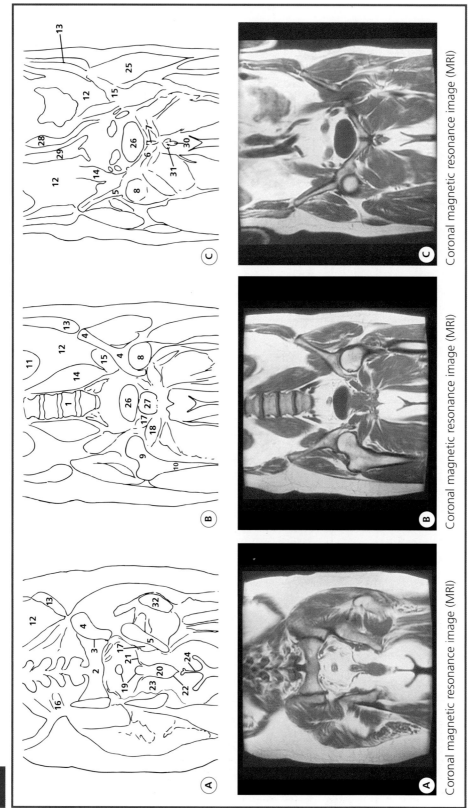

Coronal magnetic resonance image (MRI)

Coronal magnetic resonance image (MRI)

Coronal magnetic resonance image (MRI)

Section level

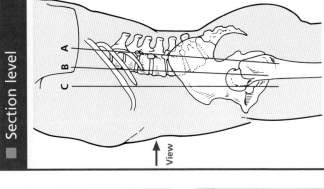

Orientation

Superior

Left

Inferior

Right

1 L4 vertebral body
2 Sacrum
3 Sacroiliac joint
4 Ilium
5 Ischium
6 Pubis
7 Pubic symphysis
8 Femoral head
9 Neck of femur
10 Shaft of femur
11 Left kidney
12 Intra-abdominal fat

13 Anterior wall musculature
    (transversus, internal/external
    obliques)
14 Psoas major
15 Iliacus
16 Quadratus lumborum
17 Obturator internus
18 Obturator externus
19 Rectum
20 Anal canal
21 Levator ani
22 Anal sphincters

23 Ischio-rectal (ischioanal) fossa
24 Natal cleft
25 Gluteal muscles
26 Bladder
27 Prostate
28 Aorta
29 Inferior vena cava
30 Corpus spongiosum
31 Corpus cavernosum
32 Greater trochanter of femur

Notes

These three T1 MR coronal images provide a good overview of the relationships of the structures within the male pelvis. In particular, the way in which the anatomy relates to the pelvic floor is demonstrated well. So too is the way in which the anterior wall musculature merges with the bony pelvis. The copious quantity of intra-abdominal fat in men is also apparent; women have relatively much more fat in the subcutaneous tissues.

In image C, the confluence of the two common iliac veins forming the inferior vena cava (**29**) can be appreciated. So too can the continuation of the aorta (**28**) as the left common iliac artery; the right common iliac

artery cannot be seen on this image, as it lies in a more anterior position as it passes anterior to the confluence of the common iliac veins. This is an important point, as the veins usually lie posterior to the arteries in this region – this is also true for the external iliac and popliteal vessels. More superiorly in the body (brachiocephalic, pulmonary and renal), the veins lie anterior to the arteries.

Such coronal images also provide a very useful overview when assessing the musculoskeletal system. The hips and sacroiliac joints are seen well, although smaller fields of view are used for more detailed imaging of a particular joint.

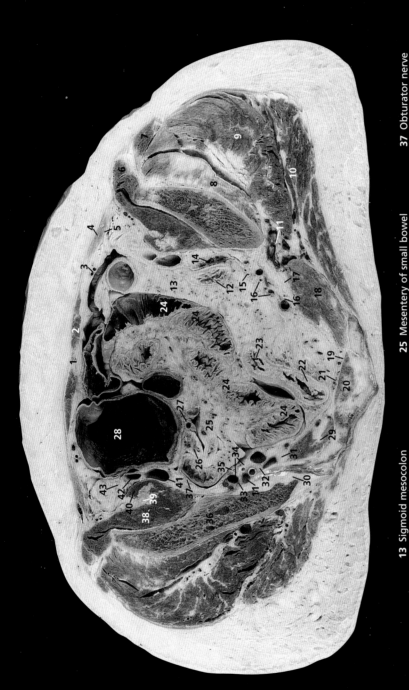

1 Linea alba
2 Rectus abdominis
3 Inferior epigastric artery and vein
4 Fused aponeurosis of external and internal oblique muscles
5 Transversus abdominis
6 Sartorius
7 Tensor fasciae latae
8 Gluteus minimus
9 Gluteus medius
10 Gluteus maximus
11 Superior gluteal artery and vein
12 Sigmoid colon

13 Sigmoid mesocolon
14 Left ovary
15 Left ureter
16 Branches of internal iliac artery and vein
17 Sciatic nerve
18 Piriformis
19 Lateral sacral artery and vein
20 Sacrum, third segment
21 Median sacral artery and vein
22 Rectum
23 Rectosigmoid junction
24 Ileum

25 Mesentery of small bowel
26 Right ovary
27 Right uterine (fallopian) tube
28 Caecum
29 Ventral ramus of third sacral nerve
30 Sacroiliac joint
31 Ventral ramus of second sacral nerve
32 Ventral ramus of first sacral nerve
33 Lumbosacral trunk
34 Uterine artery and vein
35 Right ureter
36 Ilium

37 Obturator nerve
38 Iliacus
39 Femoral nerve
40 Psoas major
41 External iliac vein
42 External iliac artery
43 Lymph node
44 Uterus (fundus)
45 Round ligament

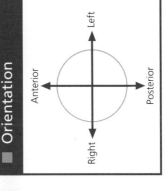

S3

View

Left

Anterior

Posterior

Right

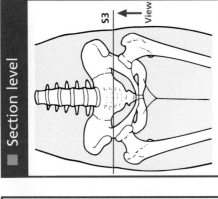

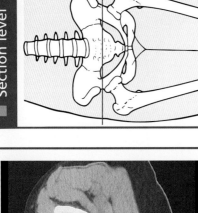

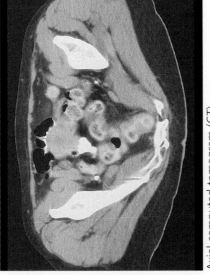

Axial computed tomogram (CT)

■ Notes

This section through the female pelvis transects the third segment of the sacrum (**20**), which delimits the commencement of the rectum (**22**) at its junction with the sigmoid colon (**23**). The rectosigmoid junction demonstrates a marked change – the rectum, unlike the colon, is free of appendices epiploicae, and the taenia coli disappear from its wall.

The left ovary is seen at (**14**) and the right ovary at (**26**); in this elderly subject, they are atrophic.

Along the internal iliac vessels (**16**) lies a rich lymphatic plexus, together with the internal iliac lymph nodes. These receive afferents from all the pelvic viscera, the deeper parts of the perineum and the muscles of the buttock.

Their efferents pass through the common iliac nodes.

The sciatic nerve (**17**) at its origin is lying on piriformis (**18**). Its important relationships can be traced in subsequent sections as it emerges through the greater sciatic foramen below piriformis to cross, in turn, obturator internus tendon with its accompanying gemelli, quadratus femoris and, finally, adductor magnus. It is covered superficially by gluteus maximus and is crossed by the long head of biceps.

Note that a degree of scoliosis in this subject explains the asymmetry of the sciatic nerve and other structures on the two sides of this section.

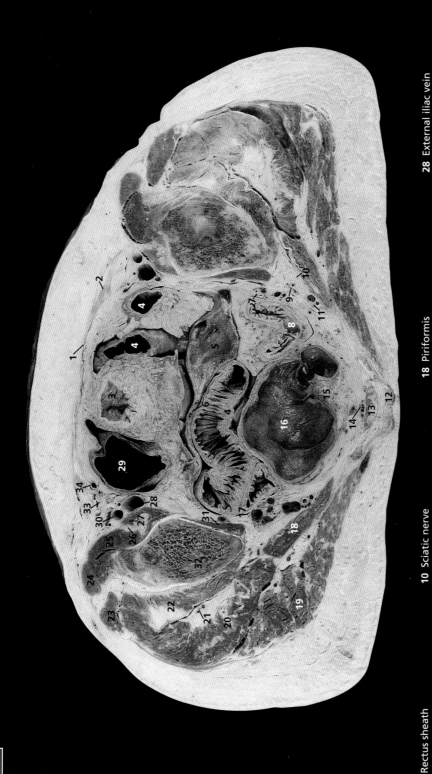

1 Rectus sheath
2 Transversus abdominis
3 Fundus of bladder
4 Ileum
5 Fundus of uterus
6 Broad ligament
7 Left ureter
8 Sigmoid colon
9 Inferior gluteal artery vein and nerve

10 Sciatic nerve
11 Internal pudendal artery, vein and pudendal nerve
12 Superior sacral cornu
13 Sacrum, fifth segment
14 Median sacral artery and vein
15 Mesorectum with superior rectal artery and vein
16 Rectum
17 Right ureter

18 Piriformis
19 Gluteus maximus
20 Gluteus medius
21 Superior gluteal artery and vein
22 Gluteus minimus
23 Tensor fasciae latae
24 Sartorius
25 Iliacus
26 Femoral nerve
27 Psoas major

28 External iliac vein
29 Caecum
30 External iliac artery
31 Obturator internus
32 Ilium
33 Round ligament
34 Inferior epigastric artery and vein

Section level

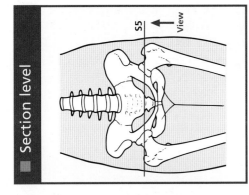

Orientation

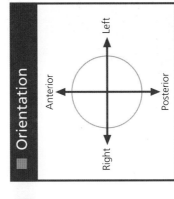

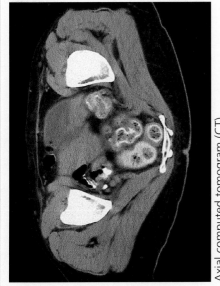

Axial computed tomogram (CT)

Notes

This section passes through the lowest (fifth) segment of the sacrum (**13**) and shaves through the fundus of the bladder (**3**) and of the uterus (**5**), together with the upper part of the broad ligament (**6**).

There is wide normal variation in the relative positions of the pelvic organs. For example, on the CT images, the fundus of the uterus was first encountered in the image on page 185. On this CT image, the body of the uterus is traversed. Conversely, the rectosigmoid junction lies at a more caudal level on the CT images than on the sections.

The rectum, from its narrow lumen at its origin, shown in the previous section, has widened into its patulous ampulla (**16**). Between the posterior aspect of the rectum (covered by its fascia propria) and the fascia covering the anterior aspect of the sacrum (**13**), the presacral fascia, is the connective tissue plane, which is developed in the surgical mobilization of the rectum and its vascular pedicle.

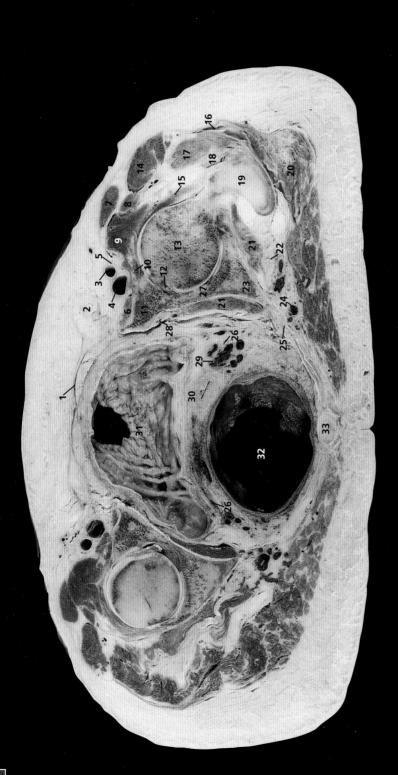

1 Inguinal ligament
2 Femoral hernia containing
  extraperitoneal fat
3 Femoral artery
4 Femoral vein
5 Femoral nerve
6 Pectineus
7 Sartorius
8 Rectus femoris
9 Iliacus

10 Psoas major tendon
11 Pubic component of acetabulum
12 Ligamentum teres
13 Head of femur
14 Tensor fasciae latae
15 Iliofemoral ligament
16 Iliotibial tract
17 Gluteus medius
18 Tendon of gluteus minimus
19 Greater trochanter

20 Gluteus maximus
21 Obturator internus
22 Sciatic nerve
23 Ischial spine
24 Inferior gluteal artery vein and
   nerve
25 Sacrospinous ligament
26 Ureter
27 Acetabulum
28 Obturator artery, vein and nerve

29 Uterine artery and vein
30 Internal os of cervix
31 Bladder
32 Ampulla of rectum
33 Coccyx

34 Ischial component of acetabulum
35 Sigmoid colon
36 Vault of vagina (with tampon)

Section level

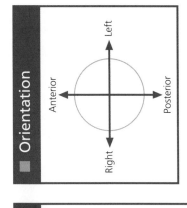

Orientation

Left

Anterior

Posterior

Right

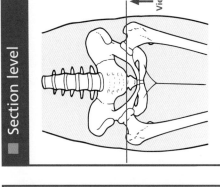
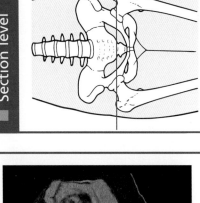

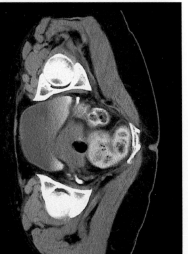

Axial computed tomogram (CT)

Notes

This section passes through the coccyx (**33**) and transects the femoral head (**13**). In this elderly subject, the uterus is atrophic; note the small size of the cervix, here divided through its internal os (**30**).

Some CT units prepare all female patients undergoing pelvic CT by giving dilute iodinated contrast medium per rectum, as here; this renders the lumen of the rectosigmoid opaque. Sometimes a tampon is present in the vagina; the air trapped by its fibres is readily recognized (**36**). This allows appreciation of the level of the vaginal vault and the external os of the cervix (**30**), even though neither structure is demonstrated directly.

The uterine artery (**29**) arises from the internal iliac artery, runs medially on levator ani towards the cervix of the uterus, and crosses above and in front of the ureter (**26**) above the lateral vaginal fornix to reach the side of the uterus, where it ascends in the broad ligament. The corresponding uterine veins (**29**), usually two in number, drain a uterine plexus along the lateral side of the uterus within the broad ligament and open into the internal iliac vein. The close relationship between the uterine vessels and the ureter is of immense importance to the gynaecological surgeon when performing a hysterectomy (see also the CT image in Axial section 4).

193

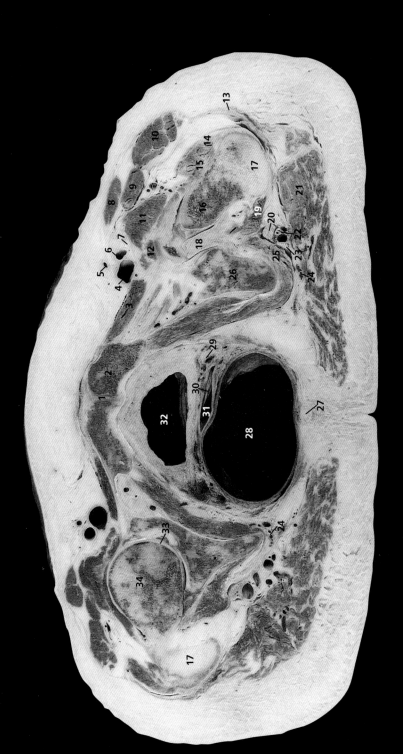

1 Pubic symphysis
2 Body of pubis
3 Pectineus
4 Femoral vein
5 Great saphenous vein
6 Femoral artery
7 Femoral nerve
8 Sartorius
9 Rectus femoris
10 Tensor fasciae latae
11 Iliacus

12 Psoas major tendon
13 Iliotibial tract
14 Gluteus medius
15 Gluteus minimus
16 Neck of femur
17 Greater trochanter
18 Ischiofemoral ligament
19 Quadratus femoris
20 Sciatic nerve
21 Gluteus maximus
22 Inferior gluteal artery and vein

23 Posterior cutaneous nerve of thigh
24 Internal pudendal artery and vein
   and pudendal nerve
25 Obturator internus
26 Ischium
27 Coccyx
28 Ampulla of rectum
29 Vaginal artery and vein
30 External os of cervix
31 Vagina
32 Bladder

33 Acetabulum
34 Femoral head

35 Ureter
36 Calcified phleboliths
37 Obturator artery, vein and nerve
38 Ischial spine

Section level

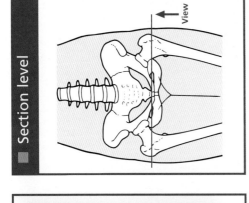

Orientation

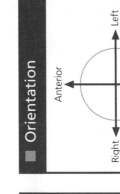

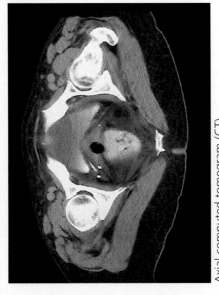

Axial computed tomogram (CT)

Notes

This section traverses the tip of the coccyx (**27**) and passes through the pubic symphysis in its upper part (**1**). Note that the vagina (**31**) is transected in its upper part so that the external os of the cervix (**30**) can be seen peeping through, with the posterior fornix of the vagina behind it. Alongside the vagina are the vaginal vessels (**29**). The vaginal artery usually corresponds to the inferior vesical artery in the male and is a branch of the internal iliac artery. It is frequently double or triple. It supplies the vagina as well as the fundus of the bladder and the adjacent part of the rectum and anastomoses with branches of the uterine artery.

This section shows well the obturator internus muscle (**25**) as it sweeps around the lesser sciatic foramen, with the sciatic nerve (**20**) lying on its superficial (posterior) face, covered posteriorly by gluteus maximus (**21**).

Many patients develop small out-pouchings, or diverticula, in the extensive plexus of small pelvic veins. These diverticula often contain calcified thrombus to form pheboliths, as demonstrated on this CT image (**36**). On plain pelvic radiographs, these may simulate ureteric calculi.

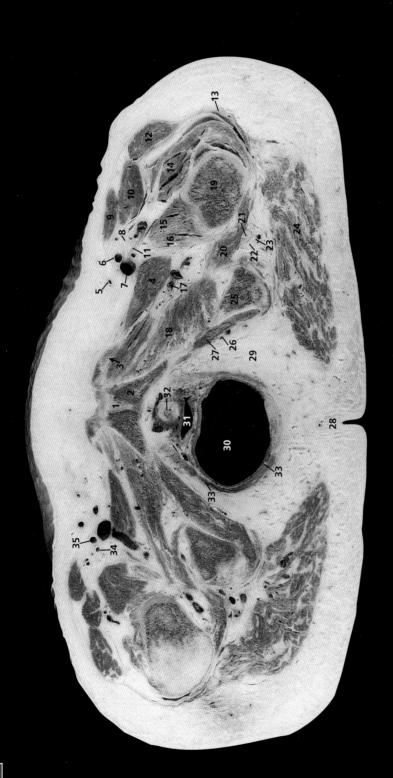

1 Symphysis pubis
2 Body of pubis
3 Adductor brevis, with adductor
  longus origin (arrowed)
4 Pectineus
5 Great saphenous vein
6 Left femoral artery
7 Femoral vein
8 Femoral nerve
9 Sartorius
10 Rectus femoris

11 Lateral circumflex femoral vein
12 Tensor fasciae latae
13 Iliotibial tract
14 Vastus lateralis
15 Iliacus
16 Psoas major tendon
17 Obturator artery and vein
18 Obturator externus
19 Femur
20 Quadratus femoris
21 Sciatic nerve

22 Posterior cutaneous nerve of thigh
23 Inferior gluteal artery and vein
24 Gluteus maximus
25 Ischial tuberosity
26 Pudendal (Alcock's) canal,
   containing internal pudendal artery
   and vein and pudendal nerve
27 Obturator internus
28 Natal cleft
29 Ischiorectal fossa
30 Rectum

31 Vagina
32 Urethra
33 Levator ani
34 Right profunda femoris artery
35 Right superficial femoral artery

36 Coccyx
37 Bladder

Section level

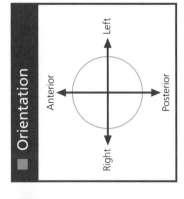

Orientation

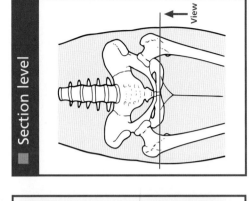

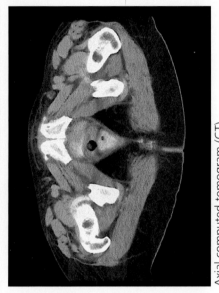

Axial computed tomogram (CT)

Notes

This section passes through the upper part of the natal cleft (**28**) and the body of the pubis (**2**). The intimate relationship between the female urethra (**32**) and vagina (**31**) is shown well; the former is actually embedded in the anterior wall of the latter.

Unusually, the lateral circumflex femoral vein (**11**) in this subject arises from the common femoral vein (**7**); more usually, the circumflex vessels arise from the profunda femoris artery and vein. The right common femoral artery

has divided into its profunda (**34**) and superficial (**35**) branches. On the left-hand side, the femoral artery (**6**) has not yet divided.

The anatomy of the ischiorectal fossa (**29**) is demonstrated well. It lies between levator ani (**33**) and obturator internus (**27**), on which can be seen the pudendal canal (**26**) and its contents. (See also Axial section 8 – male.)

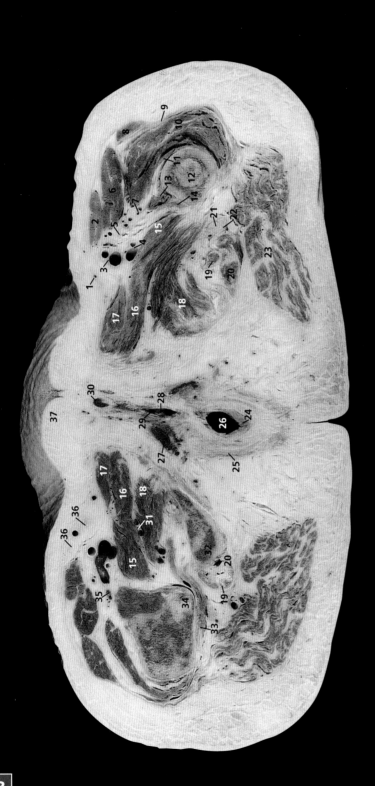

1 Great saphenous vein
2 Sartorius
3 Superficial femoral artery and vein
4 Deep femoral artery and vein
5 Femoral nerve (dividing into branches)
6 Rectus femoris
7 Lateral circumflex femoral artery and vein
8 Tensor fasciae latae
9 Iliotibial tract
10 Vastus lateralis

11 Vastus intermedius
12 Shaft of femur
13 Vastus medialis
14 Psoas major insertion to lesser trochanter with iliacus
15 Pectineus
16 Adductor brevis
17 Adductor longus
18 Adductor magnus
19 Tendon of semimembranosus
20 Origin of semitendinosus and biceps femoris muscles

21 Sciatic nerve
22 Posterior cutaneous nerve of thigh
23 Gluteus maximus
24 External anal sphincter
25 Levator ani
26 Anal canal
27 Crus of clitoris
28 Vaginal orifice
29 Urethral orifice
30 Clitoris
31 Obturator artery, vein and nerve (posterior branch)

32 Ischial tuberosity
33 Quadratus femoris
34 Lesser trochanter of femur
35 Lateral circumflex femoral vein
36 Inguinal lymph node
37 Mons pubis
38 Obturator externus
39 Ischiorectal fossa

Section level

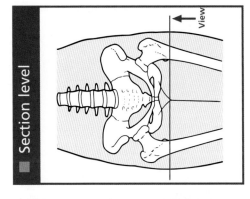

Orientation

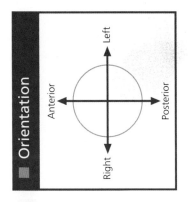

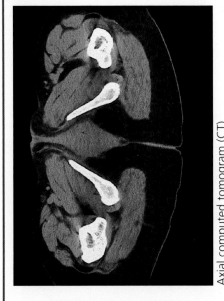

Axial computed tomogram (CT)

Notes

This section passes through mons pubis (**37**) anteriorly and the anal canal (**26**) posteriorly. Note the close relationship between the vaginal (**28**) and urethral (**29**) orifices.

The sciatic nerve (**21**), with its accompanying posterior cutaneous nerve of the thigh (**22**) immediately superficial to it, can now be seen as it lies on quadratus femoris (**33**).

199

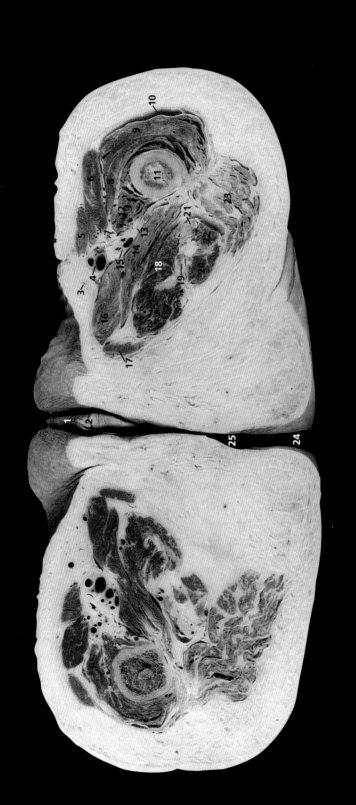

1 Prepuce of clitoris
2 Glans clitoridis
3 Great saphenous vein
4 Superficial femoral artery and vein
5 Sartorius
6 Rectus femoris
7 Femoral nerve (branch to quadratus femoris)

8 Vastus intermedius
9 Vastus lateralis
10 Iliotibial tract
11 Shaft of femur
12 Vastus medialis
13 First perforating artery and vein of profunda femoris artery and vein
14 Adductor brevis

15 Profunda femoris artery and vein
16 Adductor longus
17 Gracilis
18 Adductor magnus
19 Semimembranosus tendon
20 Semitendinosus
21 Sciatic nerve
22 Long head of biceps

23 Gluteus maximus
24 Natal cleft
25 Anal verge
26 Tensor fasciae latae

Section level

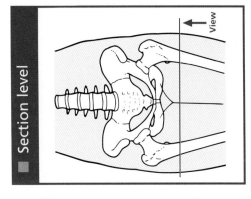

Orientation

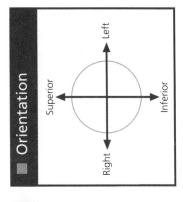

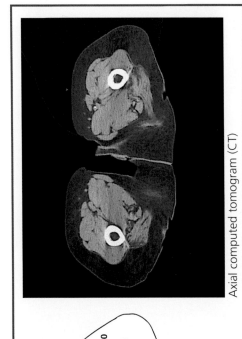

Axial computed tomogram (CT)

Notes

This section passes through the upper thigh but demonstrates the prepuce (**1**) and glans (**2**) of the clitoris. The anal verge (**25**) can be seen within the natal cleft (**24**).

The sciatic nerve (**21**) now lies on adductor magnus (**18**) and is crossed superficially by the long head of biceps (**22**).

Axial magnetic resonance
image (MRI) T1-weighted

Axial magnetic resonance
image (MRI) T2-weighted

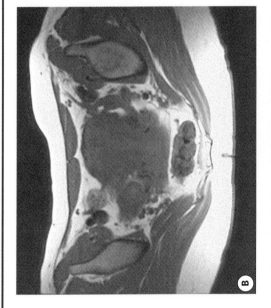

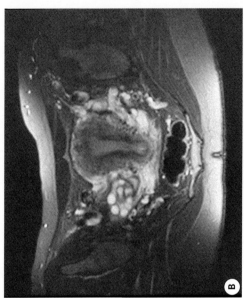

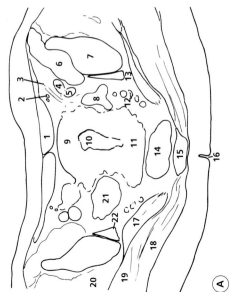

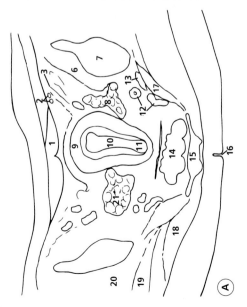

Section level

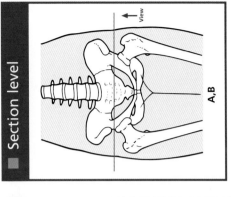

view

A,B

Orientation

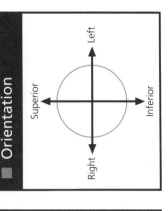

Left

Superior

Inferior

Right

Notes

T1- (A) and T2- (B) weighted axial magnetic resonance images using a pelvic phased-array coil. The design of the coil accounts for the higher signal intensity within the subcutaneous fat anteriorly and posteriorly. Note the way in which T2 weighting demonstrates the internal anatomy of the uterus and the individual follicles within the ovary.

Note how there is a normal plane of fat lateral to each ovary and internal to the ilium and obturator internus. Any enlarged obturator nodes would be seen immediately posterior to the external iliac vein and would tend to disrupt the fat plane just internal to the ilium. The way in which the external iliac artery (**4**) lies anterior to the vein (**5**) is appreciated well. The femoral nerve may be just identifiable anterior to the external iliac artery on the right, having just emerged from the gap in the iliopsoas (**6**). At the base of the gap in the medial aspect of the right iliopsoas is the low-signal-intensity iliopsoas tendon, which will continue down to the distal attachment on the lesser trochanter. In diseases of the psoas (e.g. psoas abscess), the femoral nerve (L2,3,4) is often involved. This will lead to an absent patellar tendon reflex and difficulty with full extension of the hip.

On the T1-weighted images, the epigastric vessels return low signal intensity (signal void). On T2-weighted images, they return high signal.

Note the way in which the round ligament passes lateral to the epigastric vessels en route to the inguinal canal. This course is exactly analogous to that of the vas deferens in the male patient. The round ligament contributes to keeping the uterus anteverted. Contrary to what might be thought, however, the main support for the uterus is not due to any of its ligaments; rather, it is the integrity of the pelvic-floor musculature that is important.

1 Rectus abdominis
2 Inferior epigastric vessels
3 Round ligament
4 External iliac artery
5 External iliac vein
6 Iliopsoas
7 Ilium
8 Left ovary
9 Fundus of uterus
10 Uterine cavity
11 Cervix of uterus
12 Internal iliac vessels
13 Plane of sciatic nerve
14 Rectum
15 Sacrum
16 Natal cleft
17 Piriformis
18 Gluteus maximus
19 Gluteus medius
20 Gluteus minimus
21 Right ovary
22 Obturator internus

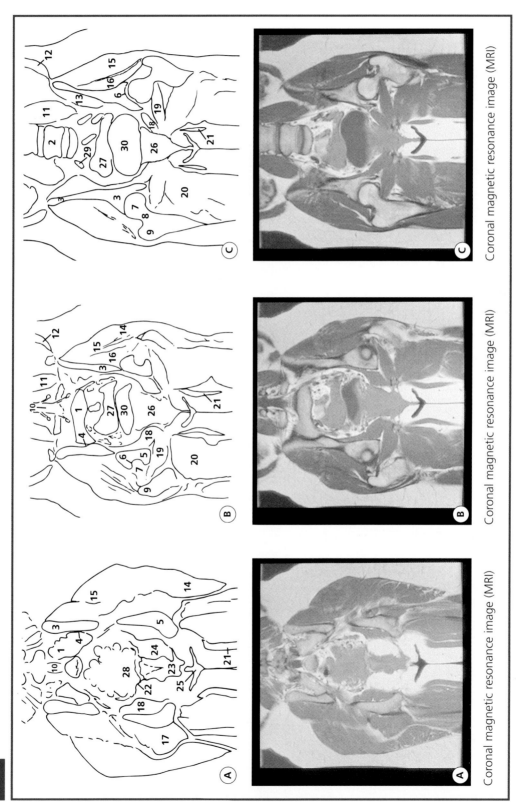

Coronal magnetic resonance image (MRI)

Coronal magnetic resonance image (MRI)

Coronal magnetic resonance image (MRI)

Section level

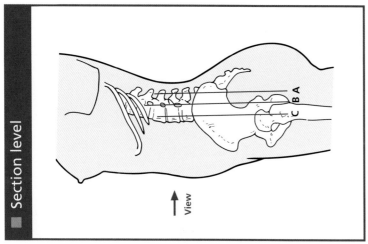

View

Orientation

Superior

Left

Inferior

Right

1 Sacrum
2 L5 vertebral body
3 Ilium
4 Sacroiliac joint
5 Ischium
6 Acetabulum
7 Femoral head
8 Femoral neck
9 Femur, greater trochanter
10 Thecal sac
11 Psoas major

12 Anterior abdominal-wall musculature
13 Iliacus
14 Gluteus maximus
15 Gluteus medius
16 Gluteus minimus
17 Quadratus femoris
18 Obturator internus
19 Obterator externus
20 Adductor group of muscles
21 Gracilis

22 Levator ani
23 Anal canal
24 Ischiorectal (ischioanal) canal
25 Natal cleft
26 Vagina
27 Uterus (body)
28 Uterus (cervix)
29 Common iliac vessels
30 Bladder

Notes

These coronal T1-weighted images elegantly demonstrate the way in which the anteverted uterine body rests on the bladder. It is important to realize that the support for the pelvic organs comes mainly from the tone in the pelvis musculature. The levator ani are important; so too are the collective contributions of all the muscles attached to the inferior bony pelvis, many of which converge directly or indirectly on the region of the perineal body. All of these muscles play a part in supporting the pelvic organs and ultimately preventing prolapse and incontinence – hence the importance of practising pelvic-floor exercises before and after pregnancy.

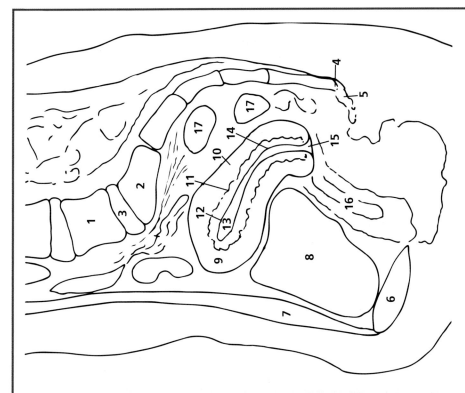

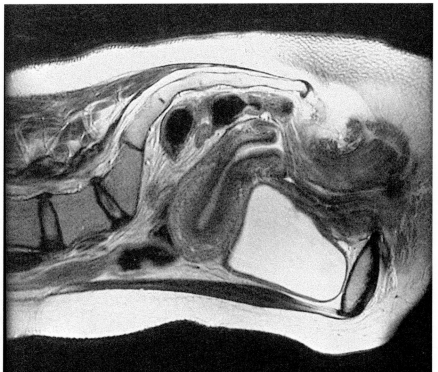

Sagittal magnetic resonance image (MRI)

Section level

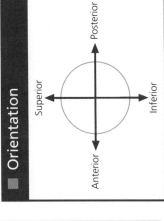

View

Orientation

Superior

Posterior

Inferior

Anterior

1 L5 vertebral body
2 S1 vertebral body
3 L5/S1 intervertebral disc
4 Lowest fixed point of sacrococcygeal region (here probably coccyx 1/2)
5 Rest of coccyx (mobile)
6 Pubic symphysis
7 Rectus abdominis
8 Bladder
9 Fundus of uterus
10 Myometrium of uterus
11 Junctional zone between myometrium and endometrium
12 Endometrium of uterus
13 Cavity of uterus
14 Internal os of uterus
15 External os of uterus
16 Vagina
17 Rectum

Notes

This midline sagittal T2-weighted magnetic resonace image illustrates many of the important features of the female pelvis. The bony dimensions can be assessed easily. The anteroposterior (AP) diameter of the pelvic inlet (from the superoposterior aspect of the pubic symphysis to the anterior aspect of the promontory on S1) is of key importance for obstetrics; ideally, this should be about 12 cm – the fetal head has a diameter of about 10.5 cm. The AP diameter of the mid-pelvis is usually somewhat larger; this is where rotation of the fetal head occurs during childbirth – much depends on the shape of the sacrum. The AP diameter of the pelvic outlet (from the inferior posterior aspect of the pubic symphysis to the anterior aspect of the lowest fixed point of the sacrum – usually the sacrococcygeal junction) should be similar to that of the inlet or sacrum; only rarely do the common anomalies at this site cause problems during childbirth.

The anatomy of the uterus is shown well. This anteverted uterus (the common arrangement) is seen clearly resting on a semi-distended bladder. The cavity is defined sharply by the endometrium, and then by the junctional zone and the myometrium peripherally. The relationship of the internal and external ostia of the cervix to the vaginal vault is shown well, as is the close relationship of the vagina and the rectum. It is important to realize that many of these relationships vary according to the degree of distension of the urinary bladder and rectum and the strength of the pelvic-floor muscles on a semi-distended bladder. The body of the uterus is usually found to be flexed forwards on the cervix, as in this section, in the so-called anteflexed position.

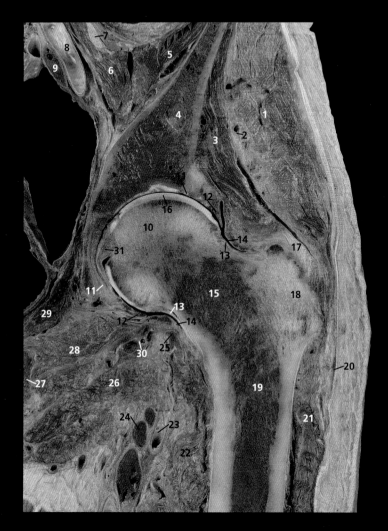

1   Gluteus medius
2   Superior gluteal
    neurovascular bundle
3   Gluteus minimus
4   Ilium
5   Iliacus
6   Psoas major
7   Femoral nerve
8   External iliac artery
9   External iliac vein
10   Head of femur
11   Rim of acetabulum
12   Acetabular labrum
13   Zona orbicularis of capsule
14   Capsule of hip joint
15   Neck of femur
16   Articular cartilage

17   Iliofemoral ligament
18   Greater trochanter
19   Shaft of femur
20   Iliotibial tract
21   Vastus lateralis
22   Vastus medialis
23   Profunda femoris artery
24   Profunda femoris vein
25   Iliopsoas tendon
26   Adductor longus
27   Ischiopubic ramus
28   Obturator externus
29   Obturator internus
30   Medial circumflex femoral
    artery and vein
31   Ligament of head of femur
    (ligamentum teres)

Section level

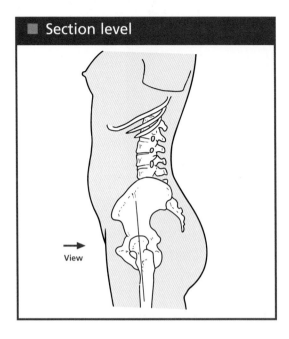

View

Orientation

Superior

Medial ← → Lateral

Inferior

Notes

This coronal section through the hip illustrates the 'ball-and-socket' arrangement of the joint. This socket is much deeper and the ball much rounder than at the shoulder. Stability is an important function here. The two powerful abductors of the hip – gluteus medius (**1**) and minimus (**3**) – have their own neurovascular bundle (the superior gluteal nerve, artery and vein), and these can be seen between the two sheets of muscle (**2**).

The ligament of the head of the femur, the ligamentum teres (**31**), is the important source of blood supply to the femoral head in the fetus and infant. It transmits the acetabular branch of the obturator artery. It becomes obliterated during early childhood, when periosteal vessels are of key importance before vessels traverse the epiphyseal plate. The blood supply to the femoral head remains of importance throughout life: avascular necrosis has many causes. The zona orbicularis of the capsule of the hip joint (**13**) transmits vessels from the lateral and medial circumflex femoral branches of the deep femoral artery (profunda femoris) to the head and neck of the femur (**10**). A subcapital fracture of the femoral head thus deprives the head of its blood supply and often leads to avascular necrosis.

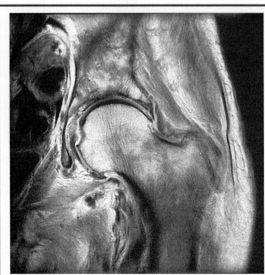

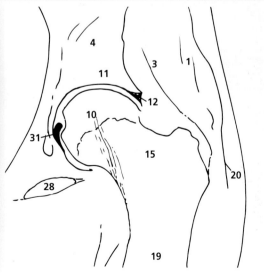

Coronal magnetic resonance image (MRI)

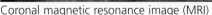

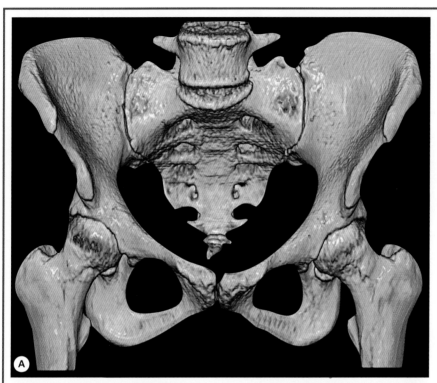

3D computed
tomogram (CT)

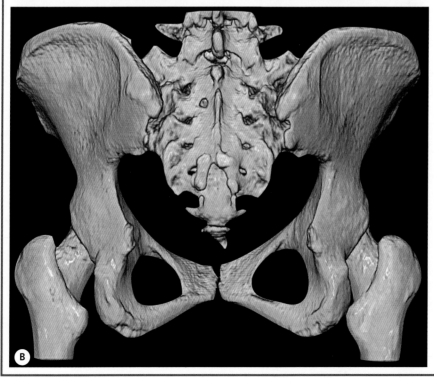

3D computed
tomogram (CT)

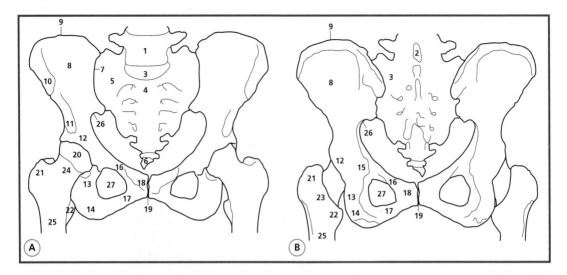

■ Orientation

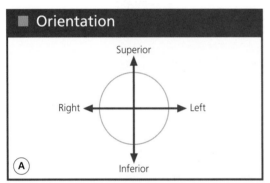

Superior

Right ← → Left

Inferior

(A)

■ Orientation

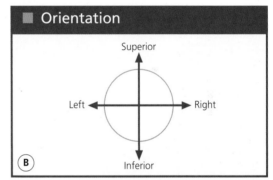

Superior

Left ← → Right

Inferior

(B)

■ Notes

Surface-shaded three-dimensional volume-rendered CT images. Because bone attenuates the X-ray beam so much, its CT attenuation value (around +1000 HU) is much greater than that of the surrounding soft tissues. Thus, the bones can be 'extracted', with no overlying artefacts, to provide information equivalent to that from a cadaveric skeleton.

These two views, anterior and posterior, show the general principles of the pelvic girdle well. Note how the femoral head (two-thirds of a hemisphere) is much better contained within the acetabular fossa than the humeral head, thereby providing stability at the expense of mobility. The obliquity of the acetabulum means that the femoral head can just be seen on the anterior view, but not posteriorly.

1 Body of fifth lumbar vertebra	8 Ilium	19 Pubic symphysis
2 Spinous process of fifth lumbar vertebra	9 Iliac crest	20 Head of femur
	10 Anterior superior iliac spine	21 Greater trochanter
3 Intervertebral disc between fifth lumbar vertebra and first segment of sacrum	11 Anterior inferior iliac spine	22 Lesser trochanter
	12 Acetabulum	23 Intertrochanteric crest
	13 Ischium	24 Neck of femur
4 Promontory of sacrum	14 Ischial tuberosity	25 Shaft of femur
5 Upper surface of latter part of sacrum (ala)	15 Ischial spine	26 Greater sciatic notch
	16 Superior pubic ramus	27 Obturator foramen
6 Coccyx	17 Inferior pubic ramus	
7 Sacroiliac joint	18 Body of pubic bone	

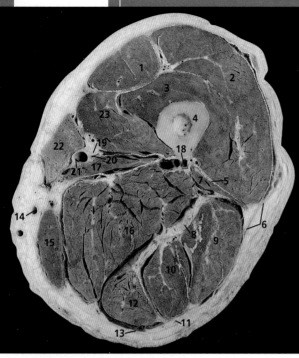

1 Rectus femoris
2 Vastus lateralis
3 Vastus intermedius
4 Femur
5 Lateral intermuscular septum
6 Iliotibial tract
7 Biceps femoris – short head
8 Sciatic nerve
9 Biceps femoris – long head
10 Semitendinosus
11 Posterior cutaneous nerve of thigh
12 Semimembranosus
13 Fascia lata (deep fascia of thigh)
14 Great saphenous vein
15 Gracilis
16 Adductor magnus
17 Adductor longus
18 Profunda femoris artery
19 Saphenous nerve
20 Femoral vein
21 Femoral artery
22 Sartorius
23 Vastus medialis

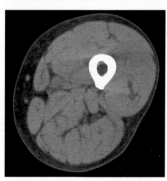

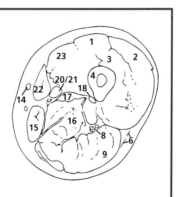

Axial computed tomogram (CT)

■ Orientation

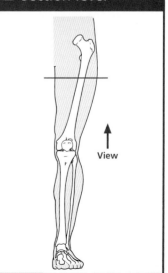

Anterior

Medial ←——→ Lateral

Posterior

■ Section level

View

■ Notes

This section passes through the upper third of the thigh and provides a useful view of the three muscular compartments of the thigh:

- The **anterior compartment**, containing quadriceps femoris, made up of the vasti (**2**, **3**, **23**) and rectus femoris (**1**), supplied by the femoral nerve.
- The **adductor compartment**, containing the three adductors (of which only adductor magnus (**16**) and adductor longus (**17**) are present at this level, brevis having already found insertion into the femoral shaft), together with gracilis (**15**). These muscles are supplied by the obturator nerve; in addition, adductor magnus receives innervation from the sciatic nerve.
- The **posterior compartment** contains the hamstrings, the biceps with its long (**9**) and short heads (**7**), semitendinosus (**10**) and semimembranosus (**12**), all supplied by the sciatic nerve.

Sartorius (**22**) lies in a separate fascial sheath.

212

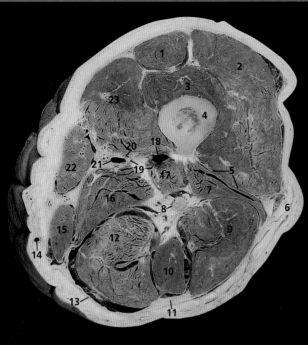

1 Rectus femoris
2 Vastus lateralis
3 Vastus intermedius
4 Femur
5 Lateral intermuscular septum
6 Iliotibial tract
7 Biceps femoris – short head
8 Sciatic nerve
9 Biceps femoris – long head
10 Semitendinosus
11 Posterior cutaneous nerve of thigh
12 Semimembranosus
13 Fascia lata (deep fascia of thigh)
14 Great saphenous vein
15 Gracilis
16 Adductor magnus – medial part
17 Adductor magnus – lateral part
18 Profunda femoris artery
19 Saphenous nerve
20 Superficial femoral vein
21 Superficial femoral artery
22 Sartorius
23 Vastus medialis

Orientation

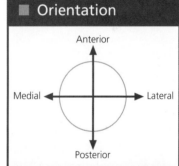

Section level

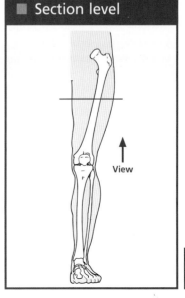

View

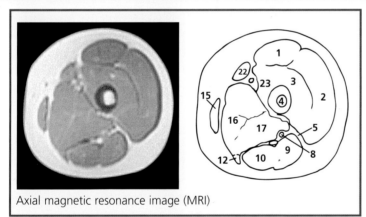

Axial magnetic resonance image (MRI)

Notes

This section passes through the mid-shaft of the femur (**4**). Note that at this level, adductor magnus is dividing into two sections. Its lateral part (**17**), which arises from the ischial ramus, forms a broad aponeurosis, which inserts along the linea aspera along the posterior border of the femoral shaft (**4**). The medial part (**16**), which arises mainly from the ischial tuberosity, descends almost vertically to a tendinous attachment to the adductor tubercle of the medial condyle of the femur. Between the two parts distally is the osseo-aponeurotic adductor hiatus, which admits the femoral vessels to the popliteal fossa.

Being a composite muscle, adductor magnus also has a composite nerve supply; the medial part is innervated by the tibial division of the sciatic nerve (**8**) and the lateral part by the obturator nerve.

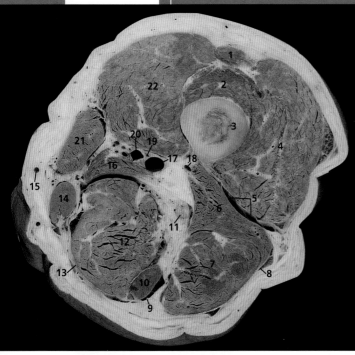

1 Rectus femoris	12 Semimembranosus
2 Vastus intermedius	13 Fascia lata (deep
3 Femur	fascia of thigh)
4 Vastus lateralis	14 Gracilis
5 Lateral	15 Great saphenous
intermuscular	vein
septum	16 Adductor magnus
6 Biceps femoris –	17 Superficial femoral
short head	vein
7 Biceps femoris –	18 Profunda femoris
long head	artery and vein
8 Iliotibial tract	19 Saphenous nerve
9 Posterior cutaneous	20 Superficial femoral
nerve of thigh	artery
10 Semitendinosus	21 Sartorius
11 Sciatic nerve	22 Vastus medialis

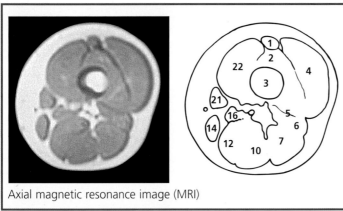

Axial magnetic resonance image (MRI)

Orientation

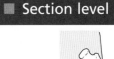

Anterior

Medial ← → Lateral

Posterior

Section level

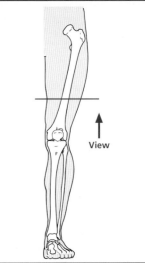

View

Notes

This section transects the lower third of the thigh. This and the previous two sections demonstrate the anatomy of the adductor, or subsartorial, canal (Hunter's canal). This is formed as a triangular aponeurotic tunnel, which leads from the femoral triangle above to the popliteal fossa below, via the hiatus in adductor magnus. The canal lies between sartorius (**21**) anteromedially, adductor longus and, more distally, adductor magnus (**16**) posteriorly and vastus medialis (**22**) anterolaterally. Its contents are the femoral artery (**20**) and vein (**17**), the saphenous nerve (**19**) and the nerve to vastus medialis until this enters and supplies this muscle.

John Hunter (1728–93) described ligation of the femoral artery within this canal in the treatment of popliteal aneurysm, and his name is now used to describe the canal.

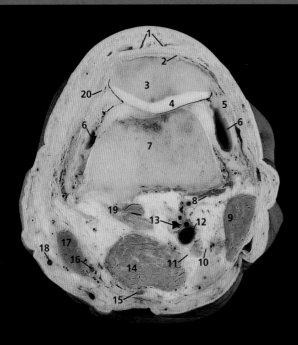

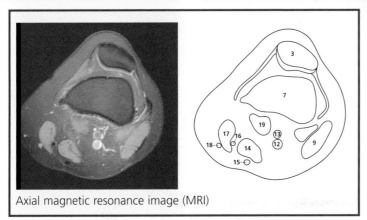

1	Prepatellar bursa	**11**	Tibial nerve
2	Tendon of	**12**	Popliteal vein
	quadriceps femoris	**13**	Popliteal artery
3	Patella	**14**	Semimembranosus
4	Articular cartilage of	**15**	Semitendinosus
	patella	**16**	Gracilis tendon
5	Lateral patellar	**17**	Sartorius
	retinaculum	**18**	Great saphenous
6	Capsule of knee		vein
	joint	**19**	Gastrocnemius
7	Femur	**20**	Tendon of vastus
8	Plantaris origin		medialis
9	Biceps femoris		
10	Common fibular	**21**	Vastus medialis
	(peroneal) nerve		

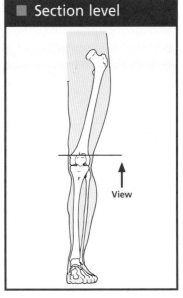

Orientation

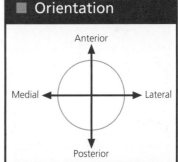

Axial magnetic resonance image (MRI)

Section level

Notes

This section passes through the upper part of the patella (**3**) and the femur just as this widens into its condyles (**7**). Note how the lateral portion of the patella (**3**) has a larger and flatter articular surface than the medial surface. This, together with the low insertion of vastus medialis (**20**) into the medial side of the patella, helps to prevent lateral dislocation of the patella. The exact alignment of the patellar depends on the relative contributions of the vasti muscles via their tendons (medial and lateral retincacula).

The sciatic nerve has now divided into the common fibular (peroneal) nerve (**10**) and tibial nerve (**11**); the latter is usually about twice the size of the former. Division usually takes place just proximal to the knee, but the sciatic nerve may divide anywhere along its course. Indeed, its division may take place at the sciatic plexus, when the common fibular (peroneal) nerve usually pierces the piriformis muscle in the greater sciatic foramen and the tibial division emerges caudal to this muscle.

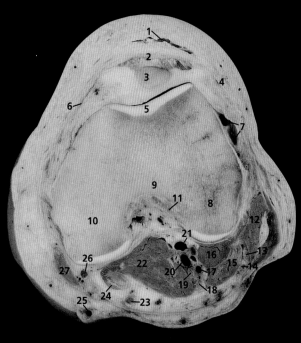

1 Prepatellar bursa	**14** Sural
2 Ligamentum	communicating
patellae	nerve
3 Patella	**15** Gastrocnemius –
4 Lateral patellar	lateral head
retinaculum	**16** Plantaris
5 Articular cartilage of	**17** Small saphenous
femur	vein – termination
6 Medial patellar	**18** Sural nerve
retinaculum	**19** Tibial nerve
7 Capsule of knee	**20** Popliteal vein
joint	**21** Popliteal artery
8 Lateral condyle of	**22** Gastrocnemius –
femur	medial head
9 Intercondylar fossa	**23** Semitendinosus
10 Medial condyle of	tendon
femur	**24** Semimembranosus
11 Anterior cruciate	tendon
ligament	**25** Great saphenous
12 Biceps femoris	vein
13 Common fibular	**26** Gracilis tendon
(peroneal) nerve	**27** Sartorius

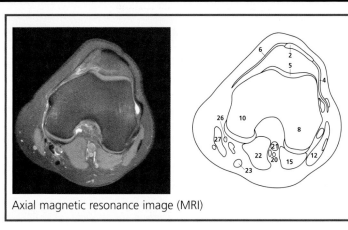

Axial magnetic resonance image (MRI)

■ Orientation

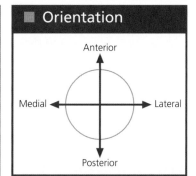

■ Section level

■ Notes

This section passes through the distal extremity of the patella (**3**) and the femoral condyles (**8**, **10**).

The anterior cruciate ligament (**11**) arises from the intercondylar fossa (**9**) of the femur laterally and slightly more proximally than the posterior cruciate ligament, whose attachment is seen better in the next cadaveric section. The anterior cruciate ligament passes downwards and forwards laterally to the posterior cruciate ligament, to attach to the anterior intercondylar area of the tibia.

The small saphenous vein (**17**), which will be seen in later sections as it lies in the superficial fascia of the back of the calf, has here pierced the deep fascia of the popliteal fossa and is about to drain into the popliteal vein (**20**). On the magnetic resonance images, these veins are joining.

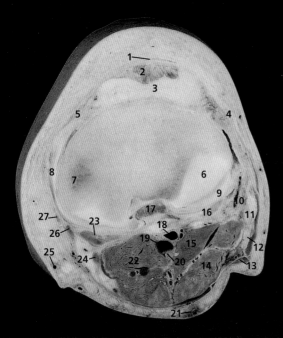

1 Infrapatellar bursa
2 Ligamentum patellae
3 Infrapatellar fat pad
4 Lateral patellar retinaculum
5 Medial patellar retinaculum
6 Sliver of cartilage over lateral condyle of tibia
7 Medial condyle of tibia
8 Medial collateral ligament
9 Lateral meniscus
10 Lateral collateral ligament
11 Tendon of biceps femoris
12 Common fibular (peroneal) nerve
13 Lateral cutaneous nerve of calf
14 Gastrocnemius lateral head
15 Plantaris
16 Popliteus
17 Posterior cruciate ligament
18 Popliteal artery
19 Popliteal vein
20 Tibial nerve
21 Small saphenous vein
22 Gastrocnemius – medial head
23 Semimembranosus tendon
24 Semitendinosus tendon
25 Great saphenous vein
26 Gracilis tendon
27 Sartorius tendon
28 Semimembranosus bursa

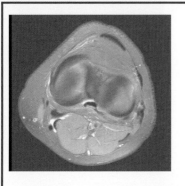

Axial magnetic resonance image (MRI)

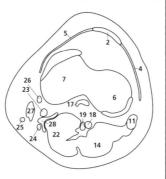

■ Orientation

Anterior

Medial ←→ Lateral

Posterior

■ Section level

View

■ Notes

This section passes through the tibial condyles (**6**, **7**). The posterior cruciate ligament (**17**) is here finding attachment to the posterior intercondylar area of the proximal articular surface of the tibia.

The popliteus tendon (**16**), which inserts on to the femur in a depression immediately distal to the lateral epicondyle, passes between the lateral meniscus (**9**) and the lateral collateral ligament (**10**) of the knee. In contrast, the medial collateral ligament (**8**) is applied closely to the medial meniscus, which lies just proximal to this plane of section. This tethering of the medial meniscus probably accounts for the much higher incidence of tears of the medial compared with the lateral meniscus.

The semimembranosus bursa contains a trace of fluid on the magnetic resonance image (**28**). It can enlarge greatly to form a popliteal cyst (a misnomer).

217

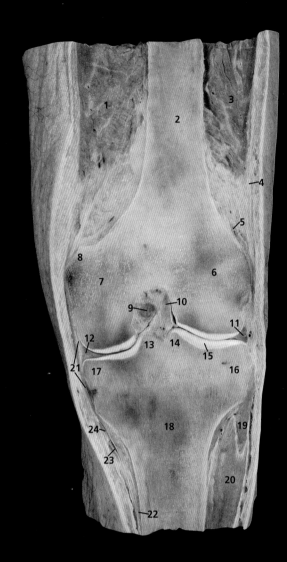

1 Vastus medialis
2 Shaft of femur
3 Vastus lateralis
4 Fascia lata
5 Superior lateral genicular artery
6 Lateral condyle of femur
7 Medial condyle of femur
8 Adductor tubercle of femur
9 Posterior cruciate ligament
10 Anterior cruciate ligament
11 Lateral meniscus
12 Medial meniscus
13 Medial intercondylar eminence/tubercle
    (also known as spine)
14 Lateral intercondylar eminence/tubercle
    (also known as spine)
15 Articular cartilage

16 Lateral condyle (plateau) of tibia
17 Medial condyle (plateau) of tibia
18 Tibia
19 Extensor digitorum longus
20 Tibialis anterior
21 Medial collateral ligament
22 Popliteus (most medial fibres)
23 Tendon of gracilis
24 Tendon of sartorius

25 Popliteus tendon
26 Lateral collateral ligament
27 Head of fibula
28 Great saphenous vein
29 Medial gastrocnemius
30 Biceps femoris

Section level

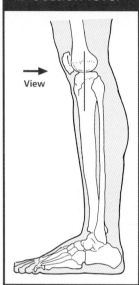

View

Notes

The posterior cruciate ligament (**9**) lies on the medial side of the anterior cruciate ligament (**10**). The former prevents posterior sliding movement of the tibia on the femur, while the latter prevents anterior displacement and resists torsional movement at the knee joint. They may be torn in violent torsional injury of the knee especially in the flexed position, when the collateral ligaments (**21**) are less tense.

It can be seen that the menisci (**11**, **12**) do little to deepen the concavity of the knee joint on either side. They do act, however, as 'shock absorbers' at the knee, for example when jumping from a height.

Note that the medial collateral ligament is continuous with the medial meniscus, whereas the lateral collateral ligament is discontinuous with the lateral meniscus. This contributes to the medial meniscus being more static and being injured more commonly; the lateral meniscus is more mobile.

Orientation

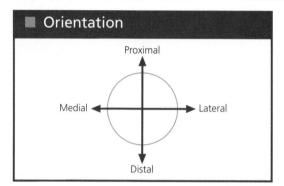

Proximal

Medial ← → Lateral

Distal

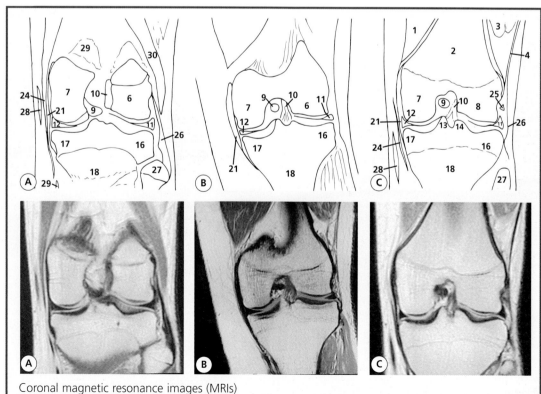

Coronal magnetic resonance images (MRIs)

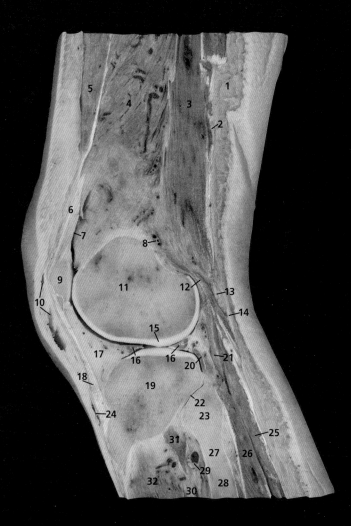

1 Superficial fascia
2 Deep fascia
3 Biceps femoris
4 Vastus intermedius
5 Vastus lateralis
6 Tendon of quadriceps femoris
7 Suprapatellar bursa
8 Lateral superior geniculate artery and vein
9 Patella
10 Prepatellar bursa
11 Lateral condyle of femur
12 Fibrous capsule of knee joint
13 Common fibular (peroneal) nerve
14 Lateral cutaneous nerve of calf
15 Articular cartilage
16 Lateral meniscus

17 Infrapatellar pad of fat extending into infrapatellar fold
18 Ligamentum patellae
19 Lateral condyle (plateau) of tibia
20 Tendon of popliteus
21 Plantaris
22 Superior tibiofibular joint
23 Head of fibula
24 Infrapatellar bursa
25 Gastrocnemius lateral
26 Soleus
27 Neck of fibula
28 Shaft of fibula
29 Anterior tibial artery and vein
30 Interosseous membrane
31 Tibialis posterior
32 Tibialis anterior

Section level

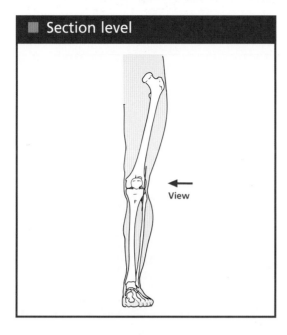

View

Orientation

Proximal

Anterior ← → Posterior

Distal

Notes

The prepatellar bursa (**10**) and infrapatellar bursa (**24**) are both subcutaneous. Either may become inflamed by continual kneeling, which produces a traumatic bursitis. A prepatellar bursa comes into contact with the ground on scrubbing the floor (hence 'housemaid's knee'), while the infrapatellar bursa does so when kneeling to pray (hence 'clergyman's knee').

The communication of the suprapatellar bursa (**7**) with the main synovial cavity of the knee is demonstrated well. It extends a hand's breadth superior to the border of the patella (**9**) and lies posterior to the quadriceps tendon (**6**). It becomes distended when there is an effusion into the knee joint. A puncture wound within a hand's breadth of the superior border of the patella must always be suspected of having penetrated the knee joint. Failure to do so may result in septic arthritis of the knee.

Plantaris (**21**) is absent in about ten per cent of subjects. Very rarely, it has two heads.

The tendon of popliteus (**20**) is connected to the lateral meniscus (**16**). It may thus retract and protect the mobile lateral meniscus during lateral rotation of the femur in flexion of the knee joint, protecting the meniscus from being crushed between the femoral and tibial condyles during this movement.

The superior tibiofibular joint (**22**) is a plane synovial joint, in contrast to the fibrous inferior tibiofibular joint.

The lateral meniscus is of even thickness throughout. Thus, a lateral sagittal slice creates a bowtie appearance to this portion of the lateral meniscus.

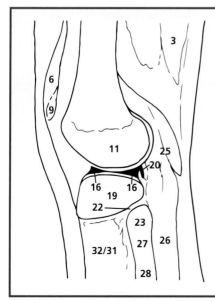

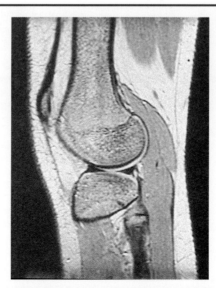

Sagittal magnetic resonance image (MRI)

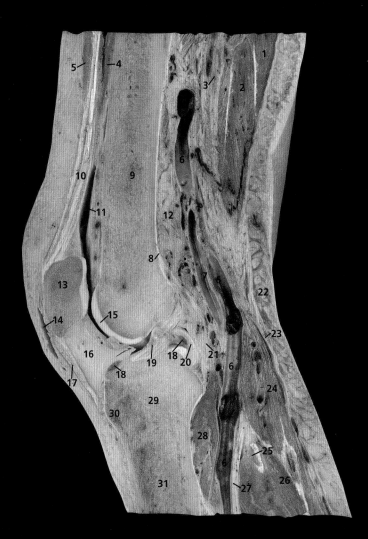

1 Semitendinosus
2 Semimembranosus
3 Sciatic nerve
4 Vastus intermedius
5 Rectus femoris
6 Popliteal vein
7 Popliteal artery
8 Popliteal surface of femur
9 Shaft of femur
10 Tendon of quadriceps femoris
11 Suprapatellar bursa
12 Popliteal pad of fat
13 Patella
14 Prepatellar bursa
15 Articular cartilage
16 Infrapatellar pad of fat (Hoffa)
   extending into infrapatellar fold

17 Ligamentum patellae
18 Medial meniscus
19 Anterior cruciate ligament
20 Posterior cruciate ligament
21 Fibrous capsule of knee joint
22 Superficial fascia
23 Deep fascia
24 Gastrocnemius
25 Tendon of plantaris
26 Soleus
27 Tibial nerve
28 Popliteus
29 Proximal end of tibia
30 Tibial tuberosity
31 Shaft of tibia

32 Transverse intermeniscal ligament

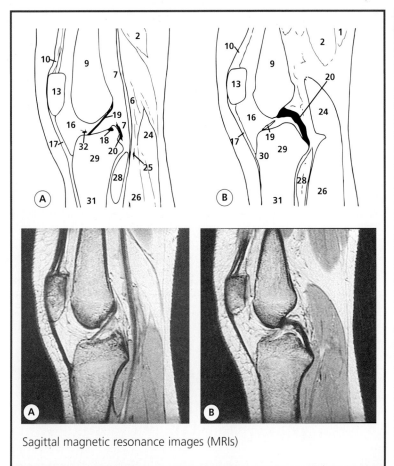

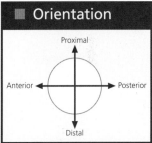

Sagittal magnetic resonance images (MRIs)

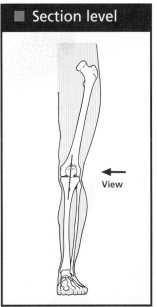

View

■ Orientation

Proximal

Anterior ◄———————► Posterior

Distal

■ Notes

The relationships in the popliteal fossa comprise the tibial nerve (**27**) most superficially, the popliteal vein (**6**) and then, more deeply, the popliteal artery (**7**). The valves in the vein are shown well. It is within these large veins that postoperative (or post-immobilization) thrombosis of the deep veins of the lower limb usually commences.

The fossa contains a large amount of fat (**12**) as well as the rather insignificant popliteal lymph nodes, usually five or six in number. Note the composition of the floor of the popliteal fossa comprises superiorly the popliteal surface of the femur (**8**), the capsule of the knee joint (**21**) and finally popliteus (**28**).

Both gastrocnemius (**24**) and soleus (**26**) contain large veins, an important component of the calf pump mechanism in venous return from the lower limb. Note also the density of the deep fascia (**23**), which assists the pumping action of the muscles.

Note that with the knee in the extended position, the anterior cruciate ligament is taut and straight; there is less tension on the posterior cruciate, which appears curved in that position. The cruciate ligaments take their names (anterior and posterior) from the site of attachment to the tibia. The anterior cruciate passes lateral to the posterior ligament.

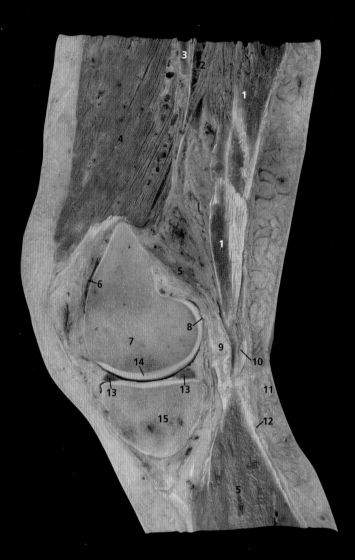

1 Semimembranosus
2 Adductor magnus
3 Femoral artery
4 Vastus medialis
5 Medial gastrocnemius
6 Suprapatellar bursa
7 Medial condyle of femur
8 Fibrous capsule of knee joint
9 Medial head/tendon of gastrocnemius
10 Tendon of semitendinosus
11 Superficial fascia
12 Deep fascia
13 Medial meniscus
14 Articular cartilage
15 Medial condyle (plateau of tibia)

■ Section level

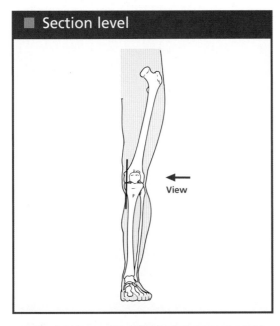

View

■ Orientation

Proximal

Anterior ← → Posterior

Distal

■ Notes

The femoral artery (**3**) passes through the hiatus in adductor magnus (**2**) to become the popliteal artery about two-thirds of the distance along a line that joins the femoral pulse at the groin, with the adductor tubercle on the medial condyle of the femur.

The posterior third of the medial meniscus is usually a little thicker than the mid and anterior thirds, in contrast to the lateral meniscus, which is of constant thickness around its circumference. Furthermore, the posterior third frequently undergoes myxoid change during early middle age; thus, this part of the medial meniscus often appears rather heterogeneous in consistency.

This section shows the possible consequence of a fracture of the shaft of the femur at its lower extremity. The medial (**9**) and lateral heads of gastrocnemius tilt the otherwise unsupported distal femoral fragment posteriorly. This may well injure the popliteal vessels, lying immediately behind. (See also Sagittal section 2.)

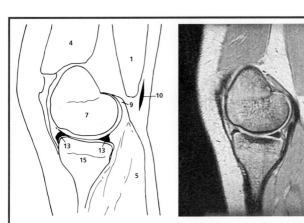

Sagittal magnetic resonance image (MRI)

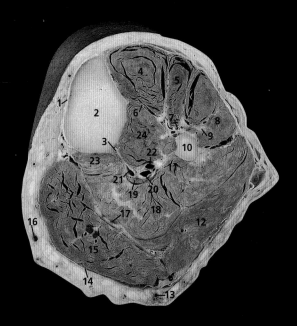

1 Subcutaneous surface of tibia
2 Tibia
3 Vertical ridge of tibia
4 Tibialis anterior
5 Extensor digitorum longus
6 Interosseous membrane
7 Anterior tibial artery and vein, with deep fibular (peroneal) nerve
8 Fibularis (peroneus) longus
9 Superficial fibular (peroneal) nerve
10 Fibula
11 Medial crest of fibula
12 Gastrocnemius – lateral head
13 Small saphenous vein
14 Deep fascia of calf
15 Gastrocnemius – medial head
16 Great saphenous vein
17 Plantaris tendon
18 Soleus
19 Tibial nerve
20 Posterior tibial artery
21 Posterior tibial vein
22 Fibular (peroneal) artery
23 Popliteus
24 Tibialis posterior

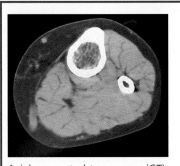

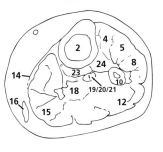

Axial computed tomogram (CT)

■ Orientation

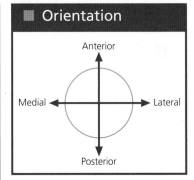

■ Section level

■ Notes

This section traverses the proximal end of the tibial shaft (**2**) and the shaft of the fibula (**10**) immediately distal to the neck of the fibula.

At this level, the common fibular (peroneal) nerve, which sweeps around the neck of the fibula deep to fibularis (peroneus) longus (**8**), has divided into its superficial fibular (peroneal) (**9**) and deep fibular (peroneal) (**7**) branches. The superficial fibular (peroneal) nerve lies deep to fibularis (peroneus) longus. The deep fibular (peroneal) nerve passes obliquely forwards, deep to extensor digitorum longus (**5**), to descend with the anterior tibial vessels (**7**).

The tendon of plantaris (**17**) lies in a well-defined tissue plane between soleus (**18**) and gastrocnemius (**12**, **15**). Fluid enters this plane following rupture of a semimembranosus bursa (Baker's cyst).

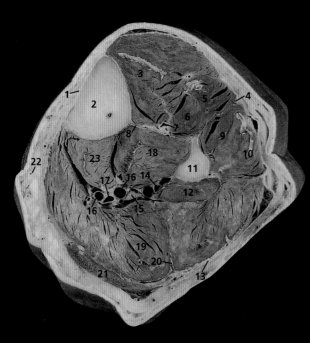

1 Subcutaneous border of tibia
2 Tibia
3 Tibialis anterior
4 Superficial fibular (peroneal) nerve
5 Extensor digitorum longus
6 Extensor hallucis longus
7 Anterior tibial artery and vein, with deep fibular (peroneal) nerve
8 Interosseous membrane
9 Fibularis (peroneus) brevis
10 Fibularis (peroneus) longus
11 Fibula
12 Flexor hallucis longus
13 Deep fascia of calf
14 Fibular (peroneal) artery, with venae comitantes
15 Tibial nerve
16 Venae comitantes of posterior tibial artery
17 Posterior tibial artery
18 Tibialis posterior
19 Soleus
20 Plantaris tendon
21 Gastrocnemius
22 Great saphenous vein
23 Flexor digitorum longus

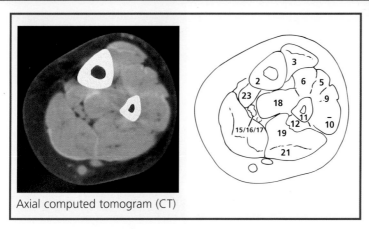

Axial computed tomogram (CT)

■ Orientation

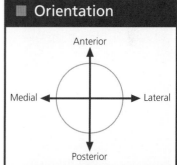

Anterior

Medial ← → Lateral

Posterior

■ Section level

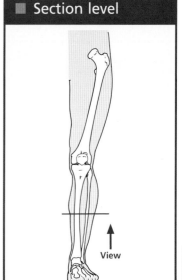

View

■ Notes

This section traverses the mid-calf. Note that the whole of the anteromedial aspect of the shaft of the tibia (**1**) is subcutaneous, covered only by skin, superficial fascia and periosteum, and crossed, in its lower part, only by the great saphenous vein (**22**) and saphenous nerve.

The neurovascular bundle of the anterior tibial vessels and deep fibular (peroneal) nerve (**7**), having descended first between extensor digitorum longus (**5**) and tibialis anterior (**3**), now runs between the latter and extensor hallucis longus (**6**), as this takes origin from the anterior aspect of the fibular shaft (**11**).

227

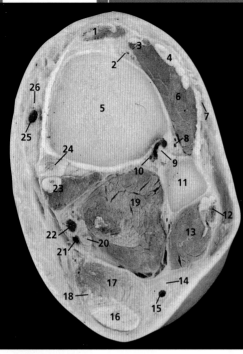

1 Tibialis anterior tendon
2 Anterior tibial artery, with venae comitantes and deep fibular (peroneal) nerve
3 Extensor hallucis longus and tendon
4 Extensor digitorum longus tendon
5 Tibia
6 Fibularis (peroneus) tertius
7 Superficial fibular (peroneal) nerve
8 Perforating branch of fibular (peroneal) artery
9 Inferior tibiofibular joint (interosseous ligament)
10 Fibular (peroneal) artery
11 Fibula
12 Fibularis (peroneus) longus tendon
13 Fibularis (peroneus) brevis
14 Sural nerve
15 Small saphenous vein
16 Tendo calcaneus (Achilles tendon)
17 Soleus
18 Plantaris tendon
19 Flexor hallucis longus
20 Tibial nerve
21 Posterior tibial vein
22 Posterior tibial artery
23 Flexor digitorum longus and tendon
24 Tibialis posterior tendon
25 Great saphenous vein
26 Saphenous nerve

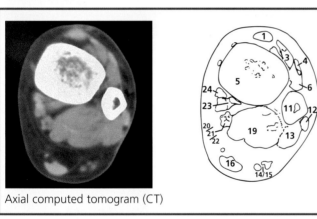

Axial computed tomogram (CT)

■ Orientation

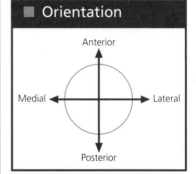

Anterior

Medial ◄——————► Lateral

Posterior

■ Section level

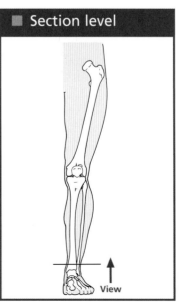

View

■ Notes

This section passes immediately above the ankle joint at the level of the inferior tibiofibular joint (**9**). This is the only fibrous joint, apart from the skull sutures, and represents the thickened distal extremity of the interosseous membrane. (See also Axial section 2.)

At this level, gastrocnemius has already become tendinous (**16**), although soleus (**17**) still displays muscle fibres. A little more distally, this too will become tendinous and fuse into the tendo calcaneus (tendo Achilles tendon).

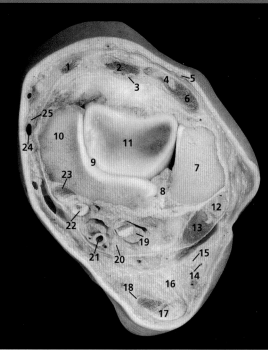

1 Tibialis anterior tendon
2 Extensor hallucis longus and tendon
3 Anterior tibial artery and venae comitantes, with deep fibular (peroneal) nerve
4 Extensor digitorum tendon
5 Superficial fibular (peroneal) nerve
6 Fibularis (peroneus) tertius and tendon
7 Lateral malleolus
8 Inferior tibiofibular joint
9 Ankle joint
10 Medial malleolus
11 Talus
12 Fibularis (peroneus) brevis tendon
13 Fibularis (peroneus) longus
14 Small saphenous vein
15 Sural nerve
16 Fat
17 Tendo calcaneus
18 Plantaris tendon
19 Flexor hallucis longus tendon
20 Tibial nerve
21 Posterior tibial artery, with venae comitantes
22 Flexor digitorum longus tendon
23 Tibialis posterior tendon
24 Great saphenous vein
25 Saphenous nerve

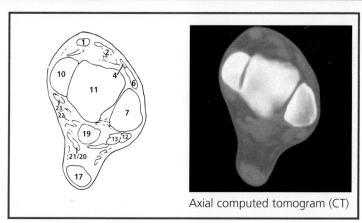

Axial computed tomogram (CT)

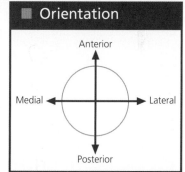

Orientation

Anterior
Medial — Lateral
Posterior

Section level

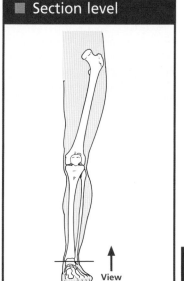

View

Notes

This section passes through the ankle joint (**9**) and the inferior tibiofibular joint (**8**). Note that this section illustrates the fibrous nature of the inferior tibiofibular joint.

Fibularis (peroneus) brevis (**12**) and fibularis (peroneus) longus (**13**) pass behind the lateral malleolus (**7**) of the fibula and will groove the bone a little more distally to form the malleolar fossa.

This section demonstrates the order of structures that pass behind the medial malleolus (**10**). These are, from the medial to the lateral side, the tendon of tibialis posterior (**23**), the tendon of flexor digitorum longus (**22**), the posterior tibial artery with its venae comitantes (**21**), the tibial nerve (**20**) and, most laterally, the tendon of flexor hallucis longus (**19**).

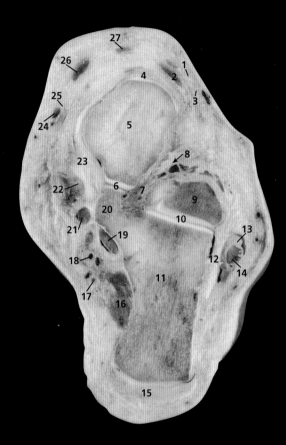

1 Extensor digitorum longus tendon
2 Extensor digitorum brevis
3 Fibularis (peroneus) tertius tendon
4 Talocalcaneonavicular joint
  (anterior talonavicular part)
5 Head of talus
6 Talocalcaneonavicular joint
  (posterior part)
7 Interosseous talocalcanean
  ligament
8 Sulcus tali (arrowed)
9 Lateral process of talus
10 Talocalcanean (subtalar) joint
11 Calcaneus
12 Capsule of talocalcanean joint
13 Fibularis (peroneus) brevis tendon
14 Fibularis (peroneus) longus tendon
15 Tendo Achilles
16 Quadratus plantae (flexor
  accessorius)

17 Lateral plantar neurovascular
  bundle
18 Medial plantar neurovascular
  bundle
19 Flexor hallucis longus tendon
20 Sustentaculum tali
21 Flexor digitorum longus tendon
22 Tibialis posterior tendon
23 Deltoid ligament of ankle
24 Great saphenous vein
25 Saphenous nerve
26 Tibialis anterior tendon
27 Extensor hallucis longus tendon

28 Tibia
29 Medial malleolus
30 Abductor hallucis
31 Abductor digiti minimi

Section level

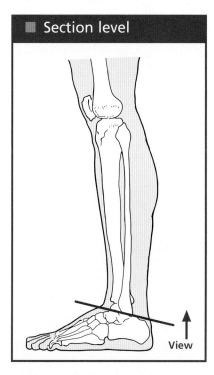

View

Orientation

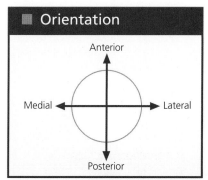

Anterior

Medial ← → Lateral

Posterior

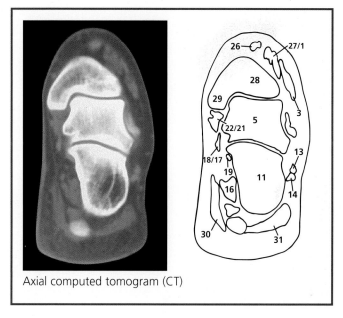

Axial computed tomogram (CT)

Notes

This section passes through the head (**5**) and lateral process (**9**) of the talus and the calcaneus (**11**). The CT image is in a more coronal plane, and hence the tibia (**28**) is seen with its articulation with the talus (**5**).

The tendon of flexor hallucis longus (**19**) passes behind the sustentaculum tali (**20**) and, more distally, grooves its inferior aspect. The sulcus tali (**8**), with its corresponding sulcus calcanei, forms the sinus tarsi and contains the strong interosseous talocalcanean ligament.

The talocalcanean joint (**10**), also termed the subtalar joint, lies between the convex posterior facet on the upper surface of the calcaneus and the concave posterior facet on the inferior surface of the talus. The talocalcaneonavicular joint is complex. It is formed by the rounded head of the talus (**5**), which fits into the concavity on the posterior aspect of the navicular, the upper surface of the plantar calcaneonavicular ligament (the spring ligament), which runs between the sustentaculum tali and the inferior aspect of the navicular, and the anterior and middle facets for the talus on the calcaneus. The anterior (**4**) and posterior (**6**) portions of this joint are shown.

A considerable degree of inversion and eversion of the foot takes place at the talocalcanean and talocalcaneonavicular joints.

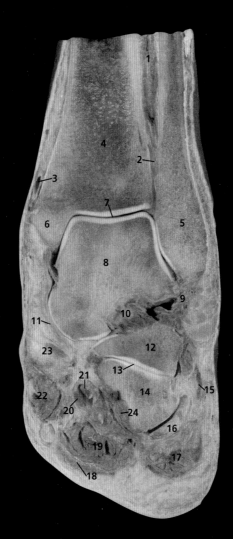

1 Tibialis posterior
2 Inferior tibiofibular joint
3 Small saphenous vein
4 Tibia
5 Lateral malleolus of fibula
6 Medial malleolus of tibia
7 Ankle joint
8 Body of talus (talar dome)
9 Lateral collateral ligament of ankle
10 Talocalcanean interosseous ligament
11 Deltoid ligament (medial collateral ligament)
12 Body of calcaneus

14 Cuboid
15 Tendon of fibularis (peroneus) brevis
16 Tendon of fibularis (peroneus) longus
17 Abductor digiti minimi
18 Plantar aponeurosis
19 Flexor digitorum brevis
20 Tendon of flexor digitorum longus
21 Tendon of flexor hallucis longus
22 Abductor hallucis
23 Tendon of tibialis posterior
24 Quadratus plantae (flexor

Section level

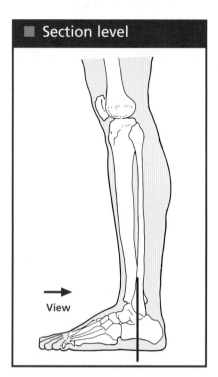

View

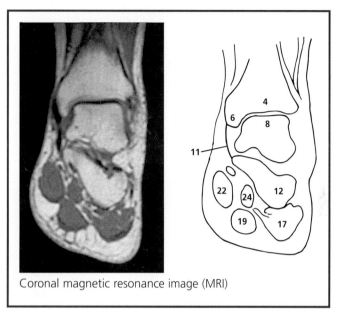

Coronal magnetic resonance image (MRI)

Orientation

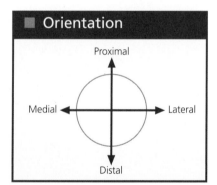

Proximal

Medial ◄──────► Lateral

Distal

Notes

By convention, the articulation between the lower end of the fibula and the tibia is described as the inferior tibiofibular joint (**2**) and is stated to be the only fibrous joint apart from those pertaining to the skull. In effect, this 'joint' represents the considerable thickening of the lowermost part of the interosseous membrane between the shafts of these two bones.

The mortice joint of the ankle (**7**) is demonstrated well. The lateral collateral ligament (**9**), especially its anterior talofibular component, is commonly injured.

The plantar aponeurosis (**18**) is thick and tough. It adheres closely to flexor digitorum brevis (**19**).

The hyaline cartilage and subchondral bone of the talar dome (**8**) is commonly damaged by relatively minor trauma. Loose fragments may break off and cause symptoms. Cystic degenerative change may follow in later life.

In spite of the fact that the talocalcanean ligament (**10**) is thick and powerful, the major part of the movements of inversion and eversion of the foot take place at this joint.

233

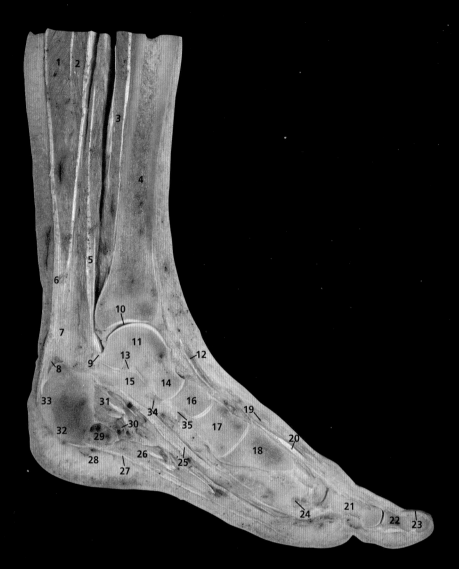

1 Gastrocnemius
2 Soleus
3 Flexor digitorum longus
4 Tibia
5 Tendon of flexor hallucis longus (posterior relation to ankle joint – see also 25)
6 Tendo calcaneus (Achilles tendon)
7 Fat deep to tendo calcaneus
8 Bursa deep to tendo calcaneous
9 Medial tubercle of posterior process of talus
10 Ankle joint
11 Body of talus
12 Tendon of tibialis anterior
13 Interosseous talocalcanean ligament
14 Head of talus
15 Sustentaculum tali
16 Navicular
17 Medial cuneiform
18 First metatarsal bone
19 Tributary of great saphenous vein
20 Extensor hallucis longus
21 Proximal phalanx of hallux
22 Distal phalanx of hallux
23 Nail bed
24 Sesamoid bone
25 Tendon of flexor hallucis longus (in foot – see also 5)
26 Abductor hallucis
27 Plantar aponeurosis
28 Dense subcutaneous fibrofatty tissue
29 Abductor digiti minimi
30 Lateral plantar artery, vein and nerve
31 Quadratus plantae (flexor accessories)
32 Medial process of tuberosity of calcaneus
33 Calcaneus
34 Plantar calcaneonavicular (spring) ligament
35 Tendon of tibialis posterior

Section level

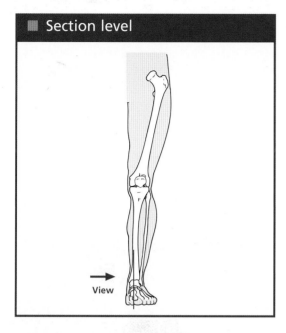

View

Orientation

Proximal

Posterior ← → Anterior

Distal

Notes

Flexor hallucis longus (**5**) is the immediate posterior relation of the ankle joint. It grooves the posterior aspect of the lower extremity of the tibia (**4**); then, distal to the capsule of the ankle joint (**10**), it grooves the posterior process of the talus between its medial (**9**) and lateral tubercle. The tendon (**25**) grooves a third bone as it passes beneath the sustentaculum tali of the calcaneus (**15**). Surprisingly, the flexor hallucis longus at this point is lateral to the flexor digitorum longus; they cross on the foot.

This section shows clearly the role of the plantar calcaneonavicular (or spring) ligament (**34**) as this passes from the sustentaculum tali (**15**) to the navicular (**16**). It supports the head of the talus (**14**). In standing, the weight of the body is borne on the medial (**32**) and lateral processes of the posterior tuberosity of the calcaneus behind, and on the heads of the metatarsals anteriorly. That of the first metatarsal, the hallux, bears two sesamoid bones (**24**), each within a tendon of flexor hallucis brevis. This section demonstrates well the dense subcutaneous fibrofatty tissue (**28**), which is developed particularly well over these two areas of contact of the foot with the ground on standing.

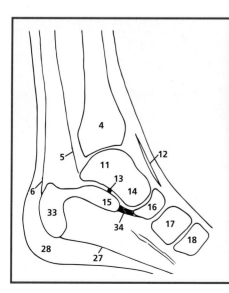

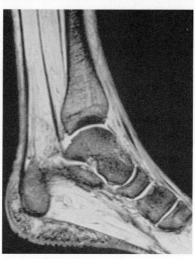

Sagittal magnetic resonance image (MRI)

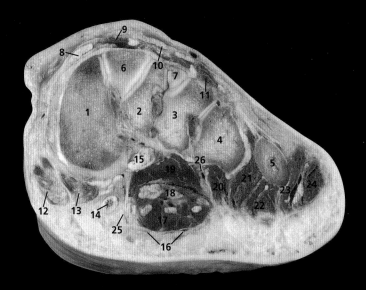

1 First metatarsal
2 Second metatarsal
3 Third metatarsal
4 Fourth metatarsal
5 Fifth metatarsal
6 Medial cuneiform
7 Fragment of lateral
   cuneiform
8 Extensor hallucis longus
   tendon
9 Extensor hallucis brevis
10 Extensor digitorum longus
   tendon
11 Extensor digitorum brevis
12 Abductor hallucis
13 Flexor hallucis brevis
14 Flexor hallucis longus
   tendon
15 Fibularis (peroneus)
   longus tendon
16 Plantar aponeurosis
17 Flexor digitorum brevis
18 Flexor digitorum longus
   tendon
19 Adductor hallucis (oblique
   head)
20 Second plantar
   interosseous
21 Third plantar interosseous
22 Flexor digiti minimi
23 Opponens digiti minimi
24 Abductor digiti minimi
25 Medial plantar artery and
   nerve
26 Lateral plantar artery and
   nerve

■ Section level

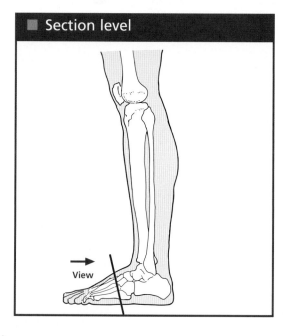

View

■ Orientation

Dorsal

Medial ◄────────► Lateral

Planter

■ Notes

This section of the lower limb passes through the forefoot and the bases of the metatarsal bones. It demonstrates the appearance of the transverse arch of the foot.

The tendon of fibularis (peroneus) longus (**15**), having grooved the inferior aspect of the cuboid, passes forward and medially to insert into the inferolateral aspect of the medial cuneiform (**6**) and the base of the first metatarsal (**1**). The sling-like action of this tendon helps maintain the transverse arch.

The medial plantar nerve (**25**) has a cutaneous distribution that closely resembles that of the median nerve of the hand – that is, the medial two-thirds of the sole of the foot and plantar aspects of the medial three and a half toes. Similarly, the lateral plantar nerve supplies the lateral third of the skin of the sole and the plantar aspects of the later one and a half toes, similar to the distribution of the ulnar nerve to the palm of the hand and fingers.

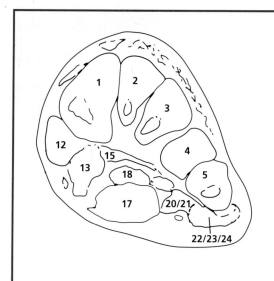

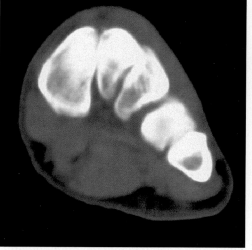

Coronal computed tomogram (CT)

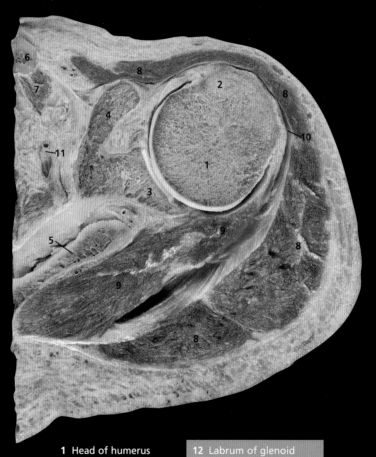

1 Head of humerus	**12** Labrum of glenoid
2 Greater tubercle of humerus	**13** Subscapularis tendon
	14 Middle glenohumeral ligament
3 Glenoid fossa of scapula	**15** Long head of biceps tendon in bicipital groove (intertubercular groove)
4 Coracoid process of scapula	
5 Spine of scapula	
6 Clavicle	
7 Subclavius	**16** Attachment of coraco-acromial and coraco-humeral ligaments
8 Deltoid	
9 Infraspinatus	
10 Subdeltoid bursa	**17** Lesser tubercle of humerus
11 Suprascapular artery and vein	**18** Transverse humeral ligament

Section level

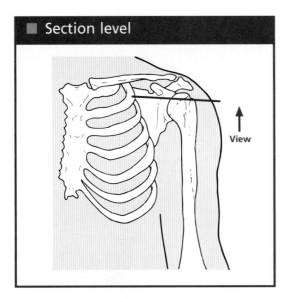

Orientation

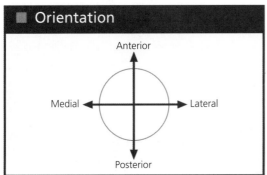

Anterior

Medial ← → Lateral

Posterior

Notes

The greater tubercle of the humerus (**2**) is the most lateral bony landmark around the shoulder. The subacromial bursa passes below the acromion and above supraspinatus to continue into the subdeltoid bursa (**10**) between the upper shaft of the humerus and the deltoid muscle (**8**).

Infraspinatus (**9**), together with supraspinatus, teres minor and subscapularis, forms a protective rotator cuff around the shoulder joint, which, as can be seen in this section, has little stability afforded by either its bony configuration or its capsular strength.

The shallow glenoid is in sharp contrast to the deep acetabulum in the hip; stability has been sacrificed for mobility in order to allow a greater range of movement.

The orientation and shape of the coracoid process is an important feature; the coraco-acromial ligament can impinge on the rotator cuff.

The tendon of subscapularis attaches mainly to the lesser tubercle, but some slips attach to the floor of the intertubercular sulcus. Furthermore, the transverse humeral ligament, which retains the long head of biceps tendon, could be regarded as fibres from the subscapular's attachment on the lesser tubercle extending on towards the greater tubercle.

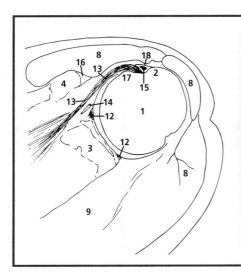

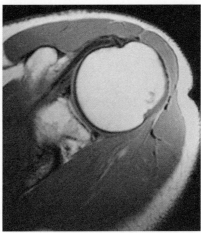

Axial magnetic resonance image (MRI)

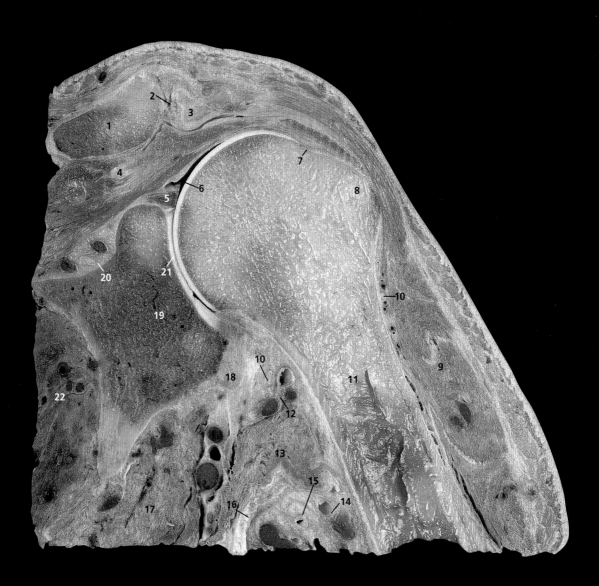

1 Clavicle
2 Acromioclavicular joint
3 Acromion of scapula
4 Supraspinatus
5 Glenoid labrum
6 Shoulder joint cavity
7 Anatomical neck of humerus
8 Greater tubercle of humerus
9 Deltoid
10 Axillary nerve accompanied by posterior circumflex humeral artery and vein
11 Shaft of humerus
12 Medial circumflex artery and vein
13 Latissimus dorsi
14 Brachial artery and vein
15 Nerves of brachial plexus
16 Tendon of teres major
17 Teres minor
18 Long head of triceps
19 Head of scapula
20 Neck of scapula
21 Glenoid fossa of scapula
22 Subscapularis
23 Long head of biceps tendon
24 Surgical neck of humerus

Section level

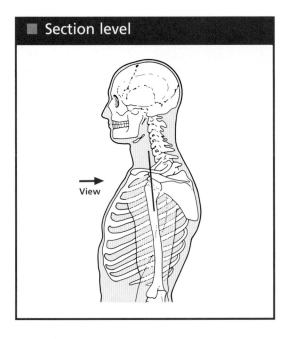

View

Orientation

Proximal

Medial ← → Lateral

Distal

Notes

The important relationship of the supraspinatus tendon (**4**) to the acromion process (**3**) and clavicle (**1**) is demonstrated well. This muscle initiates abduction of the shoulder, which is then continued powerfully by deltoid (**9**). Degenerative changes in the acromioclavicular joint frequently cause impingement on the musculotendinous junction of supraspinatus; tendonitis and a tear in the rotator cuff may follow.

Note the close relationship of the axillary nerve (**10**), together with its accompanying vessels, the posterior circumflex humeral artery and vein, to the surgical neck of the humerus (**24**). Fractures commonly occur in the region of the surgical neck; the axillary nerve may be affected. The axillary nerve may also be damaged in dislocation of the shoulder. The resultant paralysis of the deltoid muscle is demonstrated by the patient being unable to abduct the affected shoulder. There is also characteristic anaesthesia over the lateral aspect of the deltoid.

This magnetic resonance image is in a somewhat coronal oblique plane in order to demonstrate the supraspinatus muscle, tendon and insertion as a continuum.

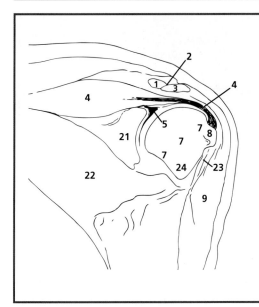

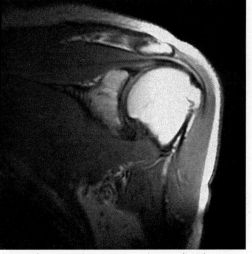

Coronal magnetic resonance image (MRI)

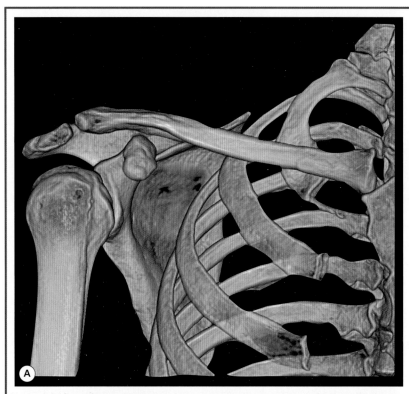

3D computed
tomogram (CT)

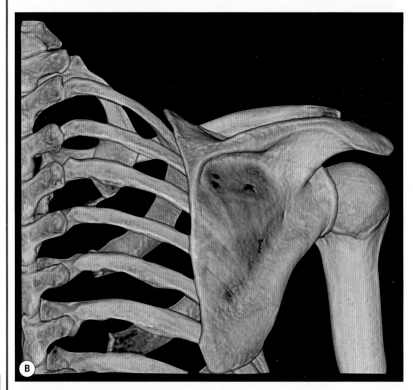

3D computed
tomogram (CT)

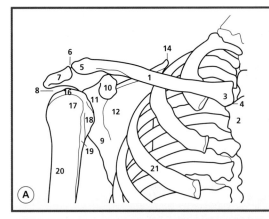

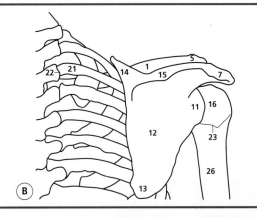

Orientation

Superior

Lateral (right) ←→ Medial

Inferior

Ⓐ

Orientation

Superior

Medial ←→ Lateral (right)

Inferior

Ⓑ

1 Shaft of clavicle	**11** Neck of scapula	**20** Shaft (proximal third) of humerus
2 Body of sternum	**12** Subscapular fossa of scapula	**21** Surgical neck of humerus
3 Sternal end of clavicle	**13** Inferior angle of scapula	**22** Costotransverse joint between third rib and transverse process of third thoracic vertebra
4 Sternoclavicular joint	**14** Superior angle of scapula	
5 Acromial end of clavicle	**15** Spine of scapula	
6 Acromioclavicular joint	**16** Head of humerus	**23** Third rib
7 Subacromial space	**17** Greater tubercle of humerus	**24** Infraspinous fossa
8 Acromion of scapula	**18** Lesser tubercle of humerus	
9 Lateral border of scapula	**19** Intertubercular sulcus of humerus	
10 Coracoid process of scapula		

Notes

Surface-shaded three-dimensional volume-rendered CT images. Because bone attenuates the X-ray beam so much, its CT attenuation value (around +1000 HU) is much greater than that of the surrounding soft tissues. Thus, the bones can be 'extracted', with no overlying artefacts, to provide information equivalent to that from a cadaveric skeleton. This subject is holding the upper arm in mild internal rotation, which means that the bicipital groove (the groove for the tendon of the long head of biceps – also known as the intertubercular suclus) (**19**) is directed medially rather than anteriorly.

The relationship of the acromioclavicular joint (**6**) to the humeral head is well appreciated, along with the important subacromial space (**8**) (normal in this subject). The rotator cuff tendons (especially supraspinatus) have to pass though this limited space. Mild congenital variations in anatomy and the inevitable degenerative changes in the acromioclavicular joint combine to impinge on this tendon. A high percentage of elderly people have damaged rotator cuffs – one of the design flaws associated with man's evolution to a biped.

Note the thinness of the scapula (**12**), which is translucent in places. The strength of the scapula lies in the border and processes; the lateral border (**9**) is especially thick and strong for the attachment of muscles.

243

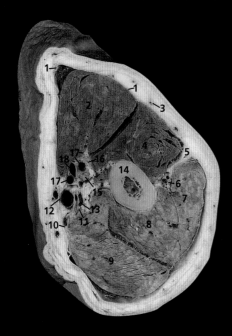

1 Deep fascia of arm
2 Biceps
3 Cephalic vein
4 Brachialis
5 Lateral intermuscular septum
6 Radial nerve, with profunda brachii artery and vein
7 Triceps – lateral head
8 Triceps – medial head
9 Triceps – long head
10 Medial intermuscular septum
11 Ulnar nerve
12 Basilic vein
13 Superior ulnar collateral artery and vein
14 Humerus shaft
15 Median nerve
16 Musculocutaneous nerve
17 Venae comitantes of brachial artery
18 Brachial artery

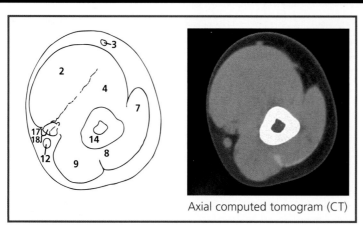

Axial computed tomogram (CT)

Orientation

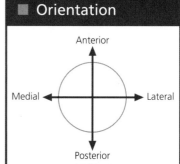

Anterior

Medial ← → Lateral

Posterior

Section level

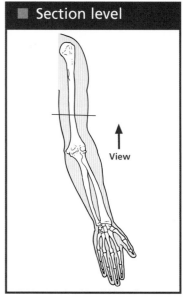

View

Notes

This section passes through the mid-shaft of the humerus (**14**). It gives a clear view of the fascial arrangements of the upper arm – the investing sheath of the deep fascia (**1**), with its lateral (**5**) and medial (**10**) intermuscular septa, which attach to the humeral shaft. These septa divide the extensor group of muscles, the triceps (**7**, **8**, **9**), from the anterior flexor group. The medial septum is pierced by the ulnar nerve (**11**) and its accompanying vessels (**13**); the lateral septum is pierced by the radial nerve with its accompanying profunda brachial artery and vein (**6**).

The median nerve (**15**) and brachial artery (**18**) bear a close relationship to each other in the upper arm, as shown in this section. Superiorly, the nerve lies on the lateral side of the artery. At the mid-humerus level, the artery is crossed superficially (sometimes deeply) by the nerve, which then descends on its medial side.

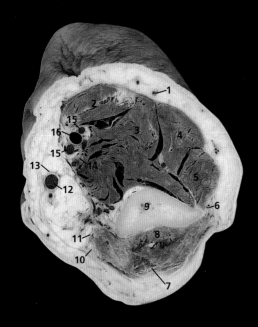

1 Cephalic vein
2 Biceps
3 Brachialis
4 Brachioradialis
5 Extensor carpi radialis longus
6 Lateral intermuscular septum
7 Triceps tendon
8 Triceps
9 Humerus

10 Ulnar nerve
11 Medial intermuscular septum
12 Basilic vein
13 Medial cutaneous nerve of forearm
14 Median nerve
15 Venae comitantes of brachial artery
16 Brachial artery

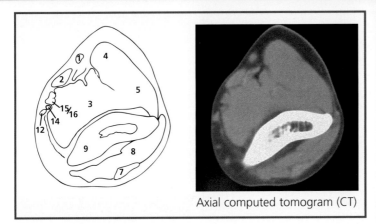

Axial computed tomogram (CT)

■ Orientation

Anterior

Medial ◀────────▶ Lateral

Posterior

■ Section level

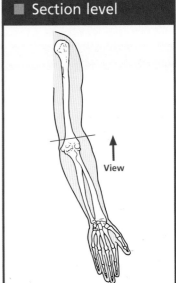

View

■ Notes

This section transects the lower end of the humeral shaft as it expands to form its medial and lateral supracondylar ridges.

The origin of extensor carpi radialis longus (**5**) is from the upper part of the lateral ridge, and this muscle arises superior to, and separate from, the remaining extensor muscles of the forearm, which originate from a common origin from the lateral epicondyle of the humerus.

The ulnar nerve (**10**), just distal to the line of this section, will pass behind the medial epicondyle of the humerus; pressure here will elicit discomfort and often paraesthesia.

245

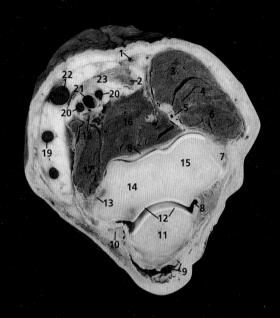

1 Cephalic vein
2 Biceps tendon
3 Brachioradialis
4 Extensor carpi radialis longus
5 Radial nerve with profunda brachii artery and vein
6 Common extensor origin
7 Lateral collateral ligament of elbow
8 Joint capsule of elbow
9 Olecranon bursa
10 Ulnar nerve
11 Olecranon process of ulna
12 Articular cartilage
13 Medial collateral ligament of elbow
14 Trochlea of humerus
15 Capitulum of humerus
16 Brachialis
17 Common flexor origin
18 Median nerve
19 Basilic vein
20 Venae comitantes of brachial artery
21 Brachial artery
22 Median cubital vein
23 Bicipital aponeurosis
24 Anconeus

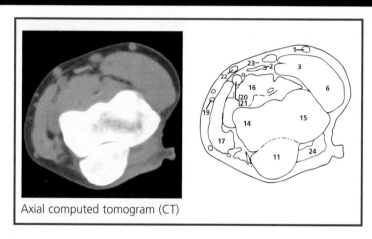

Axial computed tomogram (CT)

■ Orientation

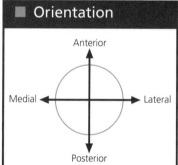

Anterior

Medial ◄——————► Lateral

Posterior

■ Section level

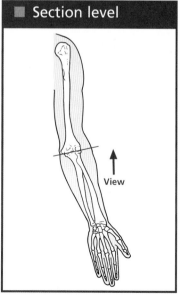

View

■ Notes

This section transects the elbow joint. The cartilage (**12**) covering the articular surfaces of the lower end of the humerus (**14**, **15**) and the olecranon process of the ulna (**11**), together with the joint cavity and collateral ligaments (**8**), are readily appreciated.

The posterior surface of the olecranon process of the ulna is separated from the skin by a bursa (**9**). This is a common site for bursitis ('student's elbow', 'miner's elbow').

The median nerve (**18**), here lying medial to the brachial artery (**21**) (see note on page 244) is well-named. It lies in the median position throughout its course in the upper arm, at the elbow, in the forearm and at the wrist as it passes into the carpal tunnel below the flexor retinaculum.

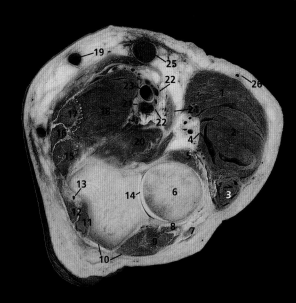

1 Brachioradialis
2 Extensor carpi radialis longus
3 Extensor carpi radialis brevis
4 Radial nerve with radial recurrent artery
5 Supinator
6 Head of radius
7 Common extensor origin
8 Annular ligament of superior radio-ulnar joint
9 Anconeus
10 Deep fascia of the forearm
11 Flexor digitorum profundus

12 Flexor carpi ulnaris
13 Ulnar nerve, with posterior recurrent ulnar artery and vein
14 Radial notch of ulna
15 Flexor digitorum superficialis
16 Palmaris longus
17 Flexor carpi radialis
18 Pronator teres
19 Basilic vein
20 Brachialis
21 Median nerve
22 Venae comitantes of brachial artery
23 Brachial artery
24 Tendon of biceps
25 Median cubital vein
26 Cephalic vein

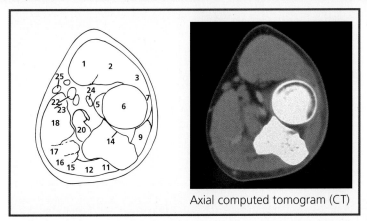

Axial computed tomogram (CT)

Orientation

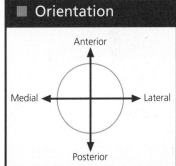

Anterior

Medial ← → Lateral

Posterior

Section level

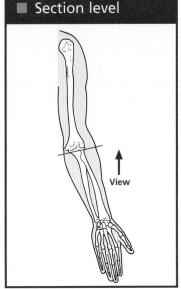

View

Notes

This section passes through the superior radio-ulnar joint between the head of the radius (**6**) and the radial notch of the ulnar (**14**). The annular ligament (**8**), which maintains the congruity of this pivot joint, is shown well. In this CT image, the hand is in the neutral position alongside the body.

The median cubital vein (**25**) passes obliquely across the front of the elbow between the cephalic vein (**26**) and the basilic vein (**19**). It is separated from the underlying brachial artery (**23**) by a condensation of the deep fascia (**10**) termed the bicipital aponeurosis. Occasionally, in high division of the brachial artery, an abnormal ulnar artery may lie immediately below the median cubital vein in the superficial fascia. This vein is therefore best avoided for intravenous injections in order to protect against inadvertent intra-arterial injection.

247

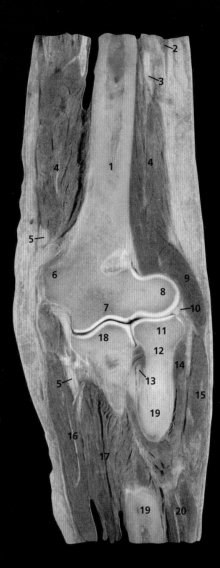

1 Shaft of humerus
2 Lateral head of triceps
3 Radial nerve
4 Medial head of triceps
5 Ulnar nerve
6 Medial epicondyle of
   humerus
7 Trochlea of humerus
8 Capitulum of humerus
9 Brachioradialis
10 Annular ligament
11 Head of radius
12 Neck of radius
13 Tendon of biceps
14 Supinator

15 Extensor carpi radialis
   longus
16 Flexor carpi ulnaris
17 Flexor digitorum
   profundus
18 Coronoid process of
   ulna
19 Shaft of radius
20 Extensor carpi radialis
   brevis

21 Olecranon fossa of
   humerus
22 Lateral epicondyle of
   humerus

Section level

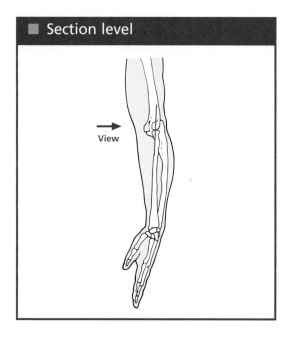

View

Orientation

Proximal

Medial ← → Lateral

Distal

Notes

The ulnar nerve (**5**) passes posterior to the medial epicondyle of the humerus (**6**), where it may be palpated. It may be injured at this site in fractures or dislocations around the elbow, or stretched in valgus deformity of this joint.

The tendon of biceps (**13**) inserts into the posterior lip of the tuberosity of the radius. It is a powerful supinator of the radio-ulnar joints and a flexor of the elbow joint.

The brachial vessels are in close anterior proximity to the elbow joint; the artery may be compromised in supracondylar fractures, which are relatively common in children.

The epicondyles have developed to provide attachment of the common extensor (lateral epicondyle) and flexor (medial epicondyle) muscle groups. Inflammation of the extensor origin on the lateral epicondyle (**22**) is known as 'tennis elbow'. This section provides an excellent view of the superior radio-ulnar joint between the head of the radius (**11**) and the radial notch of the ulna (**18**). It communicates freely with the elbow joint. Together with the inferior radio-ulnar joint, it allows the movements of pronation and supination of the forearm, which are unique to the primate upper limb.

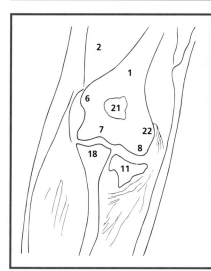

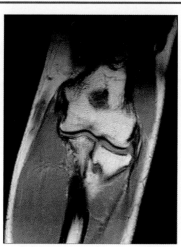

Coronal magnetic resonance image (MRI)

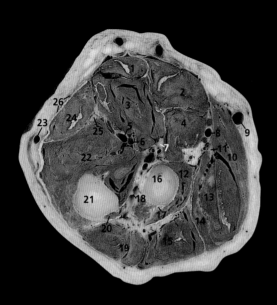

1 Palmaris longus
2 Flexor carpi radialis
3 Flexor digitorum superficialis
4 Pronator teres – humeral head
5 Ulnar artery
6 Ulnar vein
7 Median nerve, with anterior interosseous artery and vein
8 Radial artery, with venae comitantes
9 Cephalic vein
10 Brachioradialis
11 Radial nerve
12 Supinator
13 Extensor carpi radialis longus
14 Extensor carpi radialis brevis
15 Extensor digitorum
16 Radius
17 Posterior interosseous nerve
18 Posterior interosseous artery and vein
19 Extensor carpi ulnaris
20 Anconeus
21 Ulna
22 Flexor digitorum profundus
23 Basilic vein
24 Flexor carpi ulnaris
25 Ulnar nerve
26 Deep fascia of forearm

27 Pronator teres (ulnar head)

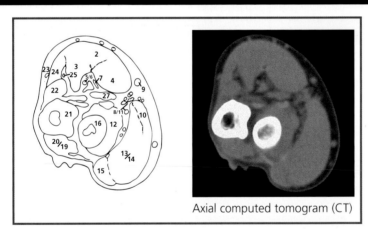

Axial computed tomogram (CT)

■ Orientation

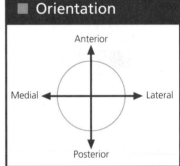

■ Section level

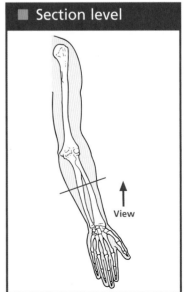

View

■ Notes

This section passes through the mid forearm. In both the section and the CT image, the forearm is viewed in the supinated position. Note how the median nerve (**7**) characteristically hugs the deep aspect of flexor digitorum superficialis (**3**). The ulnar nerve (**25**) lies sandwiched between flexor carpi ulnaris (**24**) and flexor digitorum profundus (**22**), and the radial nerve (**11**) lies beneath brachioradialis (**10**).

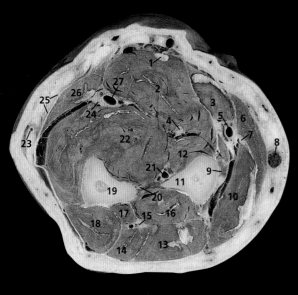

1 Palmaris longus tendon
2 Flexor digitorum superficialis
3 Flexor carpi radialis
4 Median nerve
5 Radial artery
6 Brachioradialis
7 Radial nerve
8 Cephalic vein
9 Pronator teres tendon
10 Extensor carpi radialis longus and brevis
11 Radius
12 Flexor pollicis longus
13 Extensor digitorum
14 Extensor digiti minimi
15 Posterior interosseous nerve, with artery and vein
16 Abductor pollicis longus

17 Extensor pollicis longus
18 Extensor carpi ulnaris
19 Ulna
20 Interosseous membrane
21 Anterior interosseous artery, vein and nerve
22 Flexor digitorum profundus
23 Basilic vein
24 Ulnar nerve
25 Deep fascia of forearm
26 Flexor carpi ulnaris
27 Ulnar artery with venae comitantes

28 Superficial flexor group of muscles
29 Extensor group of muscles

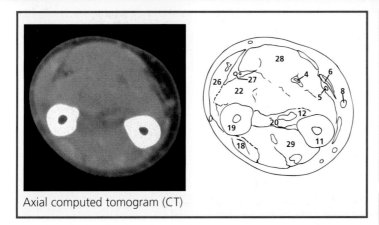

Axial computed tomogram (CT)

Orientation

Anterior

Medial ←——→ Lateral

Posterior

Section level

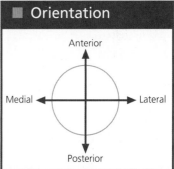

View

Notes

This section transects the supinated forearm at the junction of its upper two-thirds and lower one-third. Note that the very extensive origin of flexor digitorum profundus (**22**) is demonstrated clearly by this section. It arises from both the anterior and medial surfaces of the upper three-quarters of the ulna (**19**), from the ulnar half of the interosseous membrane (**20**) and also from the superior three-quarters of the posterior border of the ulna by an aponeurosis that is in common with that of flexor carpi ulnaris (**26**) and extensor carpi ulnaris (**18**).

251

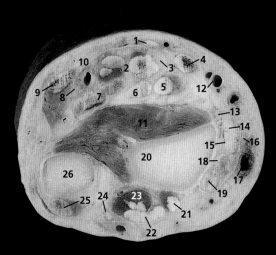

1 Palmaris longus tendon
2 Flexor digitorum superficialis tendons
3 Median nerve
4 Flexor carpi radialis tendon
5 Flexor pollicis longus tendon
6 Flexor digitorum profundus tendon to index finger
7 Flexor digitorum profundus tendon to remaining fingers
8 Ulnar nerve
9 Flexor carpi ulnaris tendon
10 Ulnar artery
11 Pronator quadratus
12 Radial artery
13 Brachioradialis insertion
14 Abductor pollicis longus tendon
15 Extensor pollicis brevis tendon
16 Radial nerve
17 Cephalic vein
18 Extensor carpi radialis longus tendon
19 Extensor carpi radialis brevis tendon
20 Radius
21 Extensor pollicis longus tendon
22 Extensor digitorum tendon
23 Extensor indicis
24 Extensor digiti minimi tendon
25 Extensor carpi ulnaris tendon
26 Ulna

27 Superficial vein

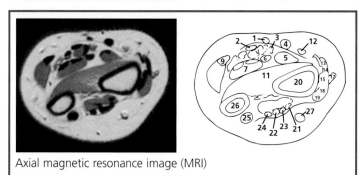

Axial magnetic resonance image (MRI)

Orientation

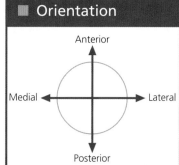

Anterior

Medial ← → Lateral

Posterior

Notes

This section transects the forearm immediately proximal to the wrist joint. The arrangement of the extensor tendons on the posterior and radial aspects of the wrist can be appreciated clearly. Note that extensor carpi ulnaris tendon (**25**) grooves the dorsal aspect of the distal ulna (**26**).

At this level, flexor digitorum profundus has given off a separate tendon to the index finger (**6**), while those for the remaining three fingers are still closely applied to each other (**7**).

Usually the cephalic vein (**17**) is easily visible at this site; here, it is a common locus for venous cannulation.

Section level

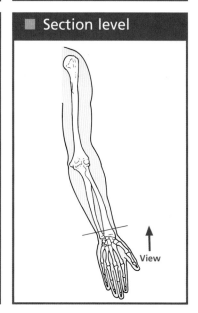

View

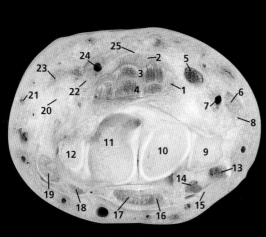

1 Flexor pollicis longus tendon
2 Median nerve
3 Flexor digitorum superficialis tendons
4 Flexor digitorum profundus tendons
5 Flexor carpi radialis tendon
6 Abductor pollicis longus tendon
7 Radial artery
8 Extensor pollicis brevis tendon
9 Styloid process of radius
10 Scaphoid
11 Lunate
12 Triquetral
13 Extensor carpi radialis longus tendon
14 Extensor carpi radialis brevis tendon

15 Extensor pollicis longus tendon
16 Extensor indicis tendon
17 Extensor digitorum tendon
18 Extensor digiti minimi tendon
19 Extensor carpi ulnaris tendon
20 Pisiform
21 Basilic vein
22 Ulnar nerve
23 Flexor carpi ulnaris tendon
24 Ulnar artery
25 Flexor retinaculum

26 Capitate
27 Hamate
28 Trapezoid
29 Trapezium

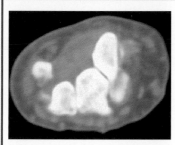

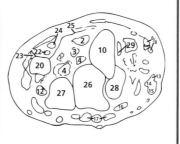

Axial computed tomogram (CT)

■ Orientation

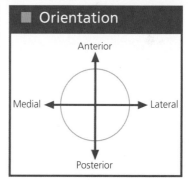

Anterior

Medial ◀——————▶ Lateral

Posterior

■ Notes

This section passes through the proximal row of carpal bones and the radial styloid process. The CT image is at a more distal level.

The radius (**9**) extends more distally than the ulna; thus, abduction of the wrist is more limited than adduction.

The pisiform bone (**20**) can be considered as a sesamoid within the termination of the tendon of flexor carpi ulnaris (**23**), which anchors via the pisohamate ligament to the hook of the hamate and via the pisometacarpal ligament to the base of the fifth metacarpal bone.

The flexor retinaculum (**25**) is a tough fibrous band across the front of the carpus, which converts its concavity into the carpal tunnel, transmitting the flexor tendons of the digits together with the median nerve (**2**). Its attachments can be seen in this section and on page 254, medially to the pisiform (**20**) and to the hook of the hamate (**27**), laterally as two laminae, the more superficial one being attached to the tubercles of the scaphoid (**10**) and the trapezium (**29**) and the deep lamina to the medial lip of the groove on the latter.

■ Section level

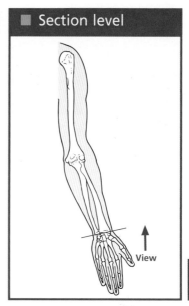

View

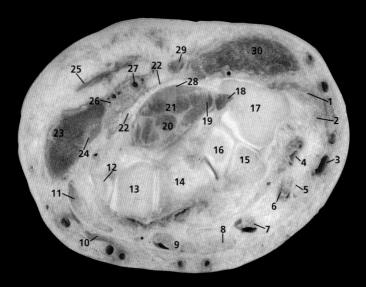

1 Abductor pollicis longus tendon
2 Extensor pollicis brevis tendon
3 Cephalic vein
4 Radial artery
5 Extensor pollicis longus tendon
6 Extensor carpi radialis longus tendon
7 Extensor carpi radialis brevis tendon
8 Extensor indicis tendon
9 Extensor digitorum tendons
10 Extensor digiti minimi tendon
11 Extensor carpi ulnaris tendon
12 Triquetral
13 Hamate
14 Capitate
15 Trapezoid
16 Scaphoid
17 Trapezium

18 Flexor carpi radialis tendon
19 Flexor pollicis longus tendon
20 Flexor digitorum profundus tendons
21 Flexor digitorum superficialis tendons
22 Flexor retinaculum
23 Muscles of hypothenar eminence
24 Pisometacarpal ligament
25 Palmaris brevis
26 Ulnar nerve
27 Ulnar artery
28 Median nerve
29 Palmaris longus tendon
30 Muscles of thenar eminence

31 Base of thumb metacarpal

Section level

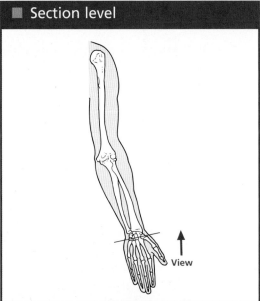

View

Orientation

Anterior

Medial ← → Lateral

Posterior

Notes

This section passes through the distal part of the carpus. The bony arch is seen well. The flexor retinaculum (**22**) has already been described (see page 253). Here, its distal attachment to the trapezium (**17**) and the hook of the hamate (**13**) can be seen. Note the tendon of flexor carpi radialis (**18**) lying in the tunnel formed by the groove on the trapezium and the two laminae of the lateral attachment of the retinaculum.

Swelling or deformity within the carpal tunnel compresses the median nerve (**28**) and produces carpal tunnel syndrome. The ulnar nerve (**26**) – part of a neurovascular bundle with the ulnar artery and its venae commitantes (**27**) – passes superficially to the flexor retinaculum and is, therefore, not implicated in this syndrome.

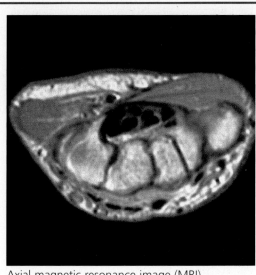

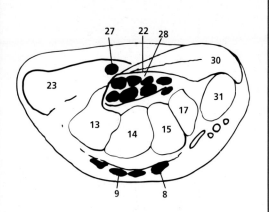

Axial magnetic resonance image (MRI)

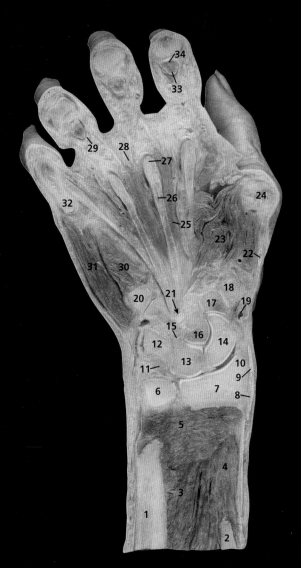

1 Shaft of ulna
2 Shaft of radius
3 Flexor digitorum profundus (see also 33)
4 Flexor pollicis longus
5 Pronator quadratus
6 Head of ulna
7 Distal end of radius
8 Abductor pollicis longus
9 Extensor pollicis brevis
10 Radial styloid process
11 Articular disc (triangular fibrocartilaginous complex, TFCC)
12 Triquetral
13 Lunate
14 Scaphoid

15 Hamate
16 Capitate
17 Trapezoid
18 Trapezium
19 Radial artery in anatomical snuffbox
20 Base of little finger bone
21 Distal opening of carpal tunnel (arrowed)
22 Extensor pollicis longus
23 Abductor pollicis
24 Head of first metacarpal
25 Second lumbrical
26 Tendon of flexor digitorum profundus
27 Tendon of flexor digitorum superficialis

28 Common digital artery, vein and nerve
29 Digital fibrous sheath of ring finger
30 Flexor digiti minimi
31 Abductor digiti minimi
32 Base of proximal phalanx of little finger
33 Tendon of flexor digitorum profundus of index finger (see also 3)
34 Tendon of flexor digitorum superficialis of index finger

35 Ulnar styloid
36 Base of index metacarpal bone

Section level

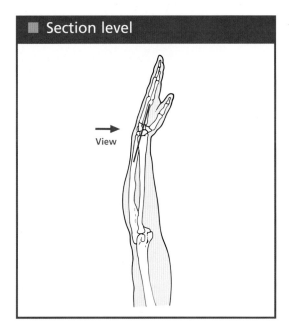

View

Orientation

Distal

Medial ← → Lateral

Proximal

Notes

Note that in the anatomical position of the wrist joint, the scaphoid (**14**) and lunate (**13**) are in contact with the distal end of the radius (**7**). The triquetral (**12**) articulates against the articular disc (**11**) only when the hand is adducted. The triquetral is, therefore, almost never injured in falls on the hand.

The pulse of the radial artery (**19**) is readily palpated in the anatomical snuffbox as the artery lies against the underlying scaphoid (**14**).

The distal end of the ulna is fractionally shorter than that of the radius. Thus, an articular disc (the triangular fibrocartilaginous complex, TFCC) runs from the ulnar styloid to the radius to complete the proximal part of the ellipsoid wrist joint. An articular disc implies two types of movement: the radius supinates and pronates around the ulna proximal to the disc. Minor variance in ulnar length probably contributes to damage to the TFCC in later life.

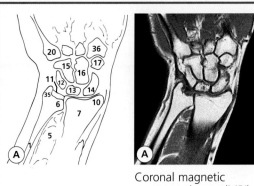

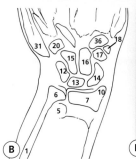

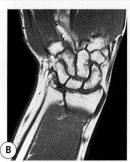

Coronal magnetic resonance image (MRI)

Coronal magnetic resonance image (MRI)

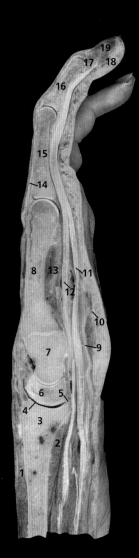

1 Extensor digitorum
2 Pronator quadratus
3 Distal end of radius
4 Wrist joint
5 Capsule of wrist joint
6 Lunate
7 Capitate
8 Metacarpal bone of
  middle finger
9 Flexor retinaculum
10 Palmar aponeurosis
11 Tendon of flexor
   digitorum superficialis
12 Tendon of flexor
   digitorum profundus
13 Adductor pollicis
14 Extensor expansion
15 Proximal phalanx of
   middle finger
16 Middle phalanx of
   middle finger
17 Distal phalanx of
   middle finger
18 Pulp space of distal
   phalanx
19 Nail bed

Section level

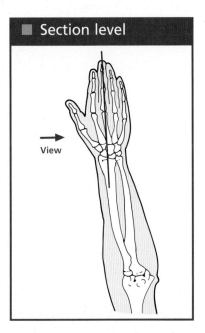

View

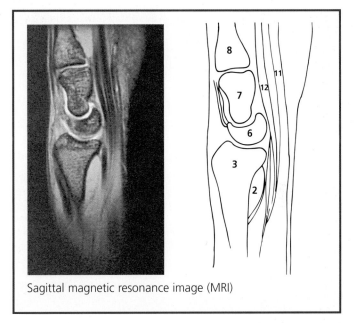

Sagittal magnetic resonance image (MRI)

Orientation

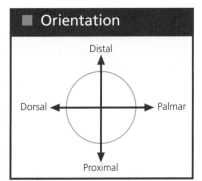

Distal

Dorsal ← → Palmar

Proximal

Notes

The 'half-moon' of the lunate (**6**) is demonstrated well in this sagittal section. This characteristic appearance enables it to be identified readily in a lateral radiograph of the hand. Lateral radiographs are needed to assess lunate or perilunate dislocations, which are often missed on anteroposterior radiographs. Note the continuous alignment of the radius, lunate, capitate and metacarpal bones.

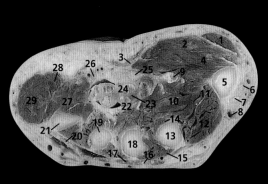

1 Abductor pollicis brevis	**17** Extensor digitorum tendon
2 Flexor pollicis brevis	**18** Third metacarpal
3 Palmar aponeurosis	**19** Fourth metacarpal
4 Oponens pollicis brevis	**20** Extensor digiti minimi tendon
5 First metacarpal	**21** Fifth metacarpal
6 Extensor pollicis brevis tendon	**22** Flexor digitorum profundus tendons
7 Extensor pollicis longus tendon	**23** Lumbrical
8 Cephalic vein	**24** Flexor digitorum superficialis tendons
9 Flexor pollicis longus tendon	**25** Median nerve
10 Adductor pollicis	**26** Ulnar artery and nerve
11 Radial artery	**27** Opponens digiti minimi
12 First dorsal interosseous	**28** Flexor digiti minimi
13 Second metacarpal	**29** Abductor digiti minimi
14 Second palmar interosseous	**30** Muscles of thenar eminence
15 Second dorsal interosseous	**31** Muscles of hypothenar eminence
16 Extensor indicis tendon	

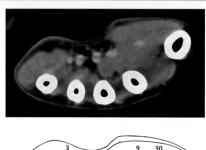

Axial computed tomogram (CT)

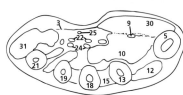

Orientation

Anterior

Medial ← → Lateral

Posterior

Section level

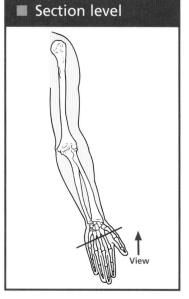

View

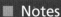

Notes

This section passes through the proximal shafts of the metacarpals.

The dense central part of the palmar aponeurosis (**3**) is triangular, its apex being continuous with the distal margin of the flexor retinaculum (see pages 253 and 254). The expanded tendon of palmaris longus (see page 252) is attached to it. It is bound strongly to the overlying skin by dense fibro-areolar tissue. Compare this with the loose superficial fascia over the extensor aspect of the hand. Oedema of the hand thus occurs only on its dorsal aspect. The lateral and medial extensions of the palmar aponeurosis are the thin superficial coverings of the thenar and hypothenar muscles, respectively.

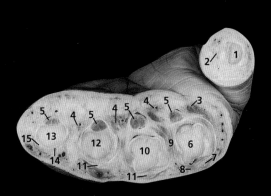

1 Proximal phalanx of thumb
2 Flexor pollicis longus tendon
3 First lumbrical
4 Neurovascular bundle
5 Flexor tendons within sheath
6 Second metacarpal head
7 Extensor digitorum tendon to index finger
8 Extensor indicis tendon
9 Interosseous muscles
10 Third metacarpal head
11 Extensor digitorum tendon
12 Fourth metacarpal head
13 Fifth metacarpal head
14 Extensor digitorum tendon to little finger
15 Extensor indicis tendon

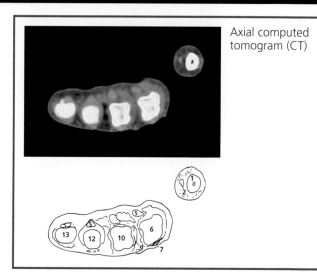

Axial computed tomogram (CT)

■ Orientation

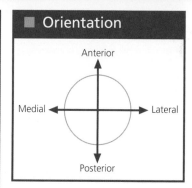

Anterior

Medial ◄─────► Lateral

Posterior

■ Section level

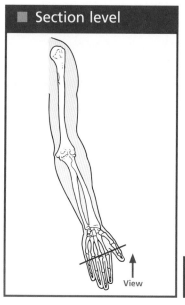

View

■ Notes

This section passes through the heads of the metacarpals of the fingers and through the proximal phalanx of the thumb (**1**). In the distal part of the palm, the digital arteries pass deeply between the divisions of the digital nerves so that, on the sides of the digits, the neurovascular bundle (**4**) has the digital nerve lying anterior to the digital artery and vein. The bundles lie adjacent to the tendon sheaths anterior to the metacarpal heads; this relationship is also maintained in the fingers. Thus, an incision along the anterior border of the bone will avoid these important structures.

The majority of entries are those mentioned in the notes section with bold numbers in brackets. These are mainly on the right (odd numbered) pages of double-page spreads. The words 'odd nos.' appearing in brackets following a page range reference are for CT or MRI images appearing over a number of consecutive odd numbered pages. Roman numerals indicate references in the preface and introduction.

abdomen xvi–xvii, 134–63
    axial section
        female 150–3
        male 134–49
    CT *see* computed tomography
accessory nerve 33
acetabulum 175, 211
Achilles tendon 228
acoustic meatus *see* auditory meatus
acoustic neuroma 61
acromioclavicular joint 99
acromion process 241
adductor compartment of thigh 212
adductor longus 185, 212
adductor magnus 185, 201, 212, 214, 225
adipose tissue *see* fat
adrenal (suprarenal) gland 151, 161
Alcock's canal *see* pudendal canal (Alcock's canal)
alveolar process of maxilla 85
alveolus (dentalis) 87
anal canal
    female 199
    male 183
anal sphincter, external 185
anal verge
    female 201
    male 185
angle of Louis 111
ankle and ankle joint 228–33, 235
annular ligament of radius 247
anorectal junction 181
anterior compartment of thigh 212
anus *see* anorectal junction *and entries under* anal
aorta 121
    abdominal xvi, 141, 145, 147, 149, 165, 187
    thoracic
        ascending 113, 115
        descending 115
aortic valve 123
aponeurosis
    epicranial 15, 53
    palmar 260
    plantar 233
appendix vermiformis 171
aqueduct of Sylvius 25
arachnoid mater 13
arm 244
arterial system, thorax 132–3
    see also specific arteries
articular cartilage, elbow joint 246

articular disc *see* disc
atlanto-axial joint 39, 87
atlanto-occipital joint 39, 57
atlas (C1) 37, 39, 59, 63, 87, 101
atrium
    left 117, 119
    right 117
    septum 117
auditory meatus/canal (acoustic meatus)
    external 33, 63
    internal 49, 61, 79
auditory nerve *see* vestibulocochlear nerve
auditory ossicles 79
auditory tube 67, 85
axial images, orientation xi–xii
axial section
    abdomen *see* abdomen
    head 10–47
    lower limb
        ankle 228–31
        knee 215–17
        leg 226–7
        thigh 212–14
    neck 82–99
    pelvis *see* pelvis
    thorax *see* thorax
    upper limb
        arm 245
        elbow 245–7
        forearm 250–1
        hand 260–1
        shoulder 238–9
        wrist 252–5
axis (C2) 37, 39, 41, 43, 53, 89, 101
    dens 37, 39, 57, 63, 77, 87, 101
azygos vein 127

basilar artery 9, 31, 49
basilic vein 247
basi-occiput 33, 83
basi-vertebral vein 159
biceps brachii tendon 249
biceps femoris
    long head 201, 212
    short head 212
bicipital groove 243
bile duct, common 139, 151
bladder
    female 191, 205
    male 175
brachial artery 244, 246, 247
brachial vein 244
brachioradialis 250
brain 2–9
    axial section 10–35
    coronal section 50–75
    images 8–9
    sagittal section 76–7
    superficial dissection 2–7
breast 123
broad ligament 191
bronchi 113, 131
buccal fat pad 75
buccinator 75, 85

cadaver preservation ix
calcaneonavicular ligament 235
calcaneus 231, 235
    sustentaculum tali of 231, 235
calcified phlebolith 195
capsule
    fibrous, knee joint 223
    internal *see* internal capsule
carotid artery
    common 93, 97, 99, 105
    external 37, 47
    internal 9, 49, 87, 91, 93
cartilage(s)
    costal 115
    elbow joint 246
    laryngeal 95, 97, 101
caudate nucleus 23, 61, 63
caval veins *see* vena cava
cavernous sinus 67
cephalic vein 109, 247, 252
cerebello-medullary cistern 57
cerebello-pontine angle syndrome 31
cerebellum 31, 55, 85
    dentate nucleus 57
    peduncles 29
    tentorium 27, 57
    tonsil 35
cerebral arteries 9
cerebral veins 57
cerebrospinal fluid 13
cervical lymph nodes 105
cervical spinal canal 101
cervical spinal cord 35, 37, 59
cervical spine 37, 45
    vertebrae *see* vertebrae
cervical vein, deep 43
cervix
    external os 195
    internal os 193
chest *see* thorax
cholecystectomy clips 133
chorda tympani 35
choroid plexus 21
cisterna ambiens 25
cisterna cerebello-medullaris 57
claustrum 23
clavicle 99, 107, 125
clinoid process, posterior 9
clitoris 201
coccyx
    female 193, 195
    male 179
collateral ligaments
    ankle, lateral 233
    elbow 246
    knee 217, 219
colliculi, inferior 27
colon xvii
    ascending 149
    descending 149, 153
    transverse 153
    see also rectosigmoid junction
colonogram, CT 154–5
commissures (corpus callosum) 19
communicating arteries 9

computed tomography (CT) ix, x
   abdomen
      axial 135–41(odd nos.), 147–53(odd
         nos.), 158, 159
      coronal 156–7
   lower limb
      ankle, axial 228, 229, 231
      foot, coronal 237
      leg, axial 226, 227
      thigh, axial 212
   neck, axial 91–9(odd nos.)
   pelvis
      3D 210
      axial, female 189–201
      axial, male 165–85
   skull/brain
      3D 8
      axial 11–19(odd nos.), 25, 29, 33–
         47(odd nos.), 69–75(odd nos.),
         81
      coronal 69–75(odd nos.), 79
   thorax 125
      axial 103–23(odd nos.), 124, 126–7
      coronal 130, 131
      sagittal 130, 131
   upper limb
      arm, axial 244
      elbow, axial 245, 246, 247
      forearm, axial 250, 251
      hand, axial 260, 261
      shoulder, 3D 242, 243
computed tomography angiography
   brain 9
   thorax 132–3
computed tomography colonogram 154–5
concha *see* nasal concha
conus medularis 141
cornea 29
corona radiata 17, 19
coronal images, orientation xii
coronal section
   head 50–75
   lower limb
      ankle 232–3
      foot 236–7
      hip 208–9
      knee 218–19
   upper limb
      elbow 249
      shoulder 240–1
      wrist/hand 256–7
coronary arteries 125
corpus callosum 19
corpus cavernosum 185
corpus spongiosum 185
costal cartilage 115
cranial nerves 31, 33, 61, 67, 79, 85, 87
cranium *see* skull
cricoid cartilage 97, 101
cruciate ligaments
   anterior 216, 219, 223
   posterior 217, 219, 223
cubital vein, median 247
cuneiform, medial 237
cutaneous nerve of thigh, lateral 199

da Vinci, Leonardo viii
De Riemer viii
deep artery of penis 185
deep fascia
   arm 244
   elbow 247
   leg 223
deltoid 239, 241
dens 37, 39, 57, 63, 77, 87, 101
dentate nucleus 57
denticulate ligament 95
descending (coronary) artery, left anterior
   125
diaphragm (and hemidiaphragm) 119, 121,
   135
   crura 137, 161
digital neurovascular bundles 261
diploic veins 11
disc (intra-articular)
   intervertebral *see* intervertebral disc
   temporomandibular joint 65
   wrist joint 257
dorsal root(s), cervical 59
dorsal root ganglion
   cervical 59
   lumbar 159
duodenum 145, 147, 149
dura mater, brain 11, 13, 15, 37, 57
dural sheath, lumbar 159

ear
   inner 78–81
   middle 79
eardrum (tympanic membrane) 63, 79
elbow 245–9
endocranium 11
epicondyles, humeral 249
epicranial aponeurosis 15, 53
epiglottis 95
ethmoid bone 75
ethmoidal sinuses 29, 71
Eustachian (auditory) tube 67, 85
extensor carpi radialis longus 245
extensor carpi ulnaris 251
   tendon 252
extensor digitorum longus 226, 227
extensor hallucis longus 227
extraocular muscles 29, 71
eye/eyeball/globe 29
   MRI 49

facial artery 47
facial bones 8
facial nerve 31, 61, 79, 85, 87
falx cerebri 13, 27, 57
fascia
   deep *see* deep fascia
   penile 185
   renal 143, 151
fast imaging sequences x
fat (adipose tissue) xvii
   in imaging
      in CT x

   suppression in MRI xi
   pericardial 137
   perirenal 151
fat pad
   buccal 75
   popliteal 223
femoral artery 225
   common 179, 197
   superficial 185, 214
femoral nerve 203
femoral vein
   common 197
   lateral circumflex 197
   superficial 185, 214
femur
   condyles 215, 216
   head 193, 209, 211
      ligament of (ligamentum teres) 177, 209
   popliteal surface 223
   shaft 183, 214
fibula, shaft 226, 227
fibular (peroneal) nerve
   common 215
   deep 226, 227
   superficial 226
fibularis (peroneus) brevis 229
fibularis (peroneus) longus 226
   tendon 237
fissures, lung 111
flaval ligaments 159
flexor carpi radialis tendon 255
flexor carpi ulnaris 250, 251
   tendon 253
flexor digitorum brevis 233
flexor digitorum longus tendon 229
flexor digitorum profundus 250, 251
   tendon 252
flexor digitorum superficialis 250
flexor hallucis longus 235
   tendon 229, 231, 235
flexor retinaculum 253, 255
foot 234–7
foramen magnum 9, 39, 59
foramen ovale (skull) 33
foramen transversarium 41, 45, 89
forearm 250–1
formalin-hardened material viii
frontal bone 11
frontal sinus 77
frontalis 53
fundus
   bladder 175, 191
   stomach 135

galea aponeurotica (epicranial aponeurosis)
   15, 53
gallbladder 153
   see also cholecystectomy clips
gastric fundus 135
gastrocnemius 223, 225, 226
   tendon 228
genioglossus 47, 91
glans of clitoris 201
globus pallidus 23, 61

glossopharyngeal nerve 33
gluteal nerve
    inferior 169
    superior 169, 209
gluteal vessels
    inferior 169
    superior 169, 171, 173, 209
gluteus maximus 169, 171, 179, 195
gluteus medius 169, 171, 209
gluteus minimus 169, 171, 209
gracilis 212
grey matter 15
gyri 17

hamate 253, 255
hamstrings 212
hand 256–61
hardening fluids viii
head
    axial section 10–47
    coronal section 50–75
    sagittal section 76–7
heart 117, 119, 124–5
helical (spiral) CT x
hemidiaphragm see diaphragm
hepatic artery 133, 139, 151
hepatic vein, right 121
hip, coronal section 208–9
history of sectional anatomy viii
Hounsfield scale x
humerus
    epicondyles 249
    greater tubercle 239
    mid-shaft 244
    neck 241
hyoid bone 67, 93
hypoglossus 93

ileum 171
iliac artery
    common 167
    external 203
    internal 173, 189
iliac crests 165
iliac vein
    external 203
    internal 189
iliopsoas 203
    see also psoas muscles
images
    imaging techniques ix, x–xi
    orientation xi–xii
incus 79
infrahyoid (strap) muscles 97, 99
infrapatellar bursa 221
infraspinatus 239
inguinal hernia, direct 177, 179
interatrial septum 117
intercostal neurovascular bundle 107
internal capsule
    anterior limb 23, 63
    posterior limb 61
interosseous membrane of forearm 251

intertubercular sulcus 243
interventricular foramen 23
intervertebral discs
    lumbar 147, 167
    lumbosacral 169
    thoracic 107, 111, 117, 119
    thoracolumbar 141
ischiorectal fossa
    female 197
    male 179, 181
ischium
    spine 177
    tuberosity 181

jaw see mandible; maxilla
jejunum 141
jugular vein
    external 93, 103
    internal 33, 35, 87, 97, 99, 105, 107

kidney xvi, 133, 139
    fascia 143, 151
knee
    axial section 215–17
    coronal section 218–19
    sagittal section 220–7

blabial mucous glands 41
labial vessels and nerves 41
labyrinthine artery 31
lacrimal gland 75
large intestine see colon; rectum
laryngeal nerve, recurrent 99, 105
laryngopharynx 93, 97, 101, 103
larynx 101, 103
    cartilages 95, 97, 101
lateral collateral ligament
    of ankle 233
    of knee 217
leg 226–7
lens 29
Leonardo da Vinci viii
levator ani
    female 197
    male 179, 181
levator palpebrae superioris 75
levator scapulae 103
ligament(s)
    of ankle 233
    of elbow 246, 247
    flaval 159
    of foot 235
    of knee 216, 217, 219, 223
    sacrospinous 177
    of uterus
        broad 191
        round 203
ligamentum denticulatum 95
ligamentum nuchae 55
ligamentum teres femoris 177, 209
ligamentum teres hepatis 153
ligamentum venosum 135

limbs
    lower 208–37
    upper 238–61
linea alba 149
lingual artery 93
lingual nerve 35
lips 41, 43, 45, 47
liver xvii, 135
    lobes 139
        caudate 153
        left 143, 153
        quadrate 151
        right 119, 147
Louis' angle 111
lower limbs 208–37
lumbar nerve, 2nd 149
lumbar spine 158–63
    intervertebral disc 147
    vertebrae see vertebrae
lumbar sympathetic chain 165
lumbar vein 145
lumbosacral discs 169
lunate 257, 259
lung 107
    fissures 111
    lower lobes 135, 137
lymph nodes
    cervical 105
    occipital 55
    pretracheal 111, 127

Macewen, Sir William viii
magnetic resonance imaging (MRI) ix
    abdomen
        axial 143, 145
        coronal 160–1
        sagittal 162–3
    ankle, coronal 233
    elbow, coronal 249
    foot, sagittal 235
    head
        axial 21, 23, 27, 29, 48–9
        coronal 51–67(odd nos.)
        sagittal 77
    hip, coronal 209
    knee
        axial 215, 216, 217
        coronal 219
        sagittal 221, 223, 225
    neck
        axial 83–9(odd nos.)
        coronal 101
    pelvis 202–7
        axial 165, 202–3
        coronal 186–7, 204–5
        female 202–7
        male 165, 186–7
        sagittal 206–7
    shoulder
        axial 239
        coronal 241
    thigh, axial 213, 214
    thorax, coronal 128–9

wrist/hand
  axial 255
  coronal 257
  sagittal 259
malleolus, medial 229
malleus 79
mandible 47, 65, 91
  canal 89
  ramus 85
mandibular nerve 33
manubriosternal joint 111
masseter 69
mastoid sinus/air cells 85
maxilla (upper jaw) 41
  alveolar process 85
maxillary artery 37
maxillary nerve 33
maxillary sinus/antrum 33, 39, 73, 83, 85
medial collateral ligament of knee 217, 219
median cubital vein 247
median nerve 244, 246, 250, 253, 255
median sacral vessels 175
mediastinum 109, 126–7
medulla oblongata 31, 59, 85
meningeal artery, middle 25
meninges 11, 53
meniscus
  lateral 217, 219, 221
  medial 219
mesenteric artery
  inferior 149, 165
  superior 133, 141, 145, 147
mesenteric vein
  inferior 165
  superior 145, 147
metacarpals 260, 261
metatarsal, first 237
Monro's foramen 23
mons pubis 199
mucous glands 69
  labial 41
muscles
  abdominal 147
  extraocular 29, 71
  strap 97, 99
  tongue 43, 67
  see also individual muscles

nasal cavity 31, 37
nasal concha
  inferior 37, 71, 83
  middle 33, 71, 73
  superior 71
nasal septum 35, 69
nasal vestibule 83
nasolacrimal duct 29, 35
nasopharynx 39, 67
natal cleft 197, 201
navicular bone (foot) 235
neck 82–101
  axial section 82–99
  sagittal section 100–1
nerve(s), *see specific nerves*

nerve roots and root sheaths
  cervical 59
  lumbar 159
neurovascular bundles
  digital (hand) 261
  intercostal 107
  superior gluteal 209
nose *see entries under* nasal
nuchal ligament 55

oblique muscles of abdomen 147
obliquus capitis inferior 39
obturator internus 179, 195, 197
occipital bone
  basilar part (basi-occiput) 33, 83
  external occipital protuberance 31
  posterior part 51
  squamous part 23
occipital lobe 55, 83, 85
occipital lymph nodes 55
occipitofrontalis 53
oculomotor nerve 67
odontoid peg (dens) 37, 39, 57, 63, 77, 87, 101
oesophagogastric junction 135
oesophagus 99, 101, 105, 117, 121
olecranon bursa 246
olecranon process 246
olfactory bulb 73
omohyoid muscle 97
optic chiasma 27
optic nerve 27, 29, 71
orbicularis oris 41
orbit 27, 29, 71
  MRI 49
oropharynx 43, 47, 91
ossicles, auditory 79
ovary 189

palate 37, 39, 69, 73, 77, 83
palatine bone 37
palatine tonsil 89
palatopharyngeal arch 43
palmar aponeurosis 260
pampiniform plexus 185
pancreas xvii, 137
  uncinate process 145
paranasal sinuses 29, 31, 33, 39, 63, 69, 71, 73, 83
  MRI 49
parathyroid gland 97
parietal bone 11, 53
parotid duct 69, 73, 83
parotid gland 45, 63, 85, 87, 89
  accessory 69, 83
patella 215, 216, 221
pedicle, L5 159
pelvicalyceal system 133
pelvis 164–207
  axial sections
    female 188–201
    male 164–85
  CT *see* computed tomography

penis 185
pericardium 119
  fat 137
  space between layers 113
pericranium (periosteum of skull) 11, 15, 53
periosteum of skull 11, 15, 53
perirenal fat 151
peroneal nerve *see* fibular nerve
peroneus brevis 229
peroneus longus *see* fibularis longus
petrous temporal bone 61, 79
phalanx, thumb 261
pharyngeal recess 83
pharynx 47, 101
  laryngeal part (laryngopharynx) 91, 95, 97, 101
  nasal part (nasopharynx) 39, 67
  oral part (oropharynx) 43, 47, 89
phlebolith, calcified 195
phrenic nerve 95, 103, 117
pia mater 13
piriformis 173, 189
pisiform bone 253
pituitary fossa 9
pituitary gland 27, 63, 77
plantar aponeurosis 233
plantar nerve, medial 237
plantaris 221
  tendon 226
pons 29, 59, 61, 83
  MRI 49
popliteal artery 223
popliteal pad of fat 223
popliteal vein 216, 227
popliteus 223
  tendon 217, 221
portal vein 139
posterior compartment of thigh 212
postnasal space 83
prepatellar bursa 221
prepuce of clitoris 201
preservation of cadavers ix
pretracheal space 127
  lymph nodes 109, 127
prevertebral fascia 47, 63
prevertebral muscles 47
proton density images x
psoas muscles 143, 149, 161
  see also iliopsoas
pterygoid muscle
  lateral 83
  medial 45
pterygopalatine fossa 33
pubis
  body 197
  symphysis 179, 195
  see also mons pubis
pudendal canal (Alcock's canal)
  female 197
  male 179
pudendal nerve 179
pudendal vessels, internal 179
pulmonary arteries 111, 127
pulmonary trunk 111
pulmonary valves 113

pulmonary vein
    superior 111
    tributaries 111
putamen 23, 61, 63

quadratus femoris 199, 212
    tendon 221
quadratus lumborum 143

radial artery 257
radial nerve 244, 250
radial notch 247, 249
radiology see images
radio-ulnar joint, superior 249
radius
    distal 253, 257
    head 247
ramus of mandible 83
rectal artery, superior 165, 167, 177
rectal vein, superior 177
rectosigmoid junction
    female 189
    male 175
rectum
    female 189, 191
    male 175
    see also anorectal junction
rectus abdominis 147
rectus capitis posterior major 55
rectus femoris 212
recurrent laryngeal nerve 97, 103
renal vein 141, 145
retromandibular vein 85
rib
    1st 125
    2nd 109
    9th 135
round ligament
    liver (ligamentum teres hepatis) 153
    uterus 203

sacral vessels, median 175
sacroiliac joint 169, 171
sacrospinous ligament 177
sacrum
    2nd segment 171
    3rd segment 173, 189
    4th segment 175
    5th segment 177, 191
    lateral mass 169
safety considerations ix
sagittal images, orientation xii
sagittal section
    foot 234–5
    head 76–7
    knee 220–7
    neck 100–1
    wrist/hand 258–9
sagittal sinus, superior 11, 55
salivary glands
    accessory/minor 41, 69
    major 45, 47, 63

saphenous nerve 185, 214
saphenous vein
    great 227
    small 216
sartorius 185, 212, 214
scalenus (scalene muscles) 47, 63, 103, 105
scalp (skin + subcutaneous tissue) 15, 53
scaphoid 253, 257
scapula 107, 243
    acromion process 241
sciatic nerve
    female 189, 195, 199, 201
    male 183
sclera 29
section(s), orientation xi–xii
sectioning ix–x
semimembranosus bursa 217
semimembranosus muscle 212
seminal vesicle 175
semispinalis capitis 43
semispinalis cervicis 43
semitendinosus 212
septum
    interatrial 117
    nasal 35, 69
septum pellucidum 21
serratus anterior 117
sesamoid bones 235
shoulder 238–43
sigmoid sinus 33
skin, cranial 15, 53
skull (cranium)
    images 8, 9
    periosteum 11, 15, 53
    sutures 21
small intestine 141, 171
soleus 223, 226
spermatic cord 179
sphenoid bone, lesser wing 69
sphenoidal sinus 29, 31, 65, 69, 77
    MRI 49
spinal accessory nerve 33
spinal canal, cervical 101
spinal cord, cervical 35, 37, 59
spine see specific regions and vertebrae
spiral CT x
spleen xvii, 121, 135
splenium of corpus callosum 19
splenius capitis 103
spring ligament 235
squamous part
    occipital bone 23
    temporal bone 25, 61
stapes 79
sternal (Louis') angle 111
sternocleidomastoid muscle 99, 103
sternocostal joint, third 123
sternohyoid muscle 97
sternothyroid muscle 97
sternum 113, 115, 117
stomach, fundus 135
straight sinus 27, 85
strap muscles 97, 99
styloid process of temporal bone 85
subacromial space 243

subarachnoid space 13, 53, 55, 57
subclavian artery 125
subclavian vein 107, 125
subcutaneous (connective) tissue, cranial 15, 53
subdeltoid process 239
subdural space 53
submandibular gland 45, 47, 63
subscapularis 111
subtalar joint 231
sulcus (sulci)
    cerebral 17, 19
    intertubercular 243
    talar 231
suprapatellar bursa 221
suprarenal (adrenal) gland 151, 161
supraspinatus tendon 241
sustentaculum tali 231, 235
sutures, cranial 21
Sylvian aqueduct 25
sympathetic chain, lumbar 165
symphysis pubis 179, 195

T1 and T2–weighted density images x
talocalcanean joint 231
talocalcanean ligament 233
talocalcaneonavicular joint 231
talus 231, 233, 235
temporal artery, superficial 17
temporal bone
    CT 78–81
    petrous ridge 61, 79
    squamous part 25, 61
    styloid process 85
    zygomatic process 67
temporal lobe 69
temporalis muscle 25
temporomandibular joint 65, 83
tendons, see specific tendons
tentorium cerebelli 27, 57
terminology xiii
testicular vein 145
testis 185
thalamus 61
thigh, axial section 212–14
thoracic vertebrae see vertebrae
thorax 103–33
    axial section
        female 122–3
        male 102–21
thumb, phalanx 261
thyroid artery, inferior 99
thyroid cartilage 95, 101
thyroid gland 97, 99
tibia 231
    condyles 217
    lower extremity 235
    shaft 226, 227
tibial artery
    anterior 226
    posterior 229
tibial nerve 215, 223, 229
tibial vein, anterior 226
tibialis anterior 227

tibialis posterior, tendon 229
tibiofibular joint
  inferior 228, 229, 233
  superior 221
tissue-specific MRI techniques x
tongue 43, 47, 67
tonsil
  cerebellar 35
  palatine 91
trachea 99, 101, 105, 111, 127
  carina 131
transverse colon 153
transverse foramen 41, 45, 76
transverse ligament of atlas 39, 63
transverse process 41, 45
transverse sinus 55, 85
transversus abdominis 147
trapezium 253, 255
trapezius 103
triangular fibrocartilaginous complex of wrist
  257
triceps 244
trigeminal nerve 31
triquetral 257
trochanter, lesser 183
tympanic cavity 79
tympanic membrane 63, 79

ulna 251
  distal 252
  olecranon process 246
  radial notch 247, 249
ulnar nerve 244, 245, 249, 250, 255
ulnar vessels 244, 255
umbilicus 165
uncinate process, pancreas 145
upper limb 238–61
ureter 173, 193

urethra
  female 197, 199
  penile 185
uterine vessels 193
uterus 191, 205, 207
  broad ligament 191
uvula 43

vagina 193, 195, 197, 199
vaginal vessels 195
vagus nerve 33, 105
vas deferens 175, 179, 185
vastus intermedius 212
vastus lateralis 212
vastus medialis 185, 212, 214, 215
veins *see specific veins*
vena cava
  inferior xvii, 121, 145, 167, 187
  superior 127
venous ligament 135
ventral nerve roots, cervical 59
ventral rami
  cervical 97
  lumbar 149, 159
ventricles (cerebral)
  fourth 29, 49
  lateral 19, 21, 51, 55
  third 21, 23
ventricles (heart)
  left 117, 119, 123
  right 117
vertebrae
  cervical 47
    C1/1st (atlas) 37, 39, 59, 63, 87, 101
    C2 *see* axis
    C3 45, 91
    C4 93
    C5 59, 95, 103

    C6 97
    C7 45, 105
  lumbar
    L2 145
    L3 149
    L4 159, 165, 167
    L5 159, 167
  sacral *see* sacrum
  thoracic
    T1–T2 107
    T4–T5 111
    T5 113
    T6 115
    T7 123
    T7–T8 117
    T8–T9 119
    T9 121
    T10 135
    T11 137
  thoracolumbar, T12–L1 141
vertebral arteries 33, 39, 41, 45, 59, 87, 99
vertebral canal (spinal canal), cervical 101
vertebral vein 91
vestibule of nose 83
vestibulocochlear (auditory) nerve 31, 61, 79
  MRI 49
vitreous humour 29
vocal folds 97, 101

white matter 15
wrist 252–9

zona orbicularis 209
zygomatic arch 69
zygomatic process of temporal bone 67